D1468446

PERMANENT REMISSIONS

SHOWS YOU HOW PHYTONUTRIENTS CAN:

- arrest the development of cancer cells
- block testosterone and estrogen from promoting cancer cell growth
- prevent tumors from spreading by choking off their blood supply
- detoxify environmental carcinogens
- reverse coronary artery disease
- reduce or eliminate the need for insulin injections for type II (adult-onset) diabetes
- boost the effectiveness of conventional cancer treatments and reduce their toxic side effects
- replace lost bone minerals in people suffering from osteoporosis

YOU'LL DISCOVER:

- the latest life-extending nutritional discoveries
- specific diets to prevent and defeat breast, prostate, stomach, and colon cancer, high blood pressure, atherosclerosis, and diabetes
- foods and supplements to enhance the effectiveness of chemotherapy, radiation, and surgery
- special disease prevention for African-Americans
- dramatic, true-life, medically documented stories of permanent remissions
- a therapeutic gourmet recipe book

And more!

◆

Let Robert Haas, M.S., and his cutting-edge nutritional plan help you maintain excellent health or achieve that state of grace known as

PERMANENT REMISSION!

Also by Robert Haas

Eat to Win
Eat to Succeed
Forever Fit (co-authored with Cher)
Eat Smart, Think Smart

PERMANENT

REMISSIONS

*Life-Extending Diet Strategies
That Can Help Prevent and Reverse
Cancer, Heart Disease, Diabetes,
and Osteoporosis*

ROBERT HAAS, M.S.

Recipes Designed by Kristin Massey

POCKET BOOKS
New York   London   Toronto   Sydney   Tokyo   Singapore

The author of this book is not a physician and the ideas, procedures, and suggestions in this book are not intended as a substitute for the medical advice of a trained health professional. All matters regarding your health require medical supervision. Consult your physician before adopting the suggestions in this book, as well as about any condition that may require diagnosis or medical attention.

In addition, statements made by the author regarding certain products are based on the author's research, and do not constitute an endorsement of any product, service, or organization by the author or publisher, each of whom specifically disclaims any responsibility for any liability, loss, or risk, personal or otherwise, which is incurred as a consequence, directly or indirectly, of the use and application of any of the contents of this book or any of the products mentioned herein.

POCKET BOOKS, a division of Simon & Schuster Inc.
1230 Avenue of the Americas, New York, NY 10020

Copyright © 1997 by Robert Haas, M.S.

Originally published in hardcover in 1997 by Pocket Books

All rights reserved, including the right to reproduce
this book or portions thereof in any form whatsoever.
For information address Pocket Books, 1230 Avenue
of the Americas, New York, NY 10020

Library of Congress Cataloging-in-Publication Data

Haas, Robert, 1948–
    Permanent remissions : life-extending diet strategies that can help
prevent and reverse cancer, heart disease, diabetes, and
osteoporosis / Robert Haas : recipes designed by Kristin Massey.
        p.   cm.
    Includes bibliographical references and index.
    ISBN: 0-671-00777-7
    1. Diet therapy—Popular works.   I. Massey, Kristin.   II. Title.
RM217.H23   1997
615.8'54—dc21   97-34766
                                                            CIP

First Pocket Books trade paperback printing December 1998

10 9 8 7 6 5 4 3 2 1

POCKET and colophon are registered trademarks of Simon & Schuster Inc.

Text design by Stanley S. Drate/Folio Graphics Co. Inc.

Printed in the U.S.A.

To my parents

ACKNOWLEDGMENTS

I would like to thank the following people (listed in alphabetical order) who contributed their time and effort during the research, writing, and editing of this book:

Emily Bestler, for her excellent and thorough editorial comments and suggestions and for her recognition of the importance of this book

Dr. Carolyn Clifford, director of the National Cancer Institute's Diet and Cancer Branch, for supplying research information

Connie Clausen, my literary mentor, for her support, advice, and longtime friendship

Steve Diamond, for his painstaking computer programming

Kristin Massey, for helping to design the life-saving recipes in this book

All the people who graciously consented to share their success stories with my readers

CONTENTS

SECTION I

INTRODUCTION: BEFORE YOU BEGIN   *3*

1   A SECOND CHANCE AT LIFE   *9*

2   CANCER: A NEW STANDARD FOR A CURE   *31*

3   PHYTONUTRIENTS: TWENTY-FIRST CENTURY VITAMINS   *46*

4   SAVE YOUR LIFE WITH SOY   *78*

5   BEATING BREAST CANCER   *96*

6   BEATING PROSTATE CANCER   *123*

7   BEATING DIABETES MELLITUS   *144*

8   BEATING CARDIOVASCULAR DISEASE   *161*

9   BEATING OSTEOPOROSIS   *203*

SECTION II
PHYTOFOOD RECIPES

PERMANENT REMISSIONS RECIPE HINTS   223
PERMANENT REMISSIONS RECIPE LIST   227
    Breakfasts   231
    Appetizers   239
    Snacks and Sandwiches   249
    Breads   259
    Soups   271
    Salads   279
    Dressings, Sauces, and Dips   287
    Entrées   295
    Side Dishes   313
    Desserts   323
    Blender Drinks   331

SECTION III

GLOSSARY   341
APPENDIX I.   *Permanent Remissions* Computer Software   349
APPENDIX II.   Directory of Selected Cancer Associations and
                 Support Groups   351
APPENDIX III.   State-by-State Guide to Cancer Research and
                 Treatment Centers   357
APPENDIX IV.   Brand-Name Food Products: Manufacturers'
                 Addresses and Phone Numbers   365
SELECTED REFERENCES   369
INDEX   395

SECTION I

Introduction

BEFORE YOU BEGIN

Has your doctor ever handed you a prescription for tomatoes to prevent cancer from getting a foothold in your body? What about salmon and oranges to reduce your risk of heart attack and stroke? How about a soy protein cocktail to stave off diabetes and osteoporosis?

Your doctor probably doesn't know which foods and nutrients you need, let alone how much of each one you should take to prevent or reverse diseases such as cancer, heart disease, diabetes, and osteoporosis. If your own doctor doesn't know which foods can keep you healthy or help you heal, how in the world are you expected to know?

You're not, but I am. I've devoted my life to the study of nutrition and disease. After earning my master of science degree in nutrition and food science from Florida State University, I began clinical studies in people with heart disease, diabetes, hypertension, osteoporosis, and cancer. During this research, I made some important discoveries about food, vitamins, and disease-fighting plant compounds called phytonutrients.

My original research in heart disease, which began in the mid-1970s, was tested successfully in a pilot study by researchers involved in the nationwide governmental heart disease study called MRFIT (Multiple Risk Factor Intervention Trial).

In the early 1980s, I opened two nutrition clinics in South Florida where I counseled hundreds of people with life-threatening diseases. Using foods and dietary supplementation, I was able to reverse the course of such diseases as coronary artery blockage, hypertension, cancer, and diabetes. Physicians who sent me their most intractable cases were astonished to discover that for the first time, their patients got progressively better, not worse. In many cases, these patients became healthier than their physicians.

In 1984, I wrote the groundbreaking book, *Eat to Win: The Sports Nutrition Bible,* which has, to date, helped nearly 3 million athletes and active people achieve peak physical performance. Olympic champions, like Jackee Joyner Kersey, have used my dietary advice to win gold medals. To this day, my *Eat to Win*–type diet is recommended by dietitians, nutritionists, physicians, professional coaches, and trainers as the gold standard for achieving endurance, stamina, and peak physical performance. I am best known for counseling world-champion athletes such as Martina Navratilova and Ivan Lendl; motion picture and TV celebrities such as Don Johnson, Mike Nichols, Marlo Thomas; and music legends Carly Simon, Cher, and Glenn Frey.

Now I want to start working with *you.*

Why?

By the time we reach the age of 20, many of us have accumulated enough visible, artery-clogging plaque to concern even the most conservative cardiologists. By the time we're 30, millions of cells in our bodies have taken at least one step toward cancer. On the day we blow out 40 candles, many of us will have developed insulin resistance, the harbinger of diabetes mellitus; others will have borderline or overt high blood pressure. At the half-century mark, some of us will have been diagnosed with invasive cancer, had a heart attack or stroke, developed full-blown diabetes, or developed the potentially fatal bone-softening disease, osteoporosis. And millions of us will have already died from these diseases.

It doesn't have to be that way.

Chemotherapy and radiotherapy for invasive cancer generally cannot eradicate all malignant cells. In theory, these treatments are designed to selectively kill cancer cells while minimizing the death of normal cells. In reality, chemotherapy and radiotherapy kill cancer cells and rapidly dividing healthy cells and create some very unpleasant and dangerous side effects: severe nausea, hair loss, anemia, organ damage, susceptibility to infection, and even cancer itself. With chemotherapy and radiotherapy, oncologists gamble that the treatment will destroy the cancer before it destroys the patient.

It doesn't have to be that way.

African-American men and women suffer from disproportionally high rates of hypertension, predisposing them to heart attacks and strokes. African-American women enjoy lower rates of breast cancer than white Americans yet suffer from more aggressive forms of the disease and die *twice as often* from it. American black men have the highest prostate cancer rate in the world, fully two times more than white Americans, yet native Africans have very low rates of prostate cancer. And black Americans die more frequently from almost all degenerative diseases at rates far higher than other groups.

It doesn't have to be that way.

The nutritional strategies for defeating cancer and other serious diseases in *Permanent Remissions* are based on my clinical research, the findings of thousands of published research studies, and the real-life case histories of people who have achieved medically verified long-term remissions from their diseases. Critics of the life-extending dietary strategies in this book might say that without formal, scientific proof (translation: long-term human clinical trials lasting decades), these strategies remain unproven. And they're right—for the moment.

But consider this: conventional cancer treatments are *proven* to fail in about 50% of all cancer patients and almost always in those with pancreas, lung, liver, bone, and advanced breast, ovarian, and colon cancer. Twenty percent of all heart bypass surgeries fail within the first year and the operation confers no extra years of life on those who can afford the $40,000–$60,000 cost. That kind of proof is the strongest reason I know to embrace *today* the life-saving dietary strategies in this book. The preponderance of the evidence I've provided tips the scales in favor of those who believe that degenerative diseases such as cancer, heart disease, diabetes, and osteoporosis can be prevented by diet and lifestyle and defeated with a one-two knockout punch of nutrition and cutting-edge medical treatments.

In one sense, containing or defeating cancer and other serious diseases is easier than preventing them. Trying to change the eating habits of people who feel well is a daunting task that often falls on deaf ears. Most people are willing to change their way of eating only after they are diagnosed with cancer or have suffered the chest-crushing pain of a heart attack—assuming they survive it.

It doesn't have to be that way.

Preventing cancer, heart disease, diabetes, and osteoporosis has never been easier or more delicious. Although the natural foods on the *Permanent Remissions* plan have been in existence for thousands of years, many of the food products and nutrient formulas you'll find in this book did not exist even a decade ago; many are so new that you may meet them for the first time in these pages. But now, even haute cuisine aficionados and fast-food fanatics can eat to live while living to eat. A host of newly developed supermarket foods and food products brings an important element to a healthy dinner table we've never had before—*taste*.

Today, you can walk out of most supermarkets and health-food stores with a basket of foods, food products, and nutrients—the same kinds now being tested by the National Cancer Institute's (NCI's) Diet and Cancer Branch—that are as powerful as any prescription drugs. *Permanent Remissions* gives you a blueprint for using these foods and food products to build better health and to help defeat the diseases that prematurely kill most of us and our loved ones.

I did not write *Permanent Remissions* to give anyone false hope of curing a potentially fatal disease. This book offers no guarantees, no promises. What it does provide is the very latest nutritional research and dietary information that can give the body the raw materials it needs to restore good health and beat back the diseases that prematurely kill most Americans. The message of *Permanent Remissions* is simple: we now possess the knowledge to prevent, forestall, halt, contain, and in some cases, reverse the diseases of aging.

Reversing heart disease, cancer, adult-type diabetes mellitus, and osteoporosis is a task best suited for the new dietary treatment strategies I propose in this book. These protocols are designed to complement, not supplant, the disease-stopping power of conventional medical treatments. Only the combination of nutrition and medicine can help us win the war on cancer and other serious health problems. Physicians and nutritionists must work together, as part of a health-care team, to achieve these goals. In my opinion, no other approach provides more effective care for the patient. And after all, isn't that what matters most?

You don't have to wait another decade until ultraconservative medical associations give this approach their blessing. You can start today by giving a copy of this book to your doctor and getting his or her approval to begin this new way of eating. Once your physician is armed with this knowledge, your chance of a long-term or permanent remission will increase manifold.

Many people may be surprised to learn that the leading killer diseases can be contained or reversed. But containment or reversal does not require the complete elimination of the diseased cells from the body: cholesterol-clogged arteries can be partially reopened to prevent heart attacks and strokes; premalignant tumor cells can be returned to their normal, healthy state; vampirelike tumor cells, attempting to appropriate the body's blood supply in order to recolonize at distant sites, can be held in check; defective muscle and fat cells can be made more sensitive to the body's own insulin to ameliorate diabetes; a thinning skeleton can be remineralized to thwart osteoporosis.

The proof required to formally confirm the effectiveness of the *Permanent Remissions* plan still must be obtained through years of painstaking study and investigation. Research is a necessity for scientists, but it is a luxury for people suffering from a life-threatening disease who cannot wait for the statistical proof of a decade-long scientific study. For them, waiting may be a fatal disease.

It doesn't have to be that way.

The *Permanent Remissions* Registry

I want you to become a part of a national movement to make traditional medical treatments for cancer and other life-threatening diseases safer and more effective.

The U.S. government and our national health organizations do not track cases of long-term and permanent remissions from cancer, atherosclerosis, diabetes, and other diseases. By submitting your case history, you will play an important role in changing the way conventional medicine now treats these diseases.

That's why I want you to write to me about your remission from *any* disease. If you have used diet and nutrients as part of your treatment and have successfully beaten back your health problem, I want to know about it.

All information will be held in confidence. Please include a return address on all correspondence. Please send a detailed description of your case history to me via computer or at the address below. Internet web site:

http://www.remission.com

Address for regular mail:

The Permanent Remissions Registry
P.O. Box 80-0102
Aventura, FL 33280

1

A SECOND CHANCE AT LIFE

Sheila Fuerst makes homemade vegetable soup the way her husband loves it and God intended: lots of fresh green and yellow vegetables simmered in a rich tomato-based stock. But this is no ordinary soup. This is the stuff medical miracles are made of.

Howard Fuerst, M.D., a Hollywood, Florida, physician diagnosed 5 years ago with highly malignant prostate cancer *and* coronary artery disease, loves the taste of his new medicine: "My new diet helped save my life. There's no doubt about it. I practiced conventional medicine for 42 years, oblivious to the miracle nutrients locked inside foods. Now I practice nutrition."

Why all the fuss over tomato soup? According to medical tests, Dr. Fuerst's severe prostate cancer has all but disappeared and his heart disease is in remission.

Not more than thirty miles up the road, Hal Pritchard, a retired Boca Raton resident, washes down a handful of vitamins with a soy cocktail that contains nutrients now being tested by the NCI's Diet and Cancer Research. "If I could have had this soy drink when I was a young man, I don't think I would have ever gotten sick. It knocked out my cancer and saved my life."

To Hal Pritchard's delight and his doctor's amazement, the malignant tumor that attacked his prostate gland no longer poses a threat to his life. And medical tests show that what little is left of it is no longer active. Hal attributes his remarkable recovery to a new soy cocktail loaded with cancer-bashing compounds called *phytonutrients*.

Phytonutrients

NATURE'S MOST POTENT MEDICINES

Stories of remissions from fatal diseases are considered rare, and cases of long-term survival after cancer has spread throughout the body also are much less common.

Nevertheless, they exist.

The question is, why? Why do some people beat the odds while others with similar medical conditions succumb?

I believe that I have discovered an answer to this question. I've uncovered a common thread that runs through a number of medically documented case histories of long-term survivors of cancer and other life-threatening illnesses: many of these survivors used *a new way of eating* that seems to make conventional medical treatments far more effective and safer than ever before.

Instead of relying solely on chemotherapy, radiotherapy, drugs, or surgery, most of the cancer, heart disease, and diabetes survivors you'll meet in this book beat the odds by embracing novel dietary strategies while following their doctors' prescribed treatments. In many cases, they switched to healthier diets made up of specific foods rich in phyto-nutrients (*phyto* means plant), powerful disease-fighting nutrients found in vegetables, fruits, plants, and herbs. This dietary strategy, or protocol, helped them regain their health and gave them a new lease on life because they placed their diseases in a state of suspended animation.

Phytonutrients can intervene at almost every treacherous twist of a cell's path toward malignancy. Certain phytonutrients can prevent carcinogens from forming in the body. Some drive cancerous cells back to normalcy. Others boost enzymes in the body that detoxify and re-move cancer-causing compounds. Still others prevent small but aggres-sive cancers from commandeering the body's blood supply, starving the hostile tumor cells before they can grow larger and spread throughout the body.

INDUSTRIAL-STRENGTH VITAMINS

What gives tomatoes their beautiful red-orange color and oranges, grapefruits, and limes, their wonderful citruslike flavor? What gives gar-lic and onions their characteristic aroma and taste? What makes red wine red, blueberries blue, and green beans green?

Phytonutrients.

Great chefs use phytonutrient-rich foods to add colors and flavors to their dishes. But phytonutrients can do far more than please the eye and palate: they can help prevent and reverse life-threatening diseases.

Technically, phytonutrients are not vitamins, which prevent deficiency diseases such as beriberi (a nerve disease caused by lack of vitamin B_1) and scurvy (a connective tissue disease due to lack of vitamin C). But phytonutrients, found exclusively in vegetables, fruits, and herbs, pack the power to defeat the degenerative diseases that stalk most Americans—cancer, heart disease, diabetes, and osteoporosis.

I think of phytonutrients as industrial-strength vitamins. Here's why:

- **Disease Prevention:** Recent research indicates that vitamin E and the phytonutrient *lycopene* (responsible for the red color of tomatoes) both reduce the risk of heart disease and some types of cancer. But you'd have to eat 4,000 calories a day in vitamin E–rich foods, such as seeds, wheat germ, and vegetable oils, to obtain a clinically effective dose (200–400 international units). On the other hand, you'd need to eat just 37 calories (one-half cup) of tomato sauce to get a cancer-stopping dose of lycopene. And lycopene packs *twice* the antioxidant power of vitamin E.
- **Disease Reversal:** Vitamins take a backseat to phytonutrients when it comes to halting the progression of disease and even reversing it. Phytonutrients can help turn cells headed toward cancer back to normal, healthy cells. Phytonutrients can block the cancer-promoting effects of the body's hormones, such as insulin, estrogen, and testosterone. And only phytonutrients can kill cancer cells by choking off their blood supply.

Phytonutrients are the most complex and powerful disease-fighting compounds in our foods. Vitamins keep us alive, but phytonutrients save our lives.

Permanent Remissions: A Revolutionary Concept

After the initial shock of cancer diagnosis, many people give up tobacco, alcohol, sunbathing, high-fat diets, and other harmful lifestyle choices. For some, it is too late. For others, the jury is still out.

Some people may spend long hours researching the latest in experimental cancer treatments from books and scientific articles. Others adopt various fad diets and take daily megadoses of vitamins. Still others seek out offshore clinics for more exotic therapies. Does it do any good?

To date, there is no evidence that any one of these approaches cures cancer. Any claims about the efficacy of such treatments vanish under the impartial scrutiny of scientific inquiry.

There is substantial clinical evidence, however, that diet and lifestyle changes improve your health and significantly reduce your risk of cancer, heart disease, diabetes and osteoporosis. Indeed, it is *overwhelming.* The evidence is far less convincing, but nevertheless encouraging, that certain foods and phytonutrients are beneficial for someone already diagnosed with invasive cancer. Fortunately, most cancers have a long latency period in which there is great potential to prevent the development of invasive cancer; it is during this period when phytonutrients are especially effective.

Permanent Remissions is a trailblazing book because at present, we have no conclusive proof that the information it contains can stop cancer or any other disease. The medically verified and seemingly miraculous accounts of long-term remissions in this book do not constitute scientific proof. They are clinical observations and case histories that, when taken with a large and growing body of published experimental evidence, strongly suggest that people who combined the dietary strategies I describe with conventional medical treatments achieved long-term and permanent remissions from cancer, heart disease, diabetes, and osteoporosis. We will not have *absolute* proof that this complementary therapeutic approach works until scientists have conducted formal research studies involving thousands of people over many years.

Why You Need *Permanent Remissions* Now

Should you wait for irrefutable proof before you embrace the nutritional strategies that have prolonged the lives of others? Maybe the question should be: do you have the time to wait for formal, scientific proof?

In 1850, about one of every 150 deaths in the United States was due to cancer. Today, one in four Americans will develop cancer during their lifetime and about half of them will die of it. Over 1 million people in the United States will be diagnosed with cancer this year, not to mention nearly 1.5 million who will develop cardiovascular disease and die from it prematurely. Will you be one of them?

The people you will meet in this book have confounded their doctors by reversing their diseases or at least stopping them in their tracks. Some have been able to banish any detectable trace of their disease, while others have greatly prolonged their lives even with clinical evidence that the disease is still present in their body. These survivors enjoy a higher quality of life than many other disease victims who rely solely on conventional therapy.

Chemotherapy, on average, helps only about half of all cancer patients, prolonging survival in varying degrees, *without* curing. Some tumors may show a dramatic decrease in size and a prolonged remission, but the tumor inevitably returns. It is also possible for conventional therapy to produce a rapid remission without significantly changing the overall survival of the individual. This is most often due to a high degree of tumor malignancy or to the severe side effects caused by the therapy itself.

The dietary strategies you will read about in this book can significantly improve the effectiveness and safety of chemotherapy, radiotherapy, and surgery and forestall death from potentially fatal diseases such as cancer, heart disease, and diabetes. These strategies are not meant to supplant the time-tested conventional disease treatments your doctor will prescribe. They are designed to work *with* such treatments, to augment their efficacy, and to reduce their toxic, unpleasant, and life-threatening side effects. Now, you can take charge of your health and work as a partner with your doctor, using the *Permanent Remissions* Plan—not as an alternative therapy but as a complementary one.

Some of the finest medical minds in the United States, such as Dr. Steven A. Rosenberg, an M.D., Ph.D. NCI researcher, and Harmon Eyre, M.D., an oncologist who is chief medical officer for the American Cancer Society (ACS), now believe that specific foods and the phytonutrients they contain provide a powerful treatment strategy that can reduce the death rate from many types of cancer. My research has convinced me that phytonutrients can prevent and reverse cancer, heart disease, diabetes, and osteoporosis. There are some very interesting clues that have come out of their observations of long-term survivors of cancer who have beaten the odds.

Phytonutrients used in conjunction with traditional cancer treatments hold the promise of helping the body halt the progression of cancer and other serious diseases longer than do conventional medical treatments alone and, in some cases, even long enough to help people *outlive their cancer.* We all have to die of something, but the message of this book is that death from cancer, heart disease, or diabetes can be forestalled long enough to perhaps enjoy a normal life and lifespan. You can play a role in your own cure.

Although certain phytonutrients can prevent and reverse cancer and other diseases in laboratory animals, their remarkable potential to help people achieve long-term remissions has not been widely disseminated among physicians and the general public.

Until *now.*

What Are Permanent Remissions?

Permanent remissions are not *spontaneous* remissions, in which a disease such as cancer suddenly and inexplicably disappears with little or no medical treatment. Although spontaneous remissions apparently do occur, they are random and rare events.

Permanent remissions, on the other hand, don't have to be random; they can be created by eating a special diet rich in phytonutrients and other nutrients while following a traditional course of medical therapy. In a long-term or permanent remission, the disease doesn't always completely disappear but is stopped in its tracks and prevented from worsening. Phytonutrients and related nutrients are the key to boosting the body's natural defenses so traditional medical treatments can work better.

Permanent remissions created through diet can also be thought of as *disease prevention,* since phytonutrients can act on diseased cells that haven't yet been discovered. They can battle the undetected premalignant tumor cell lurking in the breast, colon, or prostate *before* it turns into cancer. In addition, cholesterol-cleansing phytonutrients can remove potentially fatal but silent arterial plaque and decrease blood stickiness that can lead to heart attacks and strokes. Many people who are overweight or genetically predisposed to adult diabetes (type 2) can use phytonutrients to achieve permanent weight loss, fight genetic fate, and live healthy, drug-free lives. And those with osteoporosis, a bone-softening disease, can actually replace lost bone minerals by using the phytonutrients discussed in this book.

The Theory of Permanent Remissions

*If cancers don't grow beyond a millimeter in size, they won't kill you—
and to grow, they need blood vessels. Find a way to block the vessels,
and people could live with cancer for many years.*

—Dr. Harmon Eyre, oncologist and
chief medical officer for the ACS.

Achieving a long-term or permanent remission is far more involved than simply self-medicating at a salad bar, but the basic fact is
that specific phytonutrients found in vegetables, fruits, seeds, herbs,
and plants provide *the most potent force in nature* to send cancer and
other life-threatening disease into a state of suspended animation.

Phytonutrients are also the most powerful means we have to *prevent* cancer. Even if you eat a less-than-optimal diet, phytonutrients can
still help to forestall the biochemical events that turn healthy cells into
cancer cells.

Phytonutrients fight cancer in six ways. Each of the following
mechanisms helps explain how these life-saving compounds help create
long-term cancer remissions:

BLOOD VESSEL GROWTH BLOCKERS

The first mechanism of permanent remissions is revolutionary, yet
easy to understand. Like a new apartment building under construction,
tumor growth can't proceed without the proper plumbing to bring in
vital fluids and to remove toxic waste products. Most tumor cells cannot grow beyond a few millimeters unless they gain access to the body's
blood supply. The tumor's dependence on the body's own plumbing
system presents a problem, since the body's network of blood vessels is
almost complete at birth, and with few exceptions, no new blood vessel
growth takes place in adulthood.

To overcome this plumbing problem, many cancer cells produce
substances that fool the body into building new blood vessels. They
secrete enzymes that tunnel into nearby healthy tissues to make room
for new "pipelines" and they make specialized substances that trick
healthy cells into forming small blood vessels—a process that is called
angiogenesis.

A cancer cell is the perfect vampire: it remains immortal as long as it has access to the body's blood supply. Cut off the blood supply and, like Bram Stoker's fictional vampire, Count Dracula, the cancer cell withers and dies. Fortunately, phytonutrients found in such foods as soybeans and soy products (e.g., tofu, tempeh, soy meat substitutes, soy milk, and soy cocktails) can block the blood vessel growth factors made by cancer cells and can literally *starve tumors to death*.

Many researchers now believe that cancer cells can be prevented from growing and spreading by using certain phytonutrients that prevent them from stimulating new blood vessel growth.

Phytonutrients are extremely safe, which makes them quite different from conventional cancer therapy. Judah Folkman, M.D., a Harvard University physician and researcher who pioneered the field of angiogenesis, predicts that physicians will soon prescribe phytonutrient-based concentrates and drugs as long-term therapies to keep lingering cancer cells in a state of suspended animation after conventional cancer treatment has been completed. Folkman speculates that angiogenesis phytonutrients and drugs can prolong the state of suspended animation of cancer cells for 10, maybe 20, years. At that point, we are beginning to compete with the normal life span, since many cancers arise in the fifth decade of life. Folkman thinks that although we may not cure the disease this way, we can stabilize it—a process he calls *extending dormancy*.

HORMONE BLOCKERS

Many types of cancer cells, including those often found in the breast, ovary, and prostate, use the body's own reproductive hormones, such as estrogen, testosterone, and related hormonelike chemicals, to fuel their growth. Exposing cancer cells to high levels of these hormones is like feeding a bodybuilder steroids: in both cases, growth and strength will increase at an abnormal rate. Phytonutrients found in such foods as soy, cabbage, broccoli, tofu, and meat substitutes made from soy protein resemble the chemical structure of these hormones. This molecular similarity allows them to fit into the hormone receptor on breast and prostate cells—much like a key fits a lock—to fool healthy cells into thinking they're the real thing. Since they are not as powerful as the hormones, this bait-and-switch tactic actually blocks reproductive hormones from subverting normal cell growth into the accelerated growth that turns healthy breast and prostate cells cancerous.

FREE-RADICAL BLOCKERS

Phytonutrients found in tomatoes, oranges, garlic, onions, and soy products and such nutrients as coenzyme Q_{10}, alpha-lipoic acid, vitamin E, vitamin C, and the mineral selenium protect healthy cells from cancer-causing chemicals. These nutrients act as antioxidants, tying up free radicals (disease-causing molecules or atoms that have become dangerously unstable because of a missing electron) and protecting the cell's membrane, internal machinery, and DNA (deoxyribonucleic acid). They also help protect arteries from atherosclerosis due to diabetes and high-fat, high-cholesterol diets.

These antioxidants can provide a double blessing for those with cancer because they protect healthy cells from the damaging radiotherapy and toxic drugs used to treat the disease.

IMMUNE BOOSTERS

Phytonutrients in tomatoes, cabbage, watermelon, onions, soybeans, garlic, and citrus fruits can boost the immune system to help kill cancer cells that remain after surgery, chemotherapy, or radiotherapy. They also help reduce the toxic side effects of these rigorous treatments.

Phytonutrients usually provide a degree of immune system stimulation no ordinary vitamin–mineral supplement can achieve. In this sense, phytonutrients play a leading role in disease prevention. Phytonutrients (many of which also serve as antioxidants) work together to provide the most powerful stimulus to prevent cancer and rev up the body's cancer-fighting capabilities.

CARCINOGEN DETOXIFIERS

Cruciferous vegetables, such as broccoli, cabbage, kale, okra, and kohlrabi, and foods such as garlic and onions contain phytonutrients that can mitigate the tumor-promoting effects of the body's own hormones and environmental toxins, or *xenobiotics* (literally: foreign to life).

Many of these sulfur-containing phytonutrients can tame the powerful cancer-promoting hormone estradiol (chemically related to estrogen) and help eliminate it from the body. Other phytonutrients found in crucifers help detoxify the xenobiotics in the food, water, and air that we ingest.

ANTIADHESIVES

A number of naturally occurring carbohydrate-like compounds found in beans, peas, lentils, oranges, and grapefruit possess the unique ability to prevent cancer cells from adhering to the surface of healthy cells. These glue-blocking compounds appear to work as antiadhesives by blocking the binding site of cancer cells (called *lectins*) and preventing individual cancer cells from metastasizing. New and innovative food supplements and pharmaceuticals based on this antiadhesive concept have been developed to prevent cancer cells from attaching to healthy cells.

Carbohydrate science is the new frontier for innovative human therapeutics. The U.S. Food and Drug Administration (FDA) is reviewing human testing of a newly developed carbohydrate compound in patients with cancer at the M.D. Anderson Medical Center in Texas and the Graduate Hospital in Philadelphia. Preliminary results suggest that when intravenously administered, it can prevent cancer cells from metastasizing.

You won't have to wait a half-dozen more years for this compound to reach the drugstore shelf. A number of new products now contain a carbohydrate compound called *modified citrus pectin*. You can learn more about this promising compound in Chapter 3.

Phytonutrients Are Active Against Many Diseases

Phytonutrients don't just fight cancer—they can defeat heart disease, too. These disease-fighting food chemicals can help keep coronary arteries open for decades after bypass surgery by dissolving artery-clogging cholesterol and prevent the formation of dangerous blood clots—a life-saver for many people, since about 20% of the arteries reopened in bypass surgery typically close within a year.

Phytonutrients can help many people with adult-onset diabetes reduce or eliminate their dependence on insulin and other diabetic drugs. Phytonutrient-rich foods can help stabilize blood sugar and make cells more responsive to insulin produced by the body. Recent studies reveal that a majority of adult diabetics could normalize their high blood sugar levels within just 12–24 weeks of embracing a low-calorie, phytonutrient-rich diet and exercise program.

Phytonutrients found in a variety of vegetables, soy foods, and soy beverages can also prevent and reverse osteoporosis, a bone-softening disease that cripples millions of people, mostly women, and leads to hip fractures that can be lethal. I'll tell you about the phytonutrient-rich foods and nutrients that are just as effective as drugs for treating this preventable disease—but without the harmful side effects.

Phytonutrients: The Missing Link in Conventional Cancer Treatments

The truth about the effectiveness of conventional cancer treatments emerged slowly during the 1990s. Despite the optimistic public-service messages you might read or see on TV, the actual facts are sobering.

John Bailar, Ph.D., of Harvard University, who analyzed the cancer statistics from the NCI, discovered that until recently, the cancer death rate has steadily increased. In 1960, cancer claimed the lives of 270,000 people. In 1994, according to NCI data, 600,000 people died from cancer. Today, men of the baby-boomer generation have *three times the cancer rate* of their grandfathers. Not only do we have much more cancer today than 35 years ago, according to Dr. Bailar's analysis, we also have become less and less effective at curing it. Dr. Bailar, in his 1986 analysis, concluded, "Some 35 years of intense effort focused largely on improving treatment must be judged a qualified failure." Now, with 12 more years of data and experience, he sees little to change his conclusion. "The effect of new treatments for cancer on mortality has been largely disappointing," he concluded in his most recently published report.

The incidence of cancer is also on the rise. The NCI predicts over 1.2 million new cases for 1997. Basal-cell and squamous-cell skin cancers (the NCI estimates 700,000 new cases this year) are now so rampant *they are excluded from the cancer statistics.*

Although deaths from stomach cancer have declined significantly, many other cancers remain uncontrolled. Deaths from Hodgkin's lymphoma, the cancer that killed Jacqueline Kennedy Onassis, are up over 60% for men and nearly that for women. Deaths from prostate cancer have risen by 23% since 1960. Deaths from brain cancers are up over

25% for both sexes. And deaths from lung cancer are up a whopping 452% for women and 104% for men.

Clearly, these data reveal that conventional medical therapies for cancer have done little to win the war on cancer initiated by President Richard M. Nixon in 1971. *Permanent Remissions* offers medical science the chance to overcome the shortcomings of traditional treatments for cancer. These treatments, as good as they are, cannot deliver the level of effectiveness (and safety) required to win the war on cancer. *Permanent Remissions* offers a new, combined therapeutic approach to defeating cancer by using phytonutrient-rich foods and other supplements to augment the cancer-stopping power of chemotherapy, radiotherapy, vaccines, drugs, and surgery.

Heart Disease: Still the Number-One Killer

As with cancer, the statistics for heart disease are grim. One third of all U.S. deaths are caused by cardiovascular disease. Although the nation's collective cholesterol level has declined on average, heart disease is still the nation's number-one killer. Yet with all the people treated by coronary bypass surgery, angioplasty, balloon catheterization, clot-busting enzymes, and cholesterol-lowering drugs (many with potentially lethal side effects) and low-fat/low-cholesterol diets, this completely preventable disease remains the number-one killer in the United States.

What about conventional treatments for heart disease? In 1994, the U.S. government's Coronary Artery Surgery Study spent $24 million of our tax dollars studying 16,626 bypass surgery patients. From these, researchers selected 780 patients with good heart function but significant blockage of at least one coronary artery. They gave half the patients bypass surgery plus drugs. The other half were treated with nutritional and lifestyle changes plus drugs. Researchers discovered that *bypass surgery conferred no advantage at all, in either longevity or incidence of future heart attacks.*

Permanent Remissions offers people with heart disease a real alternative to bypass surgery. My research in nutrition and heart disease over the last 20 years and the research of other scientists has clearly demonstrated that a phytonutrient-based diet can reverse the artery blockage that leads to heart attacks and strokes. In certain cases, the coronary arteries that supply the heart have become so severely calcified that surgery may be required. The *Permanent Remissions* Plan can also offer people who must undergo bypass surgery and angioplasty a way to speed healing and make their surgery even more effective by preventing restenosis (blockage) of their new arteries.

Adult-Onset (Type 2) Diabetes: Reversible Yet Still Rampant

In 1980, Father John McCormick, a priest who had been a diabetic most of his adult life, was referred to my clinic by his diabetologist (a physician who specializes in treating diabetes mellitus) because Father McCormick's adult-onset (type 2) diabetes had gotten progressively worse. His physician placed him on insulin injections, but his blood sugar remained unacceptably high at 160 milligrams per deciliter.

I placed Father McCormick on a special phytonutrient diet and advised him to walk 45 minutes at a moderate pace just after dinner each night. Within 12 weeks, Father McCormick was able to gradually reduce and then eliminate his need for insulin entirely, under his doctor's supervision. His blood glucose fell into the normal range at 92 milligrams per deciliter (60–115 milligrams per deciliter is considered normal). Six months later, Father McCormick still required no insulin and by all clinical measures no longer had diabetes.

Father McCormick, like 16 million other adult Americans today, was a type 2 diabetic whose body had become insensitive to the blood sugar–clearing hormone, insulin. Many who suffer from this largely preventable disease will go blind, lose a leg to gangrene, or die from kidney failure or heart disease. Father McCormick was lucky. He learned how to use phytonutrient-rich foods to help send this disease into a permanent remission. Sadly, many diabetics continue to eat diets that keep them diabetic because their personal physicians are unaware of the remarkable healing powers locked inside of phytofoods.

I have worked with a number of type 2 diabetics who were able to normalize their blood glucose and live normal lives without the use of drugs. *Permanent Remissions* shows you how to reduce your risk of getting type 2 diabetes and how to control the disease if you already suffer from it.

Vitamins, Minerals, and
Permanent Remissions

Millions of Americans take multivitamins each day, but does doing so do any good? I'll tell you the truth about the role of vitamins, minerals, and other nutrients in fighting cancer, free of media hype and sensationalism. And the truth is this: certain nutrients can and do help the body fight cancer, heart disease, diabetes, and osteoporosis when used as part of a *total* dietary strategy. But no pill, however potent, can take the place of a phytonutrient-rich diet. The most brilliant scientists alive today cannot recreate in a pill what Mother Nature has put in oranges, tomatoes, and soybeans.

Certain vitamins, minerals, and nutrients can effectively boost the safety and cancer-stopping power of traditional cancer treatments. For example:

- Antioxidants, such as carotenoids, vitamin E, and selenium, enhance the effectiveness of radiotherapy and chemotherapy while providing protection against damage to normal cells.
- Vitamin C, vitamin E, calcium, and selenium help stop tumor cells from rejecting anticancer drugs. These same nutrients protect against heart damage caused by anticancer drugs called *anthracyclines* and they scavenge harmful free radicals produced by radiotherapy.
- Vitamins C and K enhance the tumor-killing effects of the anticancer medicine *bleomycin.*
- Selenium protects against kidney damage associated with the anticancer drug *cisplatin.* Vitamin A–like compounds called *retinoids,* given with anticancer drugs, enhance their tumor-killing effectiveness.

Table 1.1 lists the vitamins, minerals, and phytonutrients that help conventional cancer therapies achieve results beyond those possible with drugs and radiation alone. Most oncologists remain unaware of the healing potential these nutrients can provide their patients.

Permanent Remissions Is Grounded in Scientific Fact

I'll introduce you to a new way of eating, based on the latest knowledge I've gathered from my own clinical research, thousands of

TABLE 1.1

Nutrients and Phytonutrients for Use with Chemotherapy and Radiotherapy

Nutrient	Therapy	Activity
Calcium	Anthracyclines	Improves drug efficacy
Carnosine	Radiotherapy	Protects healthy cells against damage
Cartenoids	Radiotherapy, Chemotherapy	Protects healthy cells against damage; improves drug efficiency
Coenzyme Q10	Doxorubicin	Protects healthy cells against damage; improves drug efficacy
Diallyl sulfide/ disulfide	Cisplatin	Protects healthy cells against damage; improves drug efficacy
L-glutathione	Vincristine, Cancer Multi-Drug Resistance Doxorubicin	Protects healthy cells against damage; improves drug efficacy
Indole-3 carbinol	Doxorubicin, Vinblastine	Improves drug efficacy
Inositol nicotinate	Doxorubicin	Improves drug efficacy
L-taurine	Bleomycin, Radiotherapy	Protects healthy cells against damage; improves drug efficacy
N-acetylcysteine	Radiotherapy	Protects healthy cells against damage
Niacin polynicotinate	Bleomycin	Protects healthy cells against damage; improves drug efficacy
Omega-3 fatty acids	Doxorubicin, Hyperthermia, Multi-Drug Resistance	Protects healthy cells against damage; improves drug efficacy
Panax ginseng	Radiotherapy	Protects healthy cells against damage
Phosphatidylinositol	Bleomycin	Protects healthy cells against damage
Selenium	Cisplatin, Anthracyclines, Radiotherapy	Protects healthy cells against damage; improves drug efficacy
Soy phytonutrients	Methotrexate, Radiotherapy	Protects healthy cells against damage; improves drug efficacy
Vitamin A	Methotrexate	Improves drug efficacy
Vitamin D3	Cisplatin	Improves drug efficacy
Vitamin E	Doxorubicin; Bleomycin, Radiotherapy, Hyperthermia, Anthracyclines	Protects healthy cells against damage
Vitamin C	Doxorubicin, Misonidazole, Anthracyclines, Bleomycin, Radiotherapy	Protects healthy cells against damage
Vitamin K	Bleomycin	Improves drug efficacy

published scientific studies, the latest findings from the NCI's Diet and
Cancer Branch, and the research of some of this country's most innovative cancer doctors. You'll meet celebrities and ordinary Americans who
have used this new way of eating to augment the power of conventional
medical treatments and to achieve long-term and permanent remissions
from their life-threatening diseases.

All the cases of long-term and permanent remissions you'll read
about in this book have been medically documented. As I discovered,
there are far too many medically verified cases of these remarkable remissions from cancer, heart disease, and diabetes to consider them random or rare. Phytonutrients and other natural compounds can help
many cancer victims live longer and better than others who rely on
conventional medical therapies alone.

New Remission Therapies for Cancer: Twenty-first-Century Medicine Now

Each day, your immune system pumps out cancer-fighting medicines. These life-saving molecules, such as *interferons* and *interleukins,*
can direct the immune system to obliterate precancerous cells in short
order. Many of the phytonutrients that I tell you about in the following
chapters will help to stimulate the production of these and other of the
body's own miracle medicines.

As powerful as these substances are, however, a body abused by
years of poor diet, tobacco intake, alcohol intake, too much sunlight,
and exposure to environmental carcinogens such as air pollution sometimes requires heroic measures—new and experimental medical therapies.

Take the case of New Mexico Supreme Court Justice Stanley F.
Frost, which recently received national media attention. Judge Frost
was convinced that the Christmas of 1995 would be his last. But thanks
to a new concept in cancer treatment called *biochemotherapy,* he is alive
and cancer-free to celebrate more Christmases with his family.

The 54-year-old retired judge was diagnosed with metastatic melanoma in April 1995. His surgeon removed cancerous lymph nodes and
referred him to the John Wayne Cancer Institute at Saint John's Hospital, Santa Monica, for follow-up treatment.

In May 1995, the doctors there discovered cancer in Frost's left lung and brain. Chief surgeon Donald Morton, M.D., removed the lung tumor and began a treatment protocol using a new cancer vaccine he developed. The vaccine is made from irradiated cancer cells obtained from other patients and is designed to direct the body's immune system to attack melanoma cells from the patient's own tumor. An oncologist at the institute also gave Judge Frost a new treatment that combines traditional chemotherapy with interleukin-2 and alpha-interferon, natural substances ordinarily made by the body that stimulate the immune system.

Judge Frost's Christmas gift arrived in early December 1996 when he returned to the cancer institute for follow-up testing. The present came in the form of an amazing yet true medical report: *doctors found no signs of cancer.* He is in complete remission and has been since June 1996. His physician, Robert O'Day, M.D., believes that if he stays in remission for 18 months, it's unlikely the cancer will come back.

Judge Frost beat the odds. He is also optimistic that cancer researchers will continue to develop new and promising therapies. Biochemotherapy is just one of the new and innovative cancer treatments that can lead to a long-term or permanent remission. I'll tell you how you can contact the leading cancer research centers in the United States and obtain the latest information on cutting-edge cancer therapies in Appendix III (pages 357–64).

Innovative Ways to Boost the Cancer-Killing Power of Conventional Therapies

I'll show you how to enjoy phytonutrient-rich foods, phytofood products, special recipies, and dietary supplements that will augment the efficacy and safety of conventional medical therapies for cancer. Sadly, the vast majority of oncologists remain unaware that diet and nutrition play such a vital role in stopping cancer cells from growing and spreading. Many cancer specialists don't know, for example, that the type of fat that you eat can radically alter the effectiveness of certain cancer treatments. Here's an example of how dietary fat can augment cancer treatments:

The fats (called omega-3 fatty acids) in a salmon steak you may have eaten last month are now part of the cell membranes that surround the cells in your body. Normal cells and cancer cells alike incorporate dietary fats into their membranes, essentially mirroring the fat profile of your diet.

You can use this phenomenon to modify the physical and chemical composition of cancer cell membranes. This strategy can help those with cancer because certain fatty acids and oils, such as the omega-3 fatty acids found in salmon, mackerel, tuna, and other seafood, can sensitize malignant cells to at least two conventional cancer therapies: *hyperthermia,* a treatment that raises the body temperature to kill heat-sensitive cancer cells, and the commonly prescribed chemotherapy drug, doxorubicin.

Modifying dietary fat intake to enhance the effectiveness of certain cancer therapies is just one of many life-saving nutritional strategies you will learn about in *Permanent Remissions.* I will show you and your physician how to use this information to decrease your risk of suffering a serious illness and increase your chances of surviving one.

What Your Doctor Didn't Learn in Medical School about Nutrition

Doctors receive little medical school training in nutrition. Any nutrition courses that your own physician *might* have enrolled in were most likely undervalued by the medical faculty and poorly taught. Sadly, nutrition has never played a significant role in the medical curricula in U.S. medical schools.

Why has the medical establishment neglected one of the most essential and critically important health topics in the education of our physicians? When will our nation's healers be properly trained in the science of nutrition—a specialty that can prevent and reverse the most devastating of degenerative diseases?

Charles L. Sanders, Ph.D., a professor at the University of Washington and Washington State University who has written over 120 peer-reviewed publications in experimental cancer research and toxicology since 1966, believes there are three reasons why physicians have overlooked the possibility of treating their cancer patients with powerful nutrients:

1. The use of dietary compounds in the treatment of cancer is a relatively new area of study for the medical community. Many physicians

mistakenly believe that there are insufficient published scientific data on the basis of which to recommend nutritional therapies for their patients.

2. Most physicians lack the confidence and knowledge to counsel their patients on lifestyle and dietary modifications for cancer control.

3. Physicians who use alternative therapies in treating cancer may find their peers attempting to revoke their license to practice medicine.

Thousands of published scientific studies clearly demonstrate the benefit of dietary factors in disease prevention and therapy. One of the goals of *Permanent Remissions* is to make this information available to physicians and help them implement this life-saving information.

Many health experts point to the powerful influence of the pharmaceutical industry, food-processing conglomerates, and conservative physician-dominated medical associations as the primary reasons for this shameful lack of nutritional training in medical schools. These authorities suspect that such organizations see a danger to their interests and profits if the general public were to embrace healthier dietary practices and lifestyles. As Dr. Sanders points out, published research has consistently shown that physicians' prescribing habits tend to follow drug companies' promotional efforts and not necessarily the conclusions of scientific experts or authoritative panels.*

I take a less cynical view. I believe that most physicians pay little attention to nutrition and its role in prevention and treatment of cancer and heart disease primarily because *they have not been trained to do so.* Although conventional medicine excels in managing medical emergencies, fighting infectious diseases, and developing life-saving surgical techniques, modern medicine has failed in the prevention, management, and reversal of the chronic diseases that account for 85% of our national health-care bill.

U.S. medical schools turn out doctors who practice conventional medical techniques that have little impact on the *prevention* of cancer, heart disease, and diabetes. In almost every case, physicians treat the symptoms of disease but fail to treat the cause of these serious health problems. As Dr. Sanders notes, "This is the medical approach that is consistently reimbursed by insurance companies."

Former Surgeon General Everett C. Koop, in his 1988 *Report on Nutrition and Health,* emphasized that "dietary imbalances" are the

---

*Sanders, Charles L. *Prevention and Therapy of Cancer and Other Common Diseases: Alternative and Traditional Approaches* (Infomedix, Richland, WA, 1996).

leading preventable cause of premature disease and death. Dr. Koop recommended expanded education for physicians in the areas of nutrition and lifestyle modification.

Revolutionary Life-Saving Information for American Blacks

American blacks face a tragic national health-care crisis of their own: they die more often from almost every type of cancer and they are twice as likely to suffer from hypertension, diabetes, heart disease, and stroke as white Americans. Puzzled by these appalling statistics, I investigated the roots of black health problems to determine why:

- American black women get breast cancer less frequently than American white women yet suffer *twice* the breast cancer death rate *and* have more aggressive forms of the disease.
- American black men have the highest prostate cancer rate in the world and suffer higher rates of invasive prostate cancer than native Africans or American whites.
- American black women have a higher obesity rate than American white women.
- Native Africans have normal blood pressure that does not rise with age, while twice as many American blacks as American whites suffer from hypertension.
- The overall cancer death rate among American blacks has *increased by 16%* since 1966.

I wondered about other apparent racial differences in disease rates that have perplexed health experts. For example, why do more American black women than men suffer from diabetes and why is the prevalence of diabetes higher in American black women than in American white women?

In some instances, genetics can play an important role in accounting for differences in disease rates among various racial and ethnic groups. For example, researchers believe that Ashkenazi Jewish women (those of Eastern European descent) suffer a higher rate of breast cancer than other women of the same age because many carry a mutated gene that predisposes them to the disease. But what has not been made clear, to this point, is why American blacks suffer a disproportionate amount of degenerative diseases relative to American whites. Are dissimilar disease rates due to genetics, environment, quality of health care, or cultural beliefs and practices? As I discovered, all of these variables contribute to the racial disparities in disease and mortality rates.

Early disease detection, better health education, and access to adequate health care can significantly reduce the higher rates of cancer and other diseases American black men and women suffer when compared to other groups. But there are important dietary changes that can significantly reduce the trend toward higher disease rates among American blacks.

Permanent Remissions contains revolutionary and life-saving information that can help millions of American blacks reduce their excessive death rates from cancer, heart disease, hypertension, and diabetes. Just as importantly, this new information can help millions avoid these diseases altogether.

The *Permanent Remissions* Kitchen

The basic phytonutrient-rich foods and life-saving recipes that you will enjoy on the *Permanent Remissions* diet contain more than a half million naturally occurring compounds, many of which are active against cancer, heart disease, diabetes, and osteoporosis. I'm going to show you how to enjoy all of these disease-fighting compounds with a minimum investment of effort and time.

Hungry? How about a bacon-turkey club sandwich that fights cancer and heart disease *and* helps you lose weight? What about a beef taco salad that fights breast and prostate cancer while it lowers your cholesterol and body fat? Or perhaps a shrimp-wrapped-in-bacon appetizer that helps control diabetes?

I will also show you how to use the newest disease-fighting soy foods and beverages to quickly and easily prepare meals, snacks, appetizers, and desserts that will delight the most discriminating palates. These *Permanent Remissions* recipes are based on the same foods and recipes that helped the people you'll meet in this book achieve long-term remissions from cancer and other life-threatening diseases.

Computer Software That Can Save Your Life

If you or a member of your family have access to a personal computer, you can use it to help prevent and defeat a host of diet-related

diseases. I have created a software program, based on my years of clinical experience, research, and knowledge of food technology, to give
you an effective weapon against cancer, heart disease, and other health
problems. This cutting-edge health software will turn any PC into your
own personal nutritionist. It will automatically construct life-saving
meals based on your favorite phytofoods; help you lose excess body fat
that can place you at risk of developing cancer, heart disease, and diabetes; and give you the latest life-saving information available in no other
software program. See *Appendix* I (*Permanent Remissions* Computer
Software, pages 349–50) for more information on this software.

2

CANCER: A NEW STANDARD
FOR A CURE

We are within striking distance of a cure for cancer. We still have a few riddles to solve before we can declare victory, for this is one war that is being won battle by battle, a single discovery at a time. We will defeat cancer not with one magic bullet but rather with an arsenal of weapons that includes phytonutrients, cancer vaccines, and other cutting-edge medical treatments. Cancer will end, not with a bang, as Richard Nixon envisioned when he declared his "war on cancer" in 1971, but with a whimper. We won't slaughter cancer with a single blow. We will tame it.

Recently, U.S. Health Secretary Donna Shalala proclaimed, "We are starting to win the war on cancer." Her heady pronouncement, based upon a slight decrease in overall cancer death rates in the United States, is the first decline ever noted since scientists began keeping good records of the disease at the beginning of the twentieth century. Most of the gains Secretary Shalala spoke of are the result of changes in diet and lifestyle, including reduced tobacco use, reduced exposure to chemicals in the workplace, and improved detection of malignant tumors. Ironically, much of the $35 billion we've spent on Nixon's war on cancer has had little to do with these gains.

Conventional cancer treatments provide only limited effectiveness, forcing doctors to use a meager *5 years'* survival as the benchmark for a "cure." Even this weak definition of a cure hasn't improved much over the last half century: despite recent advances in the early detection and treatment of most cancers, the 5-year survival rate for Americans with cancer has remained a disappointing 51% on average—and far lower for certain types of cancer.

Why has a cure for cancer eluded a nation that has spent a king's ransom to find one, a nation that has charged its most able scientific minds with discovering a cure for a disease that will ultimately kill one quarter of all its citizens?

A New Definition of *Cure*

Phytonutrients can help us coexist peacefully with cancer even if we can't totally eliminate it. In other words, *cancer does not have to be entirely eradicated from the body to live a normal and healthy life and lifespan.* This is the new standard for a cure that makes medical sense and has a basis in other disease treatments. After all, we don't always cure diseases like diabetes and hypertension. We *control* them. Why can't we look at cancer that way?

Your doctor, untrained in nutrition, may be unaware of the latest research and clinical findings on phytonutrients and cancer; however, this book contains the biomedical references and supporting research to help your doctor understand the evidence that supports this new concept for a cure. The *Permanent Remissions* Plan uses this research as the scientific rationale for recommending specific phytonutrients to help augment the safety and effectiveness of traditional therapies.

A number of published studies involving laboratory animals and humans have demonstrated that phytonutrients possess the power to:

- Help conventional medical treatments for cancer destroy specific types of cancer cells and, in some cases, eliminate all detectable traces of the tumor
- Control tumor growth when it is not possible to destroy all detectable tumor cells
- Shrink tumors before surgery or radiotherapy
- Destroy microscopic metastases after tumors are treated with conventional therapy
- Prevent tumor cells from using the body's blood supply to grow and metastasize
- Help premalignant cells revert back to normal cells
- Make cancer cells more susceptible to chemotherapy and radiotherapy and reduce their toxic side effects

Until now, doctors have tried to overwhelm cancer with brute force, slicing and dicing it out with surgery, poisoning it with chemotherapy, freezing it with nitrogen, and zapping it with heat and radio-therapy. All too often, however, a few cells manage to survive the onslaught and develop, sometimes years later, into tumors that are impervious to treatment. The ability of the cancer cells to outmaneuver drugs and radiotherapy has long been reflected in the grim and ever-escalating cancer mortality statistics.

Phytonutrients hold the promise of being highly effective at keeping cancer in long-term remission and being much gentler to patients than current slash-and-burn conventional strategies. What seems significant about the use of phytonutrients, in addition to their cancer-stopping power, is the radical shift in cancer treatment strategy they collectively represent. Slowly but surely, researchers are beginning to speak not of completely eliminating all cancer cells from the body but of keeping them in check (Table 2.1). Many scientists now talk of reining in the cancer cell, even rehabilitating it, a task that demands the use of less toxic substances, such as phytonutrients, that can be tolerated over a lifetime.

Phytonutrients can literally force some tumors to stop growing or to shrink by choking off their blood supply. This could, theoretically, allow cancer victims to live a long and normal life; those with unde-tected tumors might never learn they had cancer. Is this really possible? Japanese men get prostate cancer at about the same rate as men living in the United States, yet many never know they have it. Practically speaking, they lead *cancer-free* lives. Their tumors remain small, silent, and noninvasive, never making themselves known.

TABLE 2.1

Suggested Classification of Cancer Treatment Outcomes

Permanent Remission: All premalignant cells or tumor cells are eradicated or pre-vented from growing beyond 1 millimeter by intake of phytonutrients and/or by conventional treatments. A permanent remission, in effect, allows those with can-cer to live a normal life and lifespan.

Long-Term Remission: Phytonutrients and/or conventional therapies reduce tumor size. Remaining cancer cells show no evidence of growth or metastasis for 5 years or more.

Stabilization: Phytonutrients are used to keep tumors in check; tumors neither shrink nor grow. This may help avert surgery and other treatments while patients and their physicians practice "watchful waiting." Periods of stabilization may last years to decades.

The unique phytonutrient content of the traditional Japanese diet can limit the growth of prostate tumors to no more than a millimeter in size, and there is strong evidence to suggest that it can do the same for other types of cancer as well. For example, the death rate from lung cancer in Japanese men is about four times lower than in U.S. men, even though Japanese men outsmoke American men by a wide margin. When native Japanese men migrate to the United States and embrace the relatively phytonutrient-poor American diet, their death rate from lung cancer soars, approaching that of U.S. men. Diet, not genetics, plays a primary role in the vast majority of prostate, breast, lung and many other types of cancer.

Phytonutrients Against Cancer: The Case of Edmund Rubin

In October 1990, Edmund Rubin showed up at his doctor's office for an annual physical exam, feeling fit and expecting a clean bill of health. What he got was totally unexpected: a diagnosis of cancer.

His doctor discovered a large mass in Rubin's abdomen. A subsequent computed tomography (CT) scan and ultrasound test revealed a large tumor on his left kidney. Rubin was scheduled for immediate surgery. The $5^{1}/_{2}$-hour surgery revealed a tumor as large as a football sitting in Rubin's body. Ominously, his surgeon found that the cancer had also spread to nearby lymph nodes—a sign that the cancer was aggressive and spreading.

Rubin's oncologist explained that this type of tumor would not respond to radiotherapy or chemotherapy. He recommended that Rubin enroll in a trial program that was about to begin to test the drug interferon. It was Rubin's only option. He took it.

After 9 months of treatment with the experimental drug, Rubin had lost 30 pounds and had suffered damage to his intestines. Even worse, the therapy didn't work: a second walnut-sized tumor appeared on his scalp over his left ear. Rubin was treated with radiotherapy, but it did no good. A pathologist found the tumor to be so aggressive that he gave Rubin no more than 6 months to live.

The last thing Edmund Rubin expected at that point was a lucky break, but he got one. It came in the form of an employee at his doctor's office who recommended that he consult Nicholas Gonzalez,

M.D., a New York City cancer specialist with a reputation of helping terminal cancer patients outlive their doctors' prognoses.

As Rubin recalls, "I had no options—nowhere else to go. So I went to see Dr. Gonzalez. I went with the attitude that whatever he wanted me to do, I was ready to comply. Thank goodness, my wife was supportive and came with me."

After 5 months on a vegetarian diet, including an occasional 5-day fruit juice fast devised by Dr. Gonzalez, Rubin began gaining back the weight he lost as a result of his interferon treatments. By 1 year, the aggressive tumor on his head—the one impervious to radiotherapy and interferon—succumbed to the diet and supplements that Rubin took religiously. The tumor regressed and all but vanished.

Conventional medicine gave Edmund Rubin 6 months to live; his phytonutrient-rich diet and supplementary nutrients gave him 6 extra years of life. Rubin is not cancer-free and he must adhere to his demanding dietary regimen for the rest of his life. But he is alive, feels well, and stops to smell the roses in his garden every day.

Dr. Gonzalez also understands the concept of a permanent remission, a term I have coined to describe the state of grace in which a tumor is not completely destroyed but is held in check for life. "It is not necessary to destroy a tumor to get the patient well. The body can contain a tumor and keep it in check like an old bird's nest," observes Gonzalez.

Morton Schneider's Story

Another Gonzalez patient, Morton Schneider, is living testament to the power of phytonutrients. One day in July 1991, while visiting with a friend, Morton Schneider, then 70, began to feel dizzy and started sweating. Believing these might be the symptoms of a heart attack, his wife urged him to go to a hospital emergency room. He reluctantly agreed, only to be given a clean bill of health by the attending physician. Nevertheless, he saw a cardiologist and brought a chest X-ray that had been taken in the hospital emergency room. Fortunately, the cardiologist had better eyesight than the emergency-room physician. He noticed a suspicious spot on Schneider's lung. Further tests revealed that it was cancer.

A surgeon removed a malignant tumor from Morton's right lung.

A CT scan had already revealed that the cancer had spread to the pancreas, liver, and adrenal glands. There were so many tumors and they were so widespread that he told Schneider that he would have essentially butchered his body had he attempted to remove them all.

Morton Schneider's surgeon was brutally frank. He said, "Morton, I can't see the necessity of putting you through the torture of chemotherapy or radiation treatment. You are not going to live much longer." Morton's oncologist was equally pessimistic; he told Schneider to wait to have chemotherapy until he developed symptoms, but that even chemotherapy would not save his life.

At that point, Morton's wife, Evelyn, a cancer survivor herself (see Evelyn's case history on page 115), investigated alternative treatments for cancer and discovered a doctor in New York City who was treating terminal cancer victims with nutrition. Just four months after his lung surgery, Morton Schneider went to see Dr. Nicholas Gonzalez.

Dr. Gonzalez likes to get cancer patients before they've had radiation or chemotherapy because he believes that in many cases these treatments may do more harm than good. Morton Schneider was such a case, having avoided these traditional treatments at his own doctor's behest.

Schneider began following Dr. Gonzalez's demanding dietary regimen (see Table 5.6, page 117) but saw no results for the first 11 months. Then, as if the hand of God came down and touched his body, some miraculous changes began to take place. Subsequent tests revealed that Schneider's cancer was slowly getting better. Instead of dying within 6 months, Morton Schneider was alive and getting well.

Today, six years later, Morton Schneider is 77 and loving life. His dietary regimen is demanding, but he believes it's a small price to pay for so great a reward. Although it is very difficult for him to give up the foods he loves—especially red meat—he continues on his demanding regimen because it has helped him live far longer than his doctors predicted. "I don't mind taking 150 capsules a day because I've beaten the odds—and I didn't have to spend $50,000 to $100,000 a year for chemotherapy and radiation treatments."

Cancer victims like Edmund Rubin and Morton Schneider didn't have the luxury of waiting around for conventional medicine to discover an effective treatment for their "untreatable" cancers. Both were given a terminal diagnosis with no treatment options. They could have sat around and waited to die, but each chose to play a key role in his own cure. Both believe that they would be dead today had they not sought an alternative treatment. Just as important, both had the will to live—an important psychological factor that studies have shown to be linked to cancer survival.

The remarkable cases of Edmund Rubin and Morton Schneider are just two examples that demonstrate the power phytonutrients and other therapies exert over cancer. Before I tell you where to find these remarkable nutrients and how to use them, I want to discuss some basics of cancer: what it is, how it arises, why it spreads, and how conventional therapies have failed to stem the cancer epidemic.

What Is Cancer?

Cancer is an abnormal growth of cells that express varying degrees of resemblance to the cells from which they originated. Cancer cells are called malignant because they acquire the ability to grow unrestrained and can invade other tissues. Normal cells grow and die in a controlled way. Cancer occurs when cells lose their internal ability to stop dividing.

Cancer actually consists of a set of more than 100 disease types. For convenience, cancer types are generally divided into five categories (Table 2.2).

All cancer begins with a single healthy cell that has been corrupted or damaged. That cell becomes two abnormal cells that become four abnormal cells and so on. It may take up to 5 years for the duplication process to occur 20 times, at which point the tumor may reach only the size of a pinhead. During this "silent" period, doctors cannot observe the cancerous tumor because it is too small to be perceived by X-rays and other imaging technologies. After many years, when the doubling process has occurred about 30 times, the tumor may have reached a size that can be felt or seen on an X-ray. The size at this point is usually about a half inch, or 1 cm, in diameter. At that stage, it contains about 1 billion cells. Some newer imaging methods, such as CT and magnetic resonance imaging (MRI), may be able to detect tumors before they reach this size.

Tumors are not always malignant. Benign tumors are composed of cells less abnormal than those of malignant tumors. Most of us already have a number of benign tumors, such as moles, freckles, and

---

TABLE 2.2

General Classification of Tumor Types

Carcinomas: Carcinomas originate in tissues that cover a surface or line internal organs. These are the most common of all cancers, found in breast, prostate, skin, lungs, and intestinal cancers.

Leukemias: These cancers originate in bone marrow, lymph nodes, and spleen. Leukemias are not solid tumors like carcinomas.

Lymphomas: These cancers originate in the lymph nodes, a group of glands found in the neck, armpits, groin, and spleen that transport and filter the body's impurities. Hodgkin's disease and non-Hodgkin's lymphomas are the two most common types of lymphoma in the United States. Burkitt's lymphoma is common in Central Africa.

Myelomas: These tumors begin in plasma cells found in the bone marrow.

Sarcomas: These tumors originate in connective tissue and muscle, attacking bones, cartilage, muscle, and lymph. Sarcomas are the rarest and most deadly tumors.

---

fatty lumps under the skin. These tumors may be cosmetic annoyances but pose no health risks. They are more "differentiated," which means they look more like the normal specialized cells of the organs or tissues in which they originated. Benign tumors may gradually push aside or displace cells and tissues, but their cells do not invade or travel through blood vessels or lymphatic vessels (the drainage system that removes toxic waste from the body) to other organs.

Cells of malignant tumors are more abnormal, are less differentiated, and are invasive and destructive. They are the cells that can kill the victim. Malignant cells invade lymphatic and blood vessels and metastasize, colonizing in distant organs. Unlike normal, healthy cells, there seems to be no limit to the number of times malignant cells can divide, making them essentially immortal.

How Cancer Arises

By the time people reach middle adulthood—and oftentimes well before then—their bodies contain millions of cells that have taken at least one step toward cancer. Although many people believe that their own genetics dooms them to cancer, only about 2%–10% of cancer is attributable to genetic or congenital factors. The vast majority of cancer patterns today reflect carcinogen exposures 2–40 years ago.

Environmental carcinogens cause 50%–90% of human cancers. Environmental carcinogens include chemical, physical, and viral agents. These agents are: ionizing radiation such as X-rays; ultraviolet radiation from the sun; tobacco, including secondhand smoke; alcoholic beverages; metals, such as cadmium, nickel, and arsenic; pesticides; aromatic amines, found in charred or cooked meats and in air pollution; chlorinated hydrocarbons, found in tap water; aflatoxins, which are molds found on peanuts and grains; the human papilloma virus, which is linked to cervical cancer; hepatitis viruses (liver cancer); Epstein-Barr virus (nasopharyngeal cancer); and human immunodeficiency virus (HIV—Kaposi's sarcoma and lymphoma).

Many carcinogens turn healthy cells into cancer cells by stimulating the formation of free radicals, which ultimately damage cellular structures and DNA (deoxyribonucleic acid). Free radicals are molecules or atoms that are electrically charged, making them highly reactive and unstable. For example, corn oil, safflower oil, and other vegetable oils (olive oil is an exception) contain a high amount of fatty acids that can be transformed by heat, oxygen, and other free radicals, resulting in the formation of more free radicals. Free radicals can attack cell membranes, artery linings, LDL (low-density lipoprotein)-cholesterol, and the cell's genetic material, setting the stage for cancer or heart disease. Even ordinary exercise and infections can generate disease-causing free radicals.

Fortunately, the body has its own built-in defense mechanisms that can tie up or quench free radicals. Many defense systems require minerals to work, such as selenium, magnesium, and zinc—all in short supply in the standard American diet. Even these powerful defenses can be overwhelmed by poor diet, tobacco, air pollution, alcohol abuse, too much sunlight, and even too much exercise. That's where phytonutrient-rich foods and supplementary antioxidant vitamins and minerals can help.

How Cancer Spreads

Metastasis—the migration of cancer cells to distant sites in the body—is what makes cancer so lethal and surgery so ineffective. Once cancer cells have dispersed throughout the body, a cure by surgery alone is no longer possible.

What allows cancer cells to leave their birthplace—the primary tumor—and roam the body, evading the immune system and escaping the biological controls that keep normal cells in place?

To metastasize successfully, malignant cells must detach from their original site, trick the body into forming new blood vessels, travel through the body's circulatory systems, including blood and lymph, to distant sites, and establish a new colony of cancer cells. Malignant cells have lost the ability to adhere to one another, as normal cells do, and to the protein latticework, known as the extracellular matrix, that fills the space between cells.

When normal cells, for any reason, have lost their ability to stick to this protein meshwork, certain genes command them to commit cellular suicide, called *apoptosis*. This programmed cell death is Mother Nature's way of preventing defective cells from turning cancerous. Somehow, cancer cells escape these controls. Most of the blame can probably be placed on oncogenes, which are mutated versions of normal genes called proto-oncogenes. Proteins made by these oncogenes send false messages to the nucleus of each cell, thereby stopping the cell from controlling its own growth and dying through apoptosis.

Once cells have lost their genetic controls, they are free to penetrate the membranes that separate cells. Many types of cancer, especially those that arise in breast, prostate, and colon, "learn" how to penetrate the basement membrane, a barrier of tissue that separates cells in these organs from the rest of the body. Basement membranes form a barrier that most normal cells cannot penetrate, but cancer cells can.

Fortunately, even if cancer cells find their way into the general circulation, the formation of metastases is not inevitable. Cancer cells still face a number of biological hurdles: they must attach to the inner lining of blood vessels, penetrate the basement membrane at the new location, invade the new tissue, and begin multiplying. Each of these obstacles taxes the tumor cell far beyond anything it faced in its original site. Many researchers believe that if wandering tumor cells do not promptly attach to a new site, they will die. It is at any of these points that phytonutrients can intervene, creating a very cancer-unfriendly environment for tumor cells (Table 2.3, Figure 2.1).

The Role of Genetics in Cancer

Studies carried out since the 1970s confirm that certain types of cancer seem to run in families, and scientists have begun to identify

TABLE 2.3

Tumor Type and Typical Metastasis Sites

Bladder: Nodes, kidney, other pelvic organs
Brain: Meninges
Breast: Bone, lung, liver, nodes, brain, meninges
Cervix: Lung, bowel, rectum, nodes, bladder
Colon: Lung, liver, nodes
Esophagus: Bone, lung, liver, nodes, adrenal glands
Head/neck: Skin, lung, nodes
Liver: Bone, lung, nodes
Kidney: Bone, lung, liver, nodes, brain
Lung: Bone, marrow, liver, nodes, kidney, brain, meninges
Melanoma: Bone, skin, lung, liver, nodes, brain
Ovary: Abdominal, cavity, uterus, liver, bowel, rectum, nodes, omentum
Pancreas: Lung, liver, bowel, rectum, nodes
Prostate: Bone, lung, liver, nodes
Sarcoma: Lung, nodes
Stomach: Bone, lung, liver, nodes
Testes: Bone, lung, liver, nodes
Thyroid: Bone, lung, nodes
Uterus: Peritoneal cavity, nodes, omentum, ovary

many of the genes that take part in the progression of cells from normalcy to cancer. Recent research has confirmed that cancer occurs in familial clusters primarily because particular classes of genes responsible for cancer are passed from parent to offspring.

All tumor cells descend from a common ancestral cell that at one point—usually decades before a tumor can be seen or felt—lost its ability to control growth through mutations to specific classes of genes.

Two classes of genes, which together only constitute a small proportion of the body's total genetic pool, play a major role in the cancer process. Ordinarily, these two types of genes play opposite roles. One set encourages cell growth, while the other suppresses it. Once this delicate balance is upset, the stage is set for the transformation of a healthy cell to a cancerous one.

For a malignant tumor to develop, mutations must occur in a number of the cell's growth-controlling genes. When this does happen, altered classes of yet other genes also contribute to the formation of the tumor by enabling the transformed cell to become invasive or capable

PATTERNS OF METASASIS

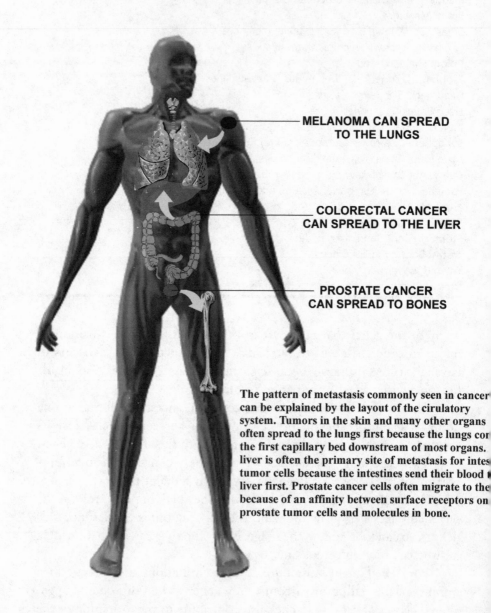

**MELANOMA CAN SPREAD
TO THE LUNGS**

**COLORECTAL CANCER
CAN SPREAD TO THE LIVER**

**PROSTATE CANCER
CAN SPREAD TO BONES**

The pattern of metastasis commonly seen in cancer
can be explained by the layout of the cirulatory
system. Tumors in the skin and many other organs
often spread to the lungs first because the lungs cor
the first capillary bed downstream of most organs.
liver is often the primary site of metastasis for intes
tumor cells because the intestines send their blood
liver first. Prostate cancer cells often migrate to the
because of an affinity between surface receptors on
prostate tumor cells and molecules in bone.

of metastasizing throughout the body. Fortunately, phytonutrients can intervene at any stage of this unchecked growth toward cancer.

Cellular Suicide: Why We Don't Get Cancer More Often

If a normal cell sustains damage that could lead to cancer, a gene called p53 instructs the cell to commit suicide. This life-saving form of cellular self-destruction helps prevent cancer from forming millions of times over the course of our lives. Scientists now believe that apoptosis failure is key to many forms of cancer.

You may have already heard about two other types of tumor-suppressor genes that can mutate and give rise to cancer: the BRAC1 gene (linked to breast cancer and ovarian cancer) and the BRAC2 gene (linked to breast cancer). These two genes account for about 5% of all premenopausal breast cancers and a substantial portion of familial ovarian cancers as well, especially among Ashkenazi Jewish women of Eastern European descent. Mutated forms of these genes can be passed from parents to offspring, creating a pattern of cancer that clearly runs in families.

The good news is that even if you inherited a mutated form of one or more tumor suppressor genes from your parents, *you are not necessarily doomed to cancer.* We now know that genes generally need to sustain multiple traumatic events, or "hits," before they allow cells to run amok and evolve into deadly tumors. This explains why people in cancer-prone families are not riddled with tumors throughout their bodies. Inheritance of just one genetic defect (first hit) predisposes a person to cancer but does not cause it directly; a second hit is usually required, usually manifested as damage caused by cigarette smoke, high-protein diets, high-fat diets, or excessive exposure to pesticides or other environmental toxins. Phytonutrients can block these carcinogenic influences from injuring a cell's delicate genetics. Moreover, phytonutrients can, in many instances, rehabilitate a damaged gene, helping a crippled cell return to a healthy and well-differentiated state.

What Makes Cancer Cells Immortal?

Normal, healthy cells usually die after a predetermined number of cell divisions or doublings, usually 50 or 60 in humans. Each cell has a built in counter, called a *telomere* (located at the tip of a chromosome, like the plastic endcap on a shoelace), that monitors the number of divisions. With each doubling, the telomere endcap shortens. At some critical threshold, the telomere instructs the cell to enter senescence; genetic chaos ensues and the cell dies its normal, programmed death.

Occasionally, a cell in this dying population escapes death by activating a gene that codes for the enzyme *telomerase,* which prevents the progressive shortening of telomeres. Human cells carry the gene for telomerase, but most of them never express it after birth (the one clear exception in humans is in the testes, which use telomerase to rebuild the telomeres of sperm cells). Once this occurs, the cell has taken the first step toward immortality. This maverick cell becomes the single malignant cell that will clone itself over and over to form a tumor that will make itself known years later in the breast, prostate, ovary, or other organ.

The Shortcomings of Traditional Cancer Therapies

Despite many advances in the early detection and treatment of most cancers, overall survival rates have not significantly changed since the 1970s. Among the organ sites with poor prognoses and low 5-year survival rates are those listed in Table 2.4.

Phytochemicals and other cutting-edge dietary treatments may offer new hope to victims of cancers with very low 5-year survival rates.

TABLE 2.4

Survival Rates of Selected Cancers

Organ Site	Approximate 5-Year Survival Rate (%)
Lung	13
Ovary	39
Stomach	16
Esophagus	9
Pancreas	3

In the following chapters, you will learn about people who used traditional medical therpay plus diet to banish the cancer.

In the next chapter, you will learn how to develop your own personal phytofood plan. This new way of eating is a departure from the U.S. government's food guide pyramid that you may have seen or perhaps even follow. The *Permanent Remissions* Phytofood Guide Pyramid (see page 51) is designed to reverse the prevailing nutritional dogma that has helped create a nation where almost seven of 10 people are overweight, a nation that loses more people to cancer, heart disease, and diabetes in 1 year than it has lost in all its wars. *Permanent Remissions* offers a new way to prevent and beat back these diseases. It also offers a new way of coexisting with cancer while living a normal life and lifespan—and a new standard for a cure.

3

PHYTONUTRIENTS: TWENTY-FIRST CENTURY VITAMINS

You sit at the breakfast table each morning, gulping down a daily multivitamin supplement, presumably to arm your body against cancer, heart disease, and other life-threatening health problems. In kitchens across the country, millions of Americans are doing the same thing. Once-a-day multivitamins are by far the most popular pills in America. But do they actually forestall disease and help any of us live longer?

Researchers at the Centers for Disease Control and Prevention (CDC) and the American Cancer Society (ACS) followed the health of nearly 1 million men and women for 7 years to discover whether people who took low-dose, garden-variety multivitamins suffered fewer deaths due to heart attacks and strokes. Those who took them regularly died from heart disease and stroke at about the same rate as those who didn't. There were no measurable differences in deaths from other causes. No studies to date show that taking once-a-day multivitamins improves the survival of well-nourished people.

The problem with conventional multivitamin supplements is one of dosage. Clinical studies clearly show that doses much higher than the recommended dietary allowances (RDAs) established by the National Research Council's (NRC's) Food and Nutrition Board are required to prevent and forestall cancer and other diseases.

In 1993, scientists at the West Virginia University School of Medicine studied the benefits of megadose vitamins for bladder cancer. Bladder cancer is an ideal type of cancer for the evaluation of preventive therapies because 88% of patients with bladder cancer whose tumors are removed surgically develop recurrent tumors.

The researchers gave one group of people a multivitamin supplement containing the RDA levels for known vitamins and minerals. Another group was given a potent multivitamin supplement containing megadoses of vitamins, including A, B₆, C, and E. This randomized, double-blind study included 65 patients with biopsy-confirmed cancer of the bladder who were already subjects in a randomized trial of immune-boosting BCG (bacillus Calmette-Guérin) therapy (a drug commonly used to treat tuberculosis). After 1 year, the overall tumor recurrence rate was 80% in the RDA group, compared to 40% in the megadose group.

The West Virginia University School of Medicine scientists concluded: "Our results clearly suggest that high doses of vitamins A, B₆, C, and E reduce the risk of recurrence in patients with transitional cell carcinoma of the bladder."

This study is representative of many others that show that megadose levels of vitamins can reduce the recurrence of cancer, especially when combined with conventional treatments. Just as important, several recent studies have shown that daily megadoses of vitamin E (200–400 international units), vitamin C (200–500 milligrams per day), and the mineral selenium (200 micrograms per day) can cut in half your risk of ever getting cancer.

Studies such as this one, which are far from conclusive, suggest that certain vitamins, taken in quantities beyond those available in ordinary foods, may provide powerful protection against disease. A diet based on phytonutrient-rich foods, however, should form the foundation of your new way of eating. Dietary supplements play an ancillary role in preventing and reversing disease. That's why they are called *supplements:* they are meant to complement and augment a healthy diet, not supplant it. Certain dietary supplements may not be appropriate for your particular needs or disease condition. That's why you should always consult with your physician before taking any dietary supplements.

At this time, the National Cancer Institute (NCI) does not recommend supplements of vitamins, minerals, herbs, or other nutrients for the prevention of cancer, but it does recommend that everyone consume a diet rich in a special class of compounds called phytochemicals. I prefer the term *phytonutrients* because these compounds, found in all plant foods, are the dietary substances that save lives. Although they have no caloric value and are technically not considered vitamins, I believe that phytonutrients play an even more important role than vitamins in preventing and reversing cancer and heart disease. In fact, I predict that phytonutrients will become the new "vitamins" of the twenty-first century.

Phytonutrients: The Real Heroes of *Permanent Remissions*

Why didn't Mother Nature just put disease-bashing phytonutrients in our bodies instead of sending us to the supermarket for them? Why did she give them to plants but not to her two-legged creatures?

One reason is that *we* have legs and plants do not. We can run from predators. Plants, on the other hand, can't run from danger. Plants rely on phytonutrients to discourage insects and animals from eating them. (Many phytonutrients are distasteful to predators; others render predators sterile and thereby reduce the predator population.) Plants also lack an immune system, so nature has given them the ability to manufacture phytonutrients that protect them against bacteria and viruses. And since plants can get cancer, too, phytonutrients play an important role in keeping them disease-free.

Plants must also make their own antioxidant phytonutrients, such as polyphenols and carotenoids, to protect their delicate cellular structures from the sun's ultraviolet radiation. Photosynthesis, a process by which plants use sunlight, carbon dioxide, and water to manufacture carbohydrates and oxygen, generates a large number of free radicals that would kill the plants were it not for the presence of protective phytonutrients. Phytonutrients also protect young seeds, guarding their ability to germinate. More than 20 classes of phytonutrient compounds found in plant foods produce anticancer activity in animals and humans. Compounds in garlic, onions, and such cruciferous vegetables as broccoli and cabbage detoxify carcinogens and prevent them from doing their dirty work. Retinoids, indoles, isothiocyanates, polyphenols, and trace minerals found in cabbage alone can inhibit breast cancer in rats. Scientists at the NCI believe that phytonutrients are active against human cancer as well.

Researchers at the NCI's Diet and Cancer Branch and at the American Heart Association (AHA) have just begun to understand how phytonutrients can halt and even reverse the growth of cancerous cells and cholesterol-filled tumors, called *plaque,* that cause a heart attack or stroke. And scientists have recently discovered that phytonutrients can help patients with adult-onset diabetes reduce or eliminate their need for insulin injections and oral medications.

Doctors have long known that if cancer cells can be stopped from spreading, nearly everyone with cancer could be cured by conventional treatments such as surgery, chemotherapy, and radiotherapy. In general, the primary cancer tumor does not kill people; it is the spread of cancer cells (called metastasis) throughout the body that kills.

Phytonutrients can and do stop tumors from growing and spreading. *The treatment strategy of combining phytonutrients with traditional cancer treatments, such as radiotherapy and chemotherapy, represents the most important advance in the treatment of cancer of the twentieth century.*

Many phytonutrients come packaged in a variety of familiar containers: broccoli, tomatoes, strawberries, oranges, lemons, grapefruit, watermelon, grapes, carrots, cabbage, garlic, and onions, to name just a few. Nearly all of them sport tongue-twisting names such as *isothiocyanates, allylic sulfides,* and *isoflavonoids.* Fortunately, you don't have to know how to pronounce them, but you do have to know where to find them and how to use them. Highly concentrated phytonutrients have been incorporated into biodesigned food products, sometimes called functional foods or nutraceuticals. These high-tech food and beverage products are currently the focus of investigation by the NCI's Diet and Cancer Branch.

Perhaps you're wondering how can ordinary foods such as tomatoes, garlic, and soy pack the kind of wallop that can knock out a ferocious and merciless killer like cancer. Never underestimate the healing power locked inside a tomato, onion, orange, or cantaloupe. *Food is the most chemically complex substance you will ever encounter.* The phytonutrient-rich foods and beverages that you will enjoy on the *Permanent Remissions* plan contain more than a half million naturally occurring compounds, many of which are active against cancer, heart disease, diabetes, and osteoporosis.

The Phytofood Pyramid Guide

A few years ago, experts at the United States Department of Agriculture (USDA), unhappy with the four-food-group arrangement and buckling under pressure from health authorities, devised a healthier and more scientific eating scheme called the USDA's Eating Right Food Guide Pyramid. The USDA plan clearly indicated that meat and dairy products should play less of a role in the American diet than had been recommended previously. This recommendation generated a collective moo and oink from dairy and meat industry associations, who promptly used all the political clout they could muster to cow the USDA into submission.

It worked. Before you can say Tutankhamen, the USDA withdrew its food guide pyramid and spent the next year and almost $1 million to redraft a new, meat- and dairy-friendly pyramid. The agency now recommended two to three daily portions of meat and dairy products, *as it had since 1958,* and increased the suggested amount of meat from 6 ounces to 5–7 ounces.

If the USDA had only your health in mind, their pyramid would look like the one depicted in Figure 3.1. I've revised this corporately corrupt food pyramid (Fig. 3.2) to portray the correct hierarchy of the world's healthiest foods—the ones that can prevent and defeat cancer, heart disease, and diabetes.

If you want to live to see your grandchildren's children, use the *Permanent Remissions* Phytofood pyramid to help you create a new way of eating for optimal health and longevity.

HOW TO USE THE *PERMANENT REMISSIONS* PHYTOFOOD PYRAMID GUIDE

The Phytofood Pyramid Guide recommends phytonutrient-rich food groups based on the number of suggested daily servings (Table 3.1).

Animal protein is restricted to small amounts of seafood rich in omega-3 fatty acids (up to two times a week) and small amounts of skim and fermented milk products (two servings a week and as called for in *Permanent Remissions* recipes—see pages 227–338). Salting foods is limited to ½ teaspoon of salt per day; tabletop sweeteners are limited to 1 tablespoon per day.

Sugar intake is derived mostly from natural sugars contained in fruits and fruit purees. A small amount of added sugar is occasionally permitted in selected recipes.

The Phytonutrient Food Guide Pyramid represents a radical departure from the USDA's Food Guide Pyramid because it:

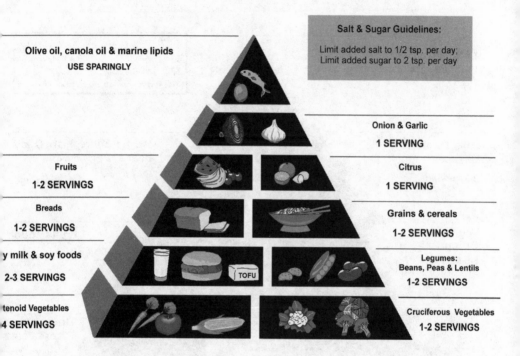

Olive oil, canola oil & marine lipids
USE SPARINGLY

Salt & Sugar Guidelines:

Limit added salt to 1/2 tsp. per day;
Limit added sugar to 2 tsp. per day

Onion & Garlic
1 SERVING

Fruits
1-2 SERVINGS

Citrus
1 SERVING

Breads
1-2 SERVINGS

Grains & cereals
1-2 SERVINGS

y milk & soy foods
2-3 SERVINGS

TOFU

Legumes:
Beans, Peas & Lentils
1-2 SERVINGS

tenoid Vegetables
4 SERVINGS

Cruciferous Vegetables
1-2 SERVINGS

PERMANENT REMISSIONS PHYTOFOOD PYRAMID

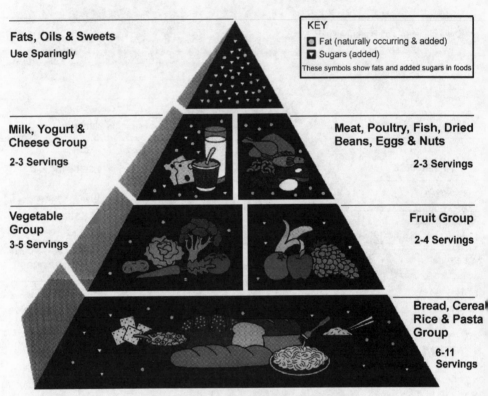

Fats, Oils & Sweets
Use Sparingly

KEY
⬚ Fat (naturally occurring & added)
▼ Sugars (added)
These symbols show fats and added sugars in foods

Milk, Yogurt & Cheese Group
2-3 Servings

Meat, Poultry, Fish, Dried Beans, Eggs & Nuts
2-3 Servings

Vegetable Group
3-5 Servings

Fruit Group
2-4 Servings

Bread, Cereal Rice & Pasta Group
6-11 Servings

USDA FOOD GUIDE PYRAMID

TABLE 3.1

Daily Phytofood Servings Guide

Phytonutrient Group	Number of servings	Totals
Friendly fats (including those from seafood)	Use sparingly*	
Garlic and onions	1	1
Citrus/other fruits	1/1–2	2–3
Whole grains/cereals	1–2/1–2	2–4
Soy foods and beverages/legumes	2–3/1–2	3–5
Carotenoid vegetables/cruciferous vegetables	3–4/1–2	4–6

*Use up to 2 teaspoons of olive oil each day or as called for in *Permanent Remissions* recipes, pages 227–338. Use dietary supplements of friendly fats as advised by your physician.

- Replaces whole grains and cereals with carotenoid- and cruciferous-rich vegetables as the pyramid foundation
- Replaces red meat, pork, and fowl with soy-based meat analogues and seafood rich in omega-3 fats
- Limits added fats primarily to monounsatured oils and omega-3 fats
- Limits dairy foods (optional) to small amounts of skim milk and fermented skim-milk products

The foundation of the Phytonutrient Food Pyramid is built upon vegetables and fruits rich in cancer-fighting carotenoids and flavonoids. It emphasizes soy foods, including the new soy meat replacement products now available in most supermarkets and natural-food stores, and soy beverages, including soy milk and soy cocktails (available in health-food stores). These foods and beverages provide the highest concentration of disease-fighting phytonutrients for the fewest calories—so important to a nation in which seven of 10 people are overweight. They are also rich sources of calcium, cholesterol-lowering fiber, and the natural spectrum of antioxidant vitamins and minerals.

Whole grains and cereals take a backseat to vegetables in the Phytonutrient Food Guide Pyramid. Why? Because complex carbohydrate foods such as bread, breakfast cereal, and pasta contain lower levels of cancer-fighting phytonutrients and are calorically denser than phytonutrient-rich vegetables and legumes. Unless you are a cancer victim fighting cachexia (loss of appetite and muscle wasting), beating back a fierce enemy such as cancer requires the most nutrition for the least calories. *A low-calorie, phytonutrient-dense diet is the fast track to a long and healthy life* (Table 3.2).

◆

TABLE 3.2

Phytonutrient Activity Chart

Phytonutrient	Food Examples	Activity
Carotenoids	Broccoli, cantaloupe, carrots, mandarin oranges, papaya, pumpkin, spinach, yellow squash, sweet potatoes	A powerful family of antioxidants that suppress or reverse cancer; reduce risk of atherosclerosis
Catechins	Green and black teas	Quench free radicals involved in cancer formation and atherosclerosis
Flavonoids	Broccoli, cabbage, carrots, citrus fruits, cucumbers, soy foods and beverages, tomatoes, yams	Block sex hormones that promote the growth of cancer cells
Indoles	Broccoli, Brussels sprouts, cabbage, cauliflower, kale, kohlrabi, mustard greens, rutabagas, turnips	Activates the body's enzymes that detoxify carcinogens; help metabolize estrogen to its harmless form
Isoflavones	Beans, peas, lentils	Block the cancer-promoting effects of sex hormones; inactivate enzymes produced by cancer cells
Isothiocyanates	Broccoli, Brussels sprouts, cabbage, cauliflower, kale, kohlrabi, mustard greens, rutabagas, turnips	Activates the body's enzymes that detoxify carcinogens; help metabolize estrogen to its harmless form
Lignans	Nuts and seeds	Quench free radicals; block sex hormones from promoting tumor formation and growth
Limonoids	Citrus fruits	Stimulate the body's enzymes that detoxify carcinogens
Monoterpenes	Broccoli, cabbage, carrots, citrus, fruits, eggplant, parsley, peppers, squash, tomatoes, yams	Quench free radicals; activate the body's enzymes to detoxify carcinogens; reduce risk of atherosclerosis
Omega-3 fatty acids	Flaxseed, walnuts, purslane	Block estrogens from promoting cancer; reduce inflammation that leads to cancer and atherosclerosis
Organosulfur Compounds	Garlic, leeks, onions, shallots	Block carcinogen formation and suppress tumor formation
Protease inhibitors	Soy foods and beverages	Block the enzymes made by cancer cells that help them spread; limit the rate of cell division; gives cells time to repair DNA damage that can lead to cancer
Sterols	Broccoli, cabbage, cucumbers, eggplant, peppers, soy foods and beverages, tomatoes, whole grains and cereals, yams	Help cells that have taken a step toward cancer revert to a normal state; help block the body from absorbing dietary cholesterol
Triterpenes	Licorice root	Block sex hormones and prostaglandins from promoting cancer

PYRAMID LEVEL ONE:
CAROTENOID-RICH FOODS AND CRUCIFEROUS VEGETABLES

Carotenoid and Cruciferous Vegetables

EAT 4–6 SERVINGS EACH DAY

What counts as a serving?

- ½ cup of tomato sauce
- ½ cup of other vegetables (cooked or raw)
- 1 cup of raw leafy vegetables such as lettuce

CAROTENOID-RICH FOODS

Mama mia! It's in the sauce.

Tomato sauce, that is. It doesn't matter if it's a supermarket brand or a simmer-all-day family recipe, all tomato sauces contain a high concentration of compounds called *carotenoids.* You're probably familiar with beta-carotene, the plant form of vitamin A. But the most powerful cancer-clobbering carotenoid is actually a compound called *lycopene.*

Lycopene is the carotenoid most efficient at quenching the type of free radicals caused by cigarette smoke and air pollution. The foods with the highest concentration of lycopene in the ordinary American diet are tomato sauce (including ketchup and tomato-based barbecue sauces), guava, watermelon, and pink grapefruit. Unlike synthetic beta-carotene dietary supplements, which contain no lycopene or any other natural carotenoids, these foods contain a spectrum of disease-fighting carotenes.

Tomatoes also contain the anticancer phytonutrients, *p-coumaric acid, chlorogenic acid, alpha-carotene, beta-carotene,* and *ascorbic acid.* This phytonutrient profile may explain why tomatoes lower the risk of cancers of the digestive tract and why people who eat a Mediterranean diet enjoy comparatively lower rates of these and other types of cancer.

For decades, scientists ignored lycopene in their studies of diet and cancer in favor of beta-carotene, another member of the carotenoid phytonutrient group found in red, yellow, green, and orange vegetables. Unfortunately, investigators in charge of several large clinical studies gave synthetic beta-carotene supplements to long-term smokers, with disastrous results. The smokers who took the beta-carotene supplements suffered higher rates of lung cancer than smokers who took no beta-carotene supplements.

Carotenoids interact with each other during digestion. Overloading the body with a single carotenoid, such as beta-carotene, can reduce the absorption of the other carotenes, such as lycopene (found in tomatoes and watermelon) *and* lower the level of vitamin E—another cancer-preventing compound—stored in the body.

Was it good science to give cigarette smokers large doses of only one synthetic carotenoid—beta-carotene—to the exclusion of all others? Since lycopene and not beta-carotene is more protective against the type of lung damage caused by cigarette smoke, the higher rates of lung cancer seen among participants in cancer studies of smokers should come as no surprise. That is why it is essential to eat a variety of carotene-rich fruits and vegetables each day.

Most of the studies that found beta-carotene to be protective against cancer in humans tracked the dietary intake of carotenoid-rich fruits and vegetables, not synthetic beta-carotene supplements. These studies revealed that beta-carotene, lycopene, and other carotenoids in fruits and vegetables work as a powerful team to fight cancer and heart disease. Dietary supplements that contain beta-carotene only, without the other naturally occurring carotenoids, provide less than optimal disease protection. That's why I recommend that if you take dietary supplements, they contain what I call a *carotenoid complex,* including alpha- and beta-carotene, lutein, lycopene, zeaxanthin, and preformed vitamin A. More research in this area is needed before we can draw any definitive conclusions about the effectiveness of carotene supplements, but one thing remains clear: dietary supplements can be used to *augment* a phytonutrient-rich diet but never to *supplant* it.

PYRAMID LEVEL ONE: CAROTENOID VEGETABLES

WHAT CAROTENOIDS DO

At least 20 major published studies demonstrate that people who eat foods with a high carotenoid content reduce their risk of cancer by 30%–50%. Here's why:

- Carotenoids keep cells in the breast healthy by curbing their growth when exposed to the estrogen-related sex hormone estradiol. Vitamin A and related compounds also enhance the immune system and direct it to release hormonelike substances that seek out and kill cancer cells.
- Carotenoids inhibit carcinogenesis in animals exposed to chemicals and the sun's UV (ultraviolet) radiation.

- Carotenoids destroy malignant cells but leave healthy cells intact. Cancer cells appear to have a leaky cell membrane, whereas normal cells have an intact one. When a carotenoid penetrates a cancer cell, the phytonutrient releases electrons that damage the cells' DNA. Healthy cells can safely break down carotenoids and prevent this damage.

Surveys show that most Americans get their carotenoids from carrots, followed by dark green leafy vegetables, sweet potatoes, oranges, and cantaloupe. Unfortunately, tomatoes are not high on this list, yet they are the richest source of carotenoids most active against lung, breast, ovarian, colon, and prostate cancer. Almost across the board, people who live in countries where tomatoes are copiously consumed enjoy much lower rates of these types of cancer than Americans.

The Mediterranean diet emphasizes tomatoes, garlic, onions, fruits, whole grains, seafood, and olive oil. It contains very small amounts of dairy foods, eggs, and sweets. People living in certain regions on the Mediterranean Sea enjoy some of the lowest rates of cancer and cardiovascular disease in the world and great longevity. Life expectancy in Greece, one of the highest in the world according to the World Health Organization (WHO), ranks second only to Japan.

The *Permanent Remissions* Plan incorporates the most powerful disease-fighting phytonutrient-rich foods from the Mediterranean and traditional Japanese diets. It also includes the latest phytonutrient "functional foods," based on the same concentrated phytonutrients now being tested by the NCI's Diet and Cancer Branch. That's why I believe the *Permanent Remissions* Plan is the world's healthiest diet.

PROMISING CAROTENOID RESEARCH

Seven major studies of carotenoid intake and cancer have established that carotenoid-rich foods are associated with reduced risk of cancer in the prostate, pancreas, lung, breast, cervix, mouth, stomach, pharynx, and bladder. A study at Johns Hopkins University found significantly lower blood levels of lycopene in patients with pancreatic cancer. In a study at Harvard University, researchers demonstrated that lycopene from tomatoes and tomato-based foods reduce prostate cancer risk better than any other fruit or vegetable.

The Harvard study, which examined 48,000 men, found that those who ate at least 10 servings a week of tomato-based foods reduced their risk of prostate cancer by 45%. However, even those who ate between 1½ and 10 servings seemed to derive some benefits. Researchers concluded that lycopene, the carotenoid that gives tomatoes their red color, was *solely responsible* for the protective effect against prostate cancer. Of 46 foods studied, three of four tomato-based foods—tomato sauce, tomatoes, and pizza (but not tomato juice)—significantly lowered the risk of prostate cancer. Of the 42 remaining fruits and vegetables examined, only strawberries were significantly associated with a reduced risk of prostate cancer.

CRUCIFEROUS VEGETABLES

Brussels sprouts, cabbage, broccoli, cauliflower, rutabagas and turnips. Yummy.

Okay, I admit most Americans aren't wild about basing their diet around these foods, but the good news is that you don't have to. Just one serving a day of cabbage (try the Cajun Coleslaw recipe on page 280) can help reduce your risk of developing breast and ovarian cancer and possibly other types as well.

Cruciferous vegetables fight cancer in at least two ways: first, by preventing estradiol, a potent form of estrogen, from subverting normal cell growth into the uncontrolled growth that leads to cancer and second, by directing the body to manufacture enzymes that detoxify chemicals in the environment called *xenobiotics* (literally: foreign to life). People who enjoy broccoli salad and coleslaw can increase the amount of these detoxifying enzymes in the liver, thereby speeding up xenobiotic metabolism and disposing of potential carcinogens.

Researchers have recently discovered that broccoli and other cruciferous veggies can overcome some cases of multidrug resistance, in which tumor cells throw off potent anticancer drugs, rendering them ineffective. For instance, a phytonutrient in broccoli called indole-3-carbinol can sensitize tumor cells to the anticancer drugs doxorubicin, and vinblastine, increasing the effectiveness of conventional chemotherapy.

PYRAMID LEVEL TWO:
SOY FOODS AND OTHER LEGUMES

Soy Products/Other Legumes and Nonfat Dairy

EAT 3–4 SERVINGS EACH DAY

What counts as a serving?

- 2 ounces of soy-based meat replacement products

- ½ cup of soy milk

- 1½ ounces of tofu

- 1 serving of Twinlab's Soy Cocktail or ecoNugenics ecogen soy powder (note: 1 serving of these products contains 50% of a day's allotment of soy)

SOYBEANS

Soybeans contain multiple cancer-fighting compounds called *isoflavones.* One of these, *genistein,* has the ability to block the development of cancer at several stages. More than 200 studies have documented the cancer-stopping power of genistein; the first study dates back to 1966, when it was identified as a compound that could block the estrogen-related hormone estradiol from binding to cells. One form of estradiol can subvert normal cell growth into uncontrolled cell division that can lead to cancer.

Phytonutrients in soy can mimic estradiol, tricking the body into producing less of the real hormone. Since several reproductive cancers depend on estradiol for growth, a reduced level of the hormone in the blood lowers the risk for these cancers. Because soy isoflavones are a thousand times weaker than estradiol, they don't have the deadly effect of estradiol made by the body. The most widely used drug in breast-cancer treatment, tamoxifen, works in a similar way. Asian women, whose diets are rich in soy, normally have lower estradiol levels than American women and enjoy half the rate of breast cancer and fewer symptoms of menopause.

Soy is so effective at regulating estradiol levels that far fewer Japanese women than American women suffer from premenstrual syndrome (PMS)—a condition caused by fluctuating hormone levels. Soy also blocks the cancer-promoting effects of testosterone-related hormones: Japanese men who eat traditional diets that contain ample amounts of soy have a much lower rate of invasive prostate cancer than

Americans. When Japanese men migrate to the United States and adopt a Western diet, their rate of invasive prostate cancer approaches that of American men.

Closer to home, Harvard researchers found that Americans in Wyoming and South Dakota who regularly ate soybeans and such soy products as tofu had less than half the risk of getting colon cancer as Americans who didn't eat soy. Other studies have linked soy consumption with reduced risk for lung, rectal, and stomach cancer. Soy has also been shown to protect against the toxicity of certain chemotherapeutic drugs. For example, soy protein can prevent the painful gastrointestinal side effects of the powerful chemotherapy drug methotrexate.

Soy milk is an excellent source of disease-fighting phytonutrients. I recommend that you use soy milk in place of cow's milk in your new way of eating. Skim milk and fermented skim-milk products, such as yogurt and buttermilk, can help the body prevent and fight cancer when used in small amounts. I recommend limiting your intake of these products to about 2 cups per week and as called for in *Permanent Remissions* recipes.

Soy plays such a vital role in the *Permanent Remissions* Plan that I've devoted a separate chapter to it. Chapter 4, Save Your Life with Soy, explains the miraculous preventive and healing powers locked inside the ordinary soybean. It also shows you how to get a healthy dose of soy from a number of new soy-based beverages and soy-based meat analogues, such as bacon, chicken, turkey, pastrami, ham, ground beef, and sausage—all available in supermarkets and health-food stores (Table 3.3).

OTHER LEGUMES

Research has shown that legumes, such as kidney beans, peas, and lentils protect against the number-one killer, heart disease. Garbanzo beans, also called chickpeas or *cecci,* fight cancer in much the same way as soybeans. All legumes contain soluble fiber that can lower the risk of colon cancer and reduce blood cholesterol levels.

Beans, peas, and lentils contain a treasure trove of disease-fighting nutrients such as fiber, selenium, chromium, magnesium, folic acid, and phytonutrients that can prevent cancer, heart disease, and diabetes. Legumes are also a low-fat and cholesterol-free food source of iron and calcium. Dozens of scientific studies have shown that legumes can reduce the risk of plaque buildup in arteries and normalize blood sugar levels in diabetics.

TABLE 3.3

Soy Meat Replacers

This New Soy Food Product	*Replaces This Traditional Food*
Soyburgers and soy crumbles	Hamburgers and ground beef
Soy hot dogs	Beef and pork hot dogs
Soy bacon and sausage	Pork sausage and bacon
Soy "milk" beverages	Cow's milk
Soy ham and soy pastrami	Luncheon and deli meats
Soy chicken and turkey	Fowl
Soy (tofu) mayonnaise	Regular mayonnaise

PYRAMID LEVEL THREE:
WHOLE GRAINS AND CEREALS

Whole Grains and Cereals

EAT 2–4 SERVINGS EACH DAY

What counts as a serving?

- 1 slice of whole-grain bread
- 1 ounce of ready-to-eat whole-grain cereal
- ½ cup of cooked cereal, rice, or pasta

All vegetables, fruits, and grains contain indigestible compounds collectively called fiber. One class of fiber, found in whole grains and cereals, mops up and hastens the elimination of the body's toxic waste. Fiber can also help reduce high levels of sex hormones that fuel the growth of hormone-sensitive tumors in the breast, ovaries, and prostate. Soluble fiber, such as that found in citrus fruit, apples, brown rice, and carrots, helps lower blood cholesterol levels and reduce the risk of cardiovascular disease.

A 1994 Gallup poll revealed that a paltry 6% of Americans consumed enough unrefined fiber-containing foods to achieve the recommended 25–35 grams of fiber suggested by most health authorities. This would require at least a doubling in dietary fiber intake for the average American, who presently consumes only about 5–10 grams of fiber each day. Studies have shown that a high-fiber diet can lower levels of circulating estrogen to reduce the risk of breast cancer. Increased dietary fiber intake also protects against cancers in the endometrium, esophagus, mouth, pharynx and stomach.

In 1960, scientists first discovered that the typical low-fiber Western diet delayed intestinal transit time, increasing the contact time between carcinogens in the diet and the colon. In the mid-1970s, British scientists observed that African natives enjoyed a much lower incidence of colon cancer, heart disease, obesity, appendicitis, diverticular disease, hiatal hernia gallstones, varicose veins, and hemorrhoids. Some health experts believe that the disease-fighting benefits of fiber are due primarily to the phytonutrients found in high-fiber foods. The truth is that fiber and phytonutrients are both indispensable to optimal health.

Plant fiber works in several ways to reduce the risk of cancer:

- Diets high in insoluble fiber can bind the sex hormones that lead to unrestrained cellular growth and cancer. By lowering the levels of certain sex hormones, fiber can prevent and slow the progression of many types of hormone-sensitive cancers, especially in the breast and prostate.
- High-fiber diets also bind bile acids that can cause colon cancer. Bile acids aid in the digestion, transportation, and elimination of fats. Dietary fiber found in wheat bran and oat bran help prevent the conversion of bile acids to secondary bile acids that can promote colorectal cancer. One study showed that adding whole-wheat and oat fiber-enriched bread to the diets of adults in Finland to double their intake of fiber reduced concentrations of secondary and total bile acids and the risk of colon cancer.
- Fermentation of vegetable fibers in the large intestine by bacteria produces significant amounts of *butyrate,* a compound that can turn premalignant cells back to normal cells. Butyrate is the preferred energy source for the cells that line the colon. Butyrate is most effective in inhibiting colon cancer in the early stages of tumor development.
- Phytic acid (inositol hexaphosphate) is found in abundance in cereals, soybeans, and other legumes. Phytic acid is primarily responsible for many of the anticancer effects of fiber. Phytic acid suppresses the development of colon cancer, liver cancer, and mammary cancer in laboratory animals.

The best advice concerning the consumption of fiber-rich foods comes from the Bible. Ezekiel 4:9 tells us: "Take unto thee wheat and barley and beans and lentils and millet and spelt and put them in one vessel and make bread out of it." Ezekiel advocates consuming a variety of fiber-rich foods to derive the maximum benefits from various types of fiber. This advice is even more relevant today, in an era when cancer, heart disease, and diabetes run rampant. In the case of fiber, variety is more than just the spice of life—it is an essential element of a long and healthy life.

PYRAMID LEVEL FOUR:
CITRUS AND OTHER FRUITS

Citrus and Other Fruits

EAT 2–3 SERVINGS EACH DAY

What counts as a serving?
- a medium apple, banana, or orange or ½ grapefruit
- ½ cup berries or chopped, cooked, or canned fruit
- ¾ cup fruit juice

Common citrus fruits, such as oranges, grapefruit, and lemons, contain a number of extremely powerful disease-fighting phytonutrients. The Florida Citrus Commission and Florida Citrus Grower's Association, aware of the latest research on citrus and cancer (and the FDA's recent decision to allow food manufacturers to make certain health claims for their products), have begun promoting the cancer-fighting capabilities of Florida orange juice in a massive print and television advertising campaign.

Oranges and other citrus fruits contain some very potent phytonutrients that can help prevent cancer and heart disease. Studies in the United States and China have shown that citrus fruits provide strong protection against esophageal cancers. People who ate citrus fruit daily had a cancer risk *more than tenfold lower* than that of those who rarely ate citrus.

Here is a list of the disease-fighting molecules that you'll get the next time you eat an orange, grapefruit, or lemon or enjoy your next glass of "liquid sunshine":

- **Citric Acid:** Citric acid, responsible to a large extent for the tart taste of citrus fruits, inhibits healthy cells from mutating into cancer cells and helps to flush carcinogens from the body.
- **Folic Acid:** Higher intakes of such folic acid-rich foods as vegetables, legumes, and whole grains are associated with a lower incidence of cancer. A deficiency of folic acid in experimental studies causes DNA damage resembling that seen in cancer cells. Folic acid is required in DNA synthesis and DNA methylation (a chemical process that helps prevent unchecked cellular growth that can lead to cancer). Folic acid works closely with vitamin B_{12} in the transportation and synthesis of

proteins, the synthesis of genetic material (DNA and RNA [ribonucleic acid]), and the formation of blood cells, the nervous system, and the immune system.

- **Limonene:** Limonene is a compound found in the oil of citrus fruit rinds, especially in oranges, lemons, limes, and grapefruit. Preliminary results from a study at the University of Wisconsin's Clinical Cancer Center indicate that limonene and related compounds cause shrinkage of mammary tumors in laboratory animals. Because of its solvent properties, limonene has been used to dissolve gallstones in humans. Animal studies suggest that orange juice protects lab animals from cancer. Dr. Najla Guthrie, Ph.D., from the University of Western Ontario in Canada found that a particular limonoid called *nomilin* was an especially powerful inhibitor of cancer in laboratory studies.

- **Quercetin and Other Bioflavonoids:** Quercetin, a disease-fighting compound found in oranges, cranberries, strawberries, apples, and grapes, exerts its anticancer effects in human breast, ovarian, leukemic, and colon cancer cells. Quercetin inhibits the growth of malignant cells in three ways by:

1. Inhibiting cell metabolism
2. Blocking estrogen binding sites on cells, reducing the growth stimulus that leads to cancer cell proliferation.
3. Triggering apoptosis in tumor cells, a condition in which a damaged cell commits suicide, thereby preventing the possibility that it could turn cancerous.

Quercetin is just one of over 20,000 compounds called *bioflavonoids*. Bioflavonoids have been identified in a variety of vegetables, including green leafy vegetables, roots, herbs, spices, onions, kale, green beans, broccoli, endive, celery, legumes, cereal grains, lettuce, tomatoes, red peppers, and broad beans. Popular bioflavonoid-containing beverages include red wine and green and black teas.

Quercetin is more effective against cancer cells when used with other bioflavonoids. For example, quercetin and *naringenin* (found in grapefruit) together inhibit breast cancer growth more effectively than do the two used apart. These compounds are also effective at removing excess iron from the body. This is important, since iron can promote cancer and heart disease by generating toxic free radicals in the liver and heart. A single glass of grapefruit juice contains enough naringenin to increase the half-life (the time a drug or nutrient stays active in the body) of the cardiac drug nifedipine.

- **Vitamin C:** This powerful water-soluble antioxidant helps regenerate vitamin E, prevent LDL (low-density lipoprotein)-cholesterol oxidation, detoxify environmental carcinogens, and assist in the body's synthesis of hormones and connective tissue, bone, and cartilage. It is required to convert folic acid into its active form in the body, and it increases the body's ability to absorb and store iron. For this reason, vitamin C should not be consumed with iron supplements. Vitamin C improves the bioavailability of the anticancer mineral selenium.

MODIFIED CITRUS PECTIN

Researchers at the Institute at Wayne State University and the University of Michigan reported the results of animal studies in which a form of pectin, a type of fiber found in oranges, grapefruits, and other noncitrus fruits, was tested to prevent the spread of prostate cancer. They found that oral doses of the modified pectin inhibited primary tumor growth and the ability of prostate cancer cells to adhere to healthy cells. This was the first report of the use of phytochemicals to prevent spontaneous prostate cancer metastasis. These preliminary findings suggest that some forms of pectin may be useful in preventing cancer cells from metastasizing to healthy tissue. Ordinary pectin, used to make jellies and jams, does not possess this cancer-stopping power. Once ordinary pectin has been chemically altered in the laboratory, however, it acquires its cancer-stopping abilities. Products containing modified citrus pectin are sold through health-food stores and mail-order companies.

PYRAMID LEVEL FIVE:
GARLIC AND ONIONS

Garlic and Onions
EAT 1 SERVING 3–4 TIMES EACH WEEK
What counts as a serving?
• 2–3 cloves fresh garlic
• 1 teaspoon powdered garlic
• 4 capsules of powdered aged garlic
• ½ cup onion, scallion, or leek

Garlic has been prescribed for centuries as a cure for everything from colds to cancer:

- Ancient Chinese writings dating back over 5,000 years reveal that garlic was used as an antibiotic and fungicide.
- The Egyptians, Greeks, and the Romans used garlic in their cooking and as a medicine.
- Heroditus wrote that Egyptians fed Hebrew slaves garlic to boost their strength and improve their health.
- Aristophanes advised athletes to eat garlic to boost their peak physical performance.
- Pliny the Elder listed garlic for dozens of uses, including tuberculosis, asthma, leprosy, and epilepsy.
- Hippocrates recommended garlic as a laxative.
- French priests in the Middle Ages used garlic to ward off the bubonic plague.
- Louis Pasteur discovered that garlic killed bacteria.
- During World War I and World War II, U.S. troops used garlic on battle wounds to prevent gangrene before penicillin became widely available.

As it turns out, many of these medicinal claims and uses for garlic have been verified by laboratory and clinical research. There have been hundreds of garlic studies, and new benefits for the bulb are being discovered all the time.

Studies that examined the dietary intakes of various populations throughout the world have shown that garlic consumption is associated with reduced mortality from cancer. Garlic inhibits the cancer-causing mold *aflatoxin* from damaging cellular DNA. Garlic reduces the formation of carcinogens in the body and facilitates their elimination from the body. A 1993 study showed that the equivalent of half a clove to one clove daily could lower cholesterol an average of 9%. A 1994 study yielded similar results.

Onions and garlic possess significant blood glucose–lowering action. The effects are similar for both raw and cooked onions. Onions make blood less sticky by blocking hormonelike chemicals called prostaglandins that can accelerate clotting and set the stage for heart attacks and strokes. Onions also block the binding of chemical carcinogens and their metabolites to DNA. Onions have been shown to enhance the body's natural antioxidant systems that protect against skin cancer. Garlic possesses cholesterol- and blood pressure–lowering actions. Too much garlic can hinder blood clotting, so people on anticoagulant medications should use garlic and garlic supplements only under a physician's supervision.

Studies at the State University of New York at Buffalo and at Brown University Medical School indicate that garlic protects against heart disease by lowering harmful LDL-cholesterol levels. Garlic discourages cholesterol from adhering to and clogging artery walls and prevents red blood cells from clumping together, which lowers the risk of blood clots. Garlic also bolsters the immune system and slows the growth of tumors by preventing abnormal cells from multiplying. Says garlic researcher Robert Lin, Ph.D., of Brown University and Harvard Medical School, "Garlic is the most promising anticancer agent we have to date."

The cancer-fighting phytonutrients in garlic and onions are not destroyed by cooking or drying. In fact, according to Dr. Lin, garlic that's been roasted, sautéed, or baked may actually be more healthful than raw: like most other phytonutrient-rich vegetables, garlic contains both pro-oxidants, which encourage the production of cancer-causing free radicals, and antioxidants. Cooking converts the pro-oxidants into disease-fighting antioxidant sulfur compounds.

Garlic use has been associated with a reduced incidence of cancer in humans, particularly for gastrointestinal cancer. A number of studies from around the world suggest that garlic and onions exert powerful anticancer/antiheart disease effects:

- A Chinese study in Shanxi Province found that people who regularly consumed large amounts of garlic and onions enjoyed lower rates of stomach cancer than those who shunned them.
- Natives of Shandong Province in China had the lowest death rate from stomach cancer, and people living in Quixia County had the highest. Residents of Shandong Province consume up to 20 grams of garlic per day, whereas those of Quixia County rarely eat garlic.
- Japanese Hawaiians who regularly eat lots of garlic and onions suffer lower rates of colorectal cancer than those who don't eat garlic.
- Quercetin, a flavonol found in onions, reduced the risk of heart attacks in Welsh men who consumed onions more than twice a week.

PYRAMID LEVEL SIX:
FRIENDLY FATS

Fat phobia has gripped the nation. Fat, say the food police, is the reason why seven of 10 Americans are overweight and have such high rates of cancer and heart disease.

The total calories we eat each day, not fat calories per se, is the reason why more Americans are fat than thin. Even a very low-fat diet will make you fat if you eat more calories than you burn. That's the skinny on fat and weight loss. But the type of fat you eat can effect your risk of cancer, heart disease, and diabetes apart from its caloric contribution to obesity.

Fat damages the body in four ways:

1. Fats suffocate cells by depriving them of oxygen. A high-fat meal can cause angina pectoris (pain in the heart) in someone who has existing coronary artery blockage because high levels of fat in the blood deprive the heart of sufficient oxygen.
2. Fats raise the level of cholesterol and uric acid in the blood, promoting atherosclerosis and gout (a form of arthritis), respectively.
3. Fats increase the risk of cancer of the prostate and colon (and possibly the breast and ovaries) by augmenting the cancer-causing effects of environmental carcinogens in our food, water, and air.
4. Fats make the body insensitive to the hormone insulin, raising blood sugar levels to dangerously high levels and fostering diabetes.

With all the damage that fats do, you may be surprised to learn that there are a few fats that actually fight cancer. These friendly fats, used judiciously and sparingly, not only can lower your risk of cancer, heart disease, and diabetes but also can help stop the progression of cancer and make radiotherapy safer and more effective at killing tumor cells and sparing healthy tissue.

COMMONLY KNOWN FRIENDLY FATS

Olive Oil

A recent survey of 820 women in Greece with breast cancer and 1,548 women who were free of cancer revealed that those who consumed plenty of vegetables, fruits, and olive oil had low rates of breast cancer. Breast cancer risk was also 25% lower among those who consumed olive oil more than once a day, the Greek study showed. Greek women who consumed the least olive oil were still ingesting much more than even the highest consumers of olive oil in the United States. The apparent protective effect of olive oil was most evident among postmenopausal women, while the protection attributed to vegetables and fruits was found in women of all ages.

In Mediterranean countries, where olive oil is widely used for cooking, breast cancer rates are 50% lower than in the United States.

Total fat intake is high in Greece, with women consuming about 42% of their calories from fat. Most of the fat consumed in Greece is mono-unsaturated olive oil. American women, on the other hand, consume about 38% of their calories from fat, but relatively little of that fat is monounsaturated. Most of the monounsaturated fats in the American diet come from meat, which is also high in artery-clogging saturated fat.

Dimitrios Trichopoulos, Ph.D., a Harvard University researcher and a coauthor of the Greek study, speculated that "American women might actually experience as much as a 50% reduction in breast cancer risk if they consumed more olive oil *in place of other fats*" [italics added].

Canola Oil

Canola oil, which now accounts for more than half of the total oil consumption in Canada, is relatively high in monounsaturates, although not nearly as high as olive oil. It also contains the omega-3 fatty acid ALA (alpha-linolenic acid). This is the same omega-3 fatty acid found in high concentrations in flaxseed (17% by weight) and can also be found in smaller concentrations in leafy vegetables and walnuts. Since there is some debate about the health effects of ALA, I recommend limiting your use of canola oil and flaxseed to occasional use in recipes. Olive oil should be your primary source of fat on the *Permanent Remissions* Plan, although there may be a few times when the taste of olive oil would not be appropriate as a recipe ingredient. In those few cases, canola oil should be your second choice.

EPA and DHA

Fish or marine oils, known as omega-3 fatty acids or EPA (eicosa-pentanoic acid) and DHA (docosahexanoic acid), inhibit the growth of transplanted tumors in laboratory animals. Recent studies show that eating as little as one or two servings of salmon each week (for a total of 8 ounces) can supply a disease-fighting dose of EPA and DHA.

If you don't eat salmon, mackerel, or tuna, you can achieve cancer-fighting levels of these friendly fats by supplementing your diet with a tablespoon of ground flaxseed, which contains fats that the body can convert into EPA. And if seafood or flaxseed don't appeal to you, ask your doctor about using an omega-3 fat dietary supplement, such as MaxEpa. This is a popular brand of fish oil that has been used in a number of clinical studies.

Friendly Fats Still Under Study

Here's a helpful guide to finding other friendly fats that scientists are currently testing against cancer. Research on these fats is still preliminary and inconclusive, but enough evidence now exists for scientists to begin evaluating them against human cancers.

GLA

A diet enriched with plant seed oils that contain gamma linolenic acid (GLA) alters the body's production of powerful hormonelike substances called prostaglandins and leukotrienes. Essentially, these oils reduce inflammation and, by doing so, seem to impede the formation and growth of tumor cells.

A Danish breast cancer study demonstrated that GLA was effective in preventing the spread of tumor cells. Women undergoing surgical and therapeutic treatment of breast cancer were given dietary supplements containing GLA plus megadoses of vitamins A, C, and E and the mineral selenium for 18 months following therapy. The women's clinical condition, extent of tumor spread, quality of life, and survival were followed during the trial. The main findings were:

1. None of the patients died during the study period (the expected number was four).
2. None of the patients showed signs of further metastases.
3. The patients' quality of life improved (no weight loss, decreased dependency on painkillers).
4. *Six patients showed partial remission of breast cancer.* A recent study revealed that 2 heaping tablespoons (about 25 grams) of freshly ground flaxseed a day may reduce the growth of breast cancer between the time of diagnosis and surgery and following surgery.

GLA can be found in trace amounts in oatmeal, but most people who want to use GLA obtain it from dietary supplements derived from borage oil. I do not recommend taking dietary supplements that contain GLA unless you have cancer and are advised to do so by a physician. The *Permanent Remissions* Plan contains a healthy dose of a number of other friendly fats shown to be effective at preventing cancer and heart disease.

CLA

First isolated 10 years ago from hamburger, conjugated linoleic acid (CLA) now appears to be present in almost all animal foods. The highest concentrations of CLA occur in red meats, milk, and cheese. CLA is formed during the cooking of foods.

Don't use this discovery as license to pig out on filet mignon and brie. CLA is one of a few cancer-fighting substances derived from animal sources, but it keeps company with some unhealthy compounds: saturated fats and cholesterol.

Several studies have demonstrated the cancer-inhibiting properties of CLA in experimental carcinogenesis and in treating cachexia, a wasting condition that occurs when the body catabolizes (burns up) muscle in response to the presence of certain types of tumor cells. Studies have shown that CLA reversed the catabolic effects of cancer without suppressing the immune system. CLA is a potent antioxidant that facilitates the entry of protein, fat, and carbohydrates into cells to be burned as energy or used for growth and maintenance.

Research studies have used supplements of concentrated CLA in laboratory animals in amounts that translate into about 3–6 grams of CLA per day for humans. U.S. dietary surveys estimate that on average, people consume about 1 g of CLA each day.

Warning: People who use CLA supplements should also eat soy foods or use a soy cocktail. (See the recipe for Super Soy Power Shake, page 337.) CLA can enhance an enzyme, called tyrosine kinase C, that cancer cells use for their metabolism. Geninstein, an active phytonutrient in soy, inhibits tyrosine kinase C. *Use CLA only under the supervision of a physician.*

ADDITIONAL FRIENDLY FAT FACTS

One of the most important benefits of omega-3 fatty acids is their ability to choke off the blood supply to small tumor cells poised to grow and spread throughout the body. Omega-3 helps precancerous cells return to a healthy state (a process called *differentiation*) and makes cancer cells more sensitive to medical treatment. Studies show that EPA and DHA slow down the life cycle of a cell during DNA duplication in lab rats. This is the time when a cell is most vulnerable to chemotherapy and radiotherapy.

Often during chemotherapy, tumors become resistant to cancer-fighting drugs. Omega-3 fatty acids such as GLA and EPA can make these refractory tumors sensitive to drug treatment. One study showed that after only 5 weeks of supplementation with omega-3, the cell membranes of leukemic cells become saturated with omega-3 fatty acids. Studies have shown that GLA and DHA can also help kill cervical cancer cells resistant to chemotherapy.

To reduce your risk of cardiovascular disease, consume one or two servings of seafood rich in omega-3 fatty acids. (Salmon should be your first choice; mackerel, sardines, swordfish, and tuna, your second choices.) This will help make your blood less sticky, thereby reducing the risk of stroke and heart attack. The results of many research studies, taken together, indicate that a diet that contains a variety of omega-3 fatty acids and other friendly fats provides optimal protection against cancer, heart disease, and diabetes.

Most published studies to date demonstrate that people who consume omega-3–rich seafood can safely lower their risk of heart disease and stroke. But obtaining omega-3 fatty acids from dietary supplements is not without risk. For example, omega-3 fatty acids may increase the susceptibility of cell membranes to destruction from oxidation unless other antioxidants, such as vitamin E, are present.

Omega-3 supplementation in healthy men has been shown to raise the level of toxic free radicals and to lower blood levels of vitamin E. Thus, increasing your intake of fish oils and all other plant-based oils (e.g., corn, safflower, peanut) increases the need for vitamin E. Concurrent supplementation with vitamin E and vitamin C (which helps regenerate vitamin E) can provide protection from fat peroxidation of fish oils and other omega-3 fatty acids. Some dietary supplement companies add vitamin E to their fish-oil supplements to protect against oxidation.

Several studies that focused on burn patients and people undergoing coronary artery bypass found no significant blood loss or changes in blood clotting after fish-oil supplementation. No adverse metabolic effects were found in patients with coronary artery disease who received 4 grams of fish-oil concentrate per day for 9 months after bypass surgery. While this research is preliminary, it does suggest that omega-3 supplements, consumed with antioxidant vitamins and in clinically tested dosages, may be used with apparent safety. More research is required before scientists can give omega-3 supplements a clean bill of health. Always consult with a physician before using these or any other dietary supplements.

LIMIT YOUR INTAKE OF ALL FATS, FRIENDLY AND UNFRIENDLY

Friendly fats provide powerful anticancer phytonutrients to the extent that you use them judiciously and sparingly. When you must use fat in a dish or recipe, choose olive oil (or canola oil in limited instances where the taste of olive oil would be undesirable) instead of corn, safflower, and peanut oils. High intakes of these latter oils have been linked to increased risk of cancer (corn and safflower oils) and heart disease (peanut oil) in laboratory animals.

Friendly fats can be part of your new *Permanent Remissions* Plan for preventing diet-related diseases as long as you faithfully follow this simple guideline: *limit total fat intake to no more than 15% of your daily calories*. Practically speaking, this translates into approximately 225 calories per day from all fats and oils—about 25 grams of fat. This amount of fat is appropriate for a healthy adult woman who weighs about 120 pounds, enjoys regular exercise, and consumes about 1,600 calories per day. A man weighing 160 pounds might eat about 30 grams of fat and 1,800 calories per day. *A phytonutrient-rich, low-calorie diet is the fast track to optimal health.*

WHAT ABOUT SUGAR AND SALT?

SUGAR

In 1971, John Yudkin, M.D., author of the book *Sweet and Dangerous,* asked, "Is there a link between sugar and cancer?" Yudkin has studied the health effects of sugar for decades and found that a high sugar intake was linked to serious health problems, such as leukemia in men and women, rectal cancer in men, and breast cancer in women. Yudkin also suspected that sugar intake was associated with cancer and heart disease. Now it seems Yudkin asked the right question.

How harmful is sugar? In the past, nagging nutritionists warned that sugar is devoid of all nutrients except calories, and dentists have decried sweets as a risk for tooth decay. Now, health experts have issued a third caution that can't be sugar-coated: two recent reports, one from the Netherlands and the other from Italy, suggest that a high sugar intake might indeed be a risk factor for certain types of cancer.

When researchers at the National Institute of Public Health and Environmental Protection in the Netherlands studied more than 100 cancer cases of gallbladder and biliary tract cancer, they discovered that sugar intake was linked to an increase in biliary tract cancer. Previous studies had shown evidence that high sugar intake was associated with gallstone formation, which itself is linked to biliary tract cancer, along with obesity.

In the other study, conducted in Italy, researchers studied food intake data gathered between 1985 and 1992 on a variety of dietary factors from people with colorectal cancer. Compared to patients who added no sugar to their beverages, the sugar-users showed an increased risk of developing colon and rectal cancers. The risks increased proportionally with amounts used.

How much sugar is too much? Some scientists would argue that any refined sugar in the diet is a risk factor for cancer, heart disease, obesity, gallstones, hypoglycemia, depression, and gout.

Most people enjoy the taste of sugar but should limit its intake because it is a highly concentrated food stripped of its fiber and nutrients. Americans consume, on average, over 2 pounds of sugar each week—about 25% of their total calories. The average American woman eats nearly her weight in sugar every year. Three fourths of the sugar we eat comes in processed foods and one fourth from pure tabletop sugar.

I've found that by limiting the use of processed foods and tabletop sweeteners, such as white or brown sugar, honey, molasses, and syrups, you can reduce your sugar intake to a reasonably safe level. This allows for the use of sugar-containing foods and condiments, such as ketchup, and an occasional sweet dessert. Whole fruit—which contains sugar—is acceptable because it contains disease-fighting phytonutrients and fiber, which helps slow the release of carbohydrates into the blood during digestion. That's why fruit and not the sugar bowl should be your primary source of sugar. If you must add sugar to coffee, tea, or other beverages, limit your consumption to 2 teaspoons a day for all tabletop sweeteners.

SALT

Many health experts now believe that salt in the American diet does not contribute substantially to hypertension for the majority of Americans. While some people who are sodium-sensitive must drastically curtail their intake of salt, most of us don't develop hypertension as a result of eating it. Why, then, is salt restricted on the *Permanent Remissions* Plan?

Salt causes edema (swelling) in the body, depriving cells of oxygen. The ratio of sodium to potassium is also adversely affected, creating an unhealthy environment inside cells. This situation can help fuel the growth of cancer cells.

Salt, when consumed in excess, increases calcium losses through urine and may decrease bone density. Studies have shown that at sodium intakes above 2,100 milligrams a day (slightly less than what's in 1 teaspoon of salt), women lose calcium each day in their urine. Women who eat the most sodium lose the most bone in their hips. If your diet in high in sodium, you'll need to increase you calcium intake significantly.

There is some added salt permitted in the *Permanent Remissions* Plan. For example, some recipes use canned tomatoes, tomato sauce, ketchup, and mustard. All of these products generally contain some salt. (Salt-sensitive individuals can choose low-sodium and sodium-free versions of these products.) I discourage adding salt to foods or to the cooking pot; however, you can safely use up to $^1/_2$ teaspoon of added salt to recipes and foods. Even limiting salt in this way, people may overconsume salt if they use too many canned or frozen foods. That's why at least one third of the calories in your new way of eating should come from fresh fruits and vegetables.

I suggest monitoring the amount of salt you can tolerate with a home blood-pressure kit, sold in most drugstores. As with sugar, less is better for everyone.

A CAUTION ABOUT ALCOHOL

Alcohol is a drug, not a food, and thus its intake is limited in the *Permanent Remissions* Plan.

You may have heard or read that the French enjoy lower rates of heart disease because they drink large amounts of wine. This so-called French paradox has prompted many physicians to recommend alcohol to some of their patients, a medical mistake with consequences that will be felt for decades.

Wine does contain phytonutrients that can help fight cancer and heart disease, but so do grapes and grape juice. These phytonutrients, known as polyphenols, are available in many fruits and vegetables, so there is no need to drink wine or other alcoholic beverages to obtain their health benefits.

Alcohol plays havoc with the body's reproductive hormones, creating a cancer-friendly environment that can increase the risk of hormone-sensitive cancers and fuel the growth of precancerous lesions. Alcohol has a toxic effect on the liver, kidneys, heart muscle, and gastrointestinal tract. Alcohol is especially irritating to the urinary bladder and prostate gland.

Like sodium, alcohol causes red blood cells to clump, forming a muddy sludge that blocks the flow of blood through small blood vessels. This creates edema, which reduces the amount of oxygen available to cells. If you suffer from angina pectoris (a painful condition in the heart caused by blockage of one of more coronary arteries), alcohol is your enemy. Just two alcoholic drinks can reduce your heart's work capacity by about 20% for up to a full day. If you have heart disease, the last thing you need is to deprive yourself of one fifth of your heart.

If you are in excellent health and exercise regularly, will a glass of wine with dinner do you any harm? No one really knows the answer; however, recent studies indicate that even a single glass of wine each day can raise a woman's risk of breast cancer.

I'm realistic enough to know that most people who love wine and other alcoholic beverages probably won't give them up until they have cancer or other life-threatening health problems (and perhaps not even then). I wouldn't want anyone to chuck the *Permanent Remissions* Plan because of a weakness for alcohol. The wealth of phytonutrients and dietary supplements in the plan will help protect you against alcohol toxicity to some extent. Drinking alcohol starts a fire and phytonutrients help put that fire out. But why start the fire in the first place?

Phytonutrients: The First Step Toward Prevention and the Next Step Toward Permanent Remissions

In the 1970s, scientists didn't know about the disease-fighting power of many of the phytonutrients you just read about in this chapter. Now that you've had a chef's tour of phytonutrients, you can better appreciate the impact that fruits, vegetables, and herbs have on disease prevention and treatment. You now have the power to take command of your health and your future. Embracing a diet based on the Phytonutrient Food Guide Pyramid should mark the first step in learning how to beat cancer, heart disease, diabetes, and osteoporosis. Taking the next step requires learning how use specific phytonutrients to beat back these diseases once they're established in the body. Phytonutrient-rich plant foods offer the first line of defense against cancer and other serious health problems. Should you develop one of these diseases, they offer an opportunity for a second chance at life.

4

SAVE YOUR LIFE WITH SOY

To many Americans, *soy* is a four-letter word.

Let's be honest. Most of us have the same attitude toward soy that we used to have about products that bore the label "made in Japan." Ironically, soy is a dietary staple in Japan and a primary reason for comparatively lower rates of prostate, breast, and ovarian cancer in Asia. The soy food intake of the Japanese also contributes to their substantially lower rates of heart disease, diabetes, and osteoporosis; average soy consumption in Japan is twenty-five-fold higher than in the United States.

Hard-core hamburger lovers turn up their noses at burgers and meat loaf extended with soy. Talk-show host Johnny Carson had a running joke for years about soy-extended ground beef, jesting that the billions of hamburgers served by McDonald's actually represented about 3 pounds of pure hamburger. (A false rumor at the time had McDonald's extending their ground beef with soy to save money.) Such undeserved disdain for soy-based meat substitutes and extenders has clearly left a bad taste for soy on the American palate. Our parents didn't serve us soy food, so most of us don't eat it or serve it to our families. And that's a shame. Because you can save your life with soy.

Newly developed soy foods that taste like hamburger, bacon, turkey, chicken, ham, and sausage and new soy cocktails are now gaining the respect of health experts and the approval of consumers. Beef lovers may call soy "mystery meat," but I call it a medical miracle.

Picking the Proper Soy Products

Soy food and beverage manufacturers such as Twin Laboratories, ecoNugenics, Edensoy, Boca Burger, Green Giant, Worthington, Swift-Eckrich, and Westbrae Natural Foods have made the ordinary soybean taste so good that nearly everyone can enjoy delicious soy cocktails, beverages, and meat substitutes that taste almost like the real thing. These new soy meat substitutes are now available in most supermarkets and health-food stores in the form of soy bacon, sausage, ground beef, hamburger patties, pastrami, and turkey. For the first time in history, you can eat "meat"—quite literally to your heart's content—while losing weight, lowering your cholesterol, and fighting deadly diseases.

Some soy products are better than others at providing high amounts of disease-fighting compounds called *isoflavones*. Unfortunately, a great deal of the isoflavone content of soy is washed out during commercial preparation of some soy meat substitutes. For example, many supermarket products made from soy protein, such as "veggie" burgers and vegetarian chili mixes, use soy protein made by alcohol extraction, a process that diminishes soy's disease-fighting isoflavone content.

Isoflavone levels in natural soy foods and products can also vary depending upon the variety of soybeans, soil, growing conditions, and type of processing (alcohol extraction versus water extraction). Because of this variability, you may want to use one of the new soy cocktails that have recently been developed, to ensure that you consume a clinically effective amount of soy isoflavones. Tables 4.1 and 4.2 show the variable isoflavone content of soy protein that is used in soy foods, beverages, and cocktails made by a growing number of manufacturers. Table 4.3 describes the phytonutrients found in soy foods.

Soy Drinks and Drink Mixes: Getting Soy into Your Diet the Easy Way

It may be difficult for many people to consume enough soy each day, especially if they cannot eat soy foods every day and because many

◆

TABLE 4.1

Range of Isoflavone Content of Supro Brand Isolated Soy Protein Products

Specific Isoflavones	Typical Range (Milligrams Per Gram of Protein)
Daidzein	0.15–0.72
Genistein	0.48–1.51
Glycitein	0.05–0.26
Total isoflavones	0.68–2.49

Source: Protein Technologies International.

TABLE 4.2

Westbrae Soy Beverage Isoflavone Chart

Soy Beverage Product	Average Milligrams of Isoflavones Per Cup
100% Organic (unsweetened)	46.4
100% Organic (original)	38.6
Plain Plus	33.3
Vanilla Plus	31.8
Carob Plus	24.7
Lite Plain	18.9
Lite Vanilla	18.4
Lite Cocoa	13.7

Source: Westbrae Natural Foods.

soy food products do not contain an optimal dose of isoflavones. Fortunately, a number of companies now make delicious protein-rich powdered beverage mixes that can make getting a healthy dose of soy phytonutrients easy and delicious. These soy beverage mixes are available in health-food stores, some supermarket chains, and by mail order (Table 4.4).

Just one serving of these isoflavone-rich soy beverage mixes each day can boost the cancer-stopping power of your diet to clinically effective levels. I highly recommend the shake described in Table 4.5 each morning for breakfast or as a light lunch or snack.

Concentrated soy beverages played a major role in helping some of the people you'll meet later in this book achieve long-term remissions from cancer and heart disease.

TABLE 4.3

Phytonutrients in Soy Foods

Isoflavones: Such isoflavones as genistein, daidzein, and glycitein, inhibit enzymes necessary for the growth of cancer cells. They are often referred to as phytoestrogens, or plant estrogens, and exhibit powerful anticancer effects against hormone-related cancers, such as breast, ovarian, prostate, and endometrial cancer. Genistein has the ability to block the development of cancer at several stages and even return precancerous cells to a normal, healthy state.

Protease Inhibitors: These block the action of proteases—enzymes—that cancer cells use to invade the body and spread to distant sites. Protease inhibitors block the activation of genes that can cause cancer. They also shield deoxyribonucleic acid (DNA) from the damaging effects of radiotherapy. Protease inhibitors are effective 2zagainst a number of health conditions, including cancer, acquired immunodeficiency syndrome (AIDS), cystic fibrosis, acute inflammation, and emphysema.

Phytosterols: Such phytosterols as ergosterol and stigmasterol help control cells from growing out of control and protect against colon and skin cancer.

Phytic Acid: Phytic acid, or phytate, is the storage form of phosphorous in plants; it acts as an antioxidant. Phytates bind with metals, such as iron, that can generate toxic free radicals that lead to cancer and cardiovascular disease.

Saponins: These possess antioxidant properties and prevent cellular mutations that can lead to cancer, especially in the colon; they also help lower blood cholesterol levels.

Cancer patients undergoing chemotherapy should ask their oncologists about using soy beverages and foods as an adjunct to therapy. Soy phytonutrients act in a synergistic manner with certain antitumor agents to inhibit cancer cell growth or induce cancer cell differentiation. For example, genistein in combination with the anticancer drug adriamycin was shown in recent laboratory studies to inhibit breast cancer cell growth.

Soy Foods and Beverages Block Angiogenesis

Angiogenesis—the process by which the body creates new blood vessels—generally marks the point of no return for small but contained tumors. Primary tumors, which are the original site of cancer in the body, rarely kill. But once the original tumor cells gain access to the body's blood supply, essentially by "tricking" nearby blood cells into

TABLE 4.4

Soy Formula Beverages

Soy Cocktails: Such as MAXILife Soy Cocktail, made by Twin Laboratories or any other soy cocktail that contains high concentration of soy isoflavones in addition to other cancer-fighting phytonutrients and antioxidants.

Soy "Milk" Beverages: Such as White Wave Silk, Edensoy, or Westbrae brands. Soy milk contains a rich supply of disease-fighting isoflavones. Just 16 ounces of soy milk per day contains enough isoflavones to equal the amount consumed by native Japanese.

ecogen: Made by ecoNugenics, contains a blend of milled and liquid soy extracts that provide a high level of soy isoflavones.

Haelan 851: Made by Haelan Products Inc., is a fermented soy beverage that doesn't have a pleasant taste but does contain a rich supply of isoflavones.

Supro: is made by Protein Technologies. Supro-based soy drinks are available to the public only in products sold through health-food stores. Read the label to discover if a product contains Supro.

TABLE 4.5

Super Soy Power Shake

Mix in a blender:
  1 serving Twinlab's MaxiLIFE Soy Cocktail
  6 ounces ice-cold fresh orange juice
  ½ medium banana or ½ cup frozen berries (optional)
  ¼ cup crushed ice
Place all ingredients into a blender and blend them on high speed for 30 seconds; serve immediately.

reaching out and embracing them, they migrate to vital organs and recolonize. Now, these tumor cells can absorb all the nutrients they need to become a solid tumor, grow, and metastasize to other parts of the body, traveling along those same blood vessels to perhaps the brain, bowel, and bones.

Nobody knows why some cancer cells can make these blood vessel–forming compounds and others can't, or why a cancer cell unable to do so may gain the ability after several years. But once the trick is learned by even a single cell within a tumor, that cell and all its progeny can do deadly damage. These cells bring in the food supply for the rest of the tumor. These are the cells that are going to kill the cancer victim.

Indeed, several studies in the past few years have hinted that people whose tumors have the greatest number of blood vessels have the highest odds of suffering a distant recurrence of their cancer. For years, cancer researchers hoped to find a way to choke off the crucial blood supply to tumor cells and starve them to death. But the biology of blood-vessel growth is so complicated that most such efforts have failed.

Recently, cancer experts have discovered that soy contains powerful antiangiogenesis compounds that can halt the enzymes used by cancer cells to trigger the growth of blood vessels in almost all tumors found in laboratory animals. *Deprived of their food supply, many tumors quickly shrink and, in some cases, disappear entirely.*

What is particularly exciting about the potential for two soy phytonutrients, genistein and daidzein, to block angiogenesis is that unlike more traditional cancer therapies, these all-natural compounds do not appear to damage normal tissue. Instead, they interfere with a step that is important *only* in the *creation* of new blood vessels. Arteries, veins, and capillaries that have existed for some time remain unaffected.

Angiogenesis Research: One Key to Achieving a Permanent Remission

Judah Folkman, director of the surgical research laboratory at Children's Hospital Medical Center of Harvard Medical School, is one of the leading angiogenesis experts in the world. He is currently testing a number of antiangiogenesis compounds that work like soy isoflavones to choke of the blood supply to tumors, shrink them to a harmless size, and keep them in a dormant state. That state of dormancy, which I believe should be the holy grail of anyone suffering from disseminated or metastatic cancer, is crucial to achieving a long-term or permanent remission.

A member of Folkman's laboratory research team at Harvard, Michael S. O'Reilly, has discovered a potent angiogenesis inhibitor, the protein *angiostatin.* This protein can prevent almost all blood-vessel growth in human prostate, breast, and colon cancers that have been implanted in laboratory animals. O'Reilly found that even when these transplants were allowed to grow to 1% of the animals' body weight, angiostatin could reduce the tumors to microscopic size and keep them dormant for as long as angiostatin was administered.

David A. Cheresh, Ph.D., and colleagues at the Scripps Institute discovered a protein that blocks the growth of blood vessels used by tumor cells to grow and metastasize. This protein interferes with molecules (called integrins) on the surface of cells lining blood vessels. Cheresh's angiogenesis inhibitor may one day become a useful adjunct to radiotherapy or chemotherapy.

Beverly A. Teicher, Ph.D., of the Dana-Farber Cancer Institute in Boston, uses combinations of angiogenesis inhibitors and chemotherapy drugs in laboratory animals with cancer. In one experiment, 42% of the animals were cured by a combination of angiogenesis inhibitors and drugs but not by either treatment alone.

This is precisely why it is so important for you to give this book to your doctor. Most cancer specialists remain unaware that angiogenesis inhibitors, such as those found in soy foods and beverages (Tables 4.6 and 4.7), work synergistically with conventional cancer treatments. The basis for this synergism is easy to understand.

There are two types of cells in a cancerous tumor—endothelial cells (these line the inside of blood vessels) and tumor cells. Each type of cell responds differently to therapy. Endothelial cells don't usually mutate like tumor cells normally do and thus do not become resistant to chemotherapy or radiotherapy. In addition, as Dr. Folkman points out, every 10–100 new tumor cells require at least one new endothelial cell. When an angiogenesis inhibitor halts the growth of one endothelial cell, the effect on tumor cells is greatly increased.

I believe that after the completion of chemotherapy or radiotherapy, soy foods and concentrated soy isoflavones, such as those found in the new generation of soy cocktails now sold in health-food stores, can be used as a long-term treatment to keep cancer in a state of extended dormancy. These are the angiogenesis inhibitors you can use *today*. They're inexpensive and you don't need a doctor's prescription to use them, although you should obtain your doctor's approval. Soy foods and beverages can be used for life to maintain a tumor's dormancy. The general lack of tumor resistance developed against soy phytonutrients and their safety make them the compounds of choice that can help you achieve a long-term or permanent remission.

How Much Soy Do You Need?

Studies involving whole soy foods are not considered as "clean" as studies using individual soy phytonutrients because it is difficult to

TABLE 4.6

Foods Derived from the Soybean

Food	Description
Miso	A fermented paste made from cooked, aged soybeans, salt, water, and koji, a cultured grain from rice or barley that contains *Aspergillus oryae* or *Aspergillus sojae;* miso is rich in friendly bacteria and digestive enzymes
Natto	Made from whole cooked soybeans fermented with *Bacillus natto* until it has a sticky consistency and a pungent odor; natto can be used in place of ordinary cheese
Soy flour	Made from finely ground roasted soybeans; contains a rich supply of protein; available in a defatted version
Soy grits	Made from coarsely ground whole dried soybeans
Soy milk	A creamy, milklike beverage made from whole soybeans by grinding soaked cooked soybeans and pressing soy "milk" out of the beans; commercial soy milks have added ingredients such as sugars, oils, and salt
Soy sauce	Made from a mixture of whole roasted soybeans, wheat flour, and fermenting agents (e.g., yeast, mold)
Soy yogurt	Made from soy milk fermented by active bacterial cultures
Tempeh	Made from whole cooked soybeans infused with a culture (a mold called *Rhizopus oryzae*) and let stand for 24 hours; forms a dense cake with a chewy meatlike texture
Textured vegetable protein	Made from defatted soy flakes that are compressed until protein fibers change structure; must be reconstituted with water before it can be used in recipes to replace ground beef
Tofu	Made from dried soybeans that have been soaked in water and then crushed and boiled; a coagulant (calcium sulfate, vinegar, or lemon juice) is added to separate curd from whey; curds are poured into molds and let sit

know precisely what it is about a particular food that causes its effect. Is soy's effect due to genistein or to its other cancer-fighting compounds? Or perhaps to some as yet unknown factors?

This bias toward isolated chemical factors in foods stems from the fact that most researchers who work with genistein are primarily molecular biologists, not nutritionists. Fortunately, several investigators are proposing large human trials with soy to see if ordinary soy foods and beverages can prevent cancer in people who are at increased risk of developing cancer (e.g., they have a family history of cancer) or delay secondary tumors in and improve survival of people already stricken with cancer.

TABLE 4.7

Brand-Name Soy Products

Brand	Products
Boca Burger	Meatless, Vegan Original Soy Burger
EdenSoy	Original Organic Soy Beverage
Green Giant	Harvest Burger Harvest Burger for Recipes
Lightlife	Meatless Smart Deli Meatless Country Ham Meatless Turkey Meatless Bologna Meatless Gimme Lean!
Morningstar Farms	Breakfast Links Breakfast Patties "Chik" Nuggets Deli Franks Breakfast Strips
Mori-Nu	Silken Tofu for shakes and sauces
Nasoya	Tofu mayonnaise Firm Tofu
Soya Kaas	Monterey Jack Style Cheese Substitute
Soyco	Lite & Less Grated Parmesan Cheese Alternative
Twinlab MaxiLIFE	Soy Cocktail Phytonutrient Cocktail
Vitasoy	Light Cocoa 1% Fat Natural Soy Drink
Westbrae	Cafe Lite Plain Lite Vanilla Lite Cocoa
Westsoy	Non Fat Soy Beverage Non Dairy Creamer
White Wave	Meatless Chicken Style Sandwich Slices Meatless Pastrami Meatless Philly Style Steak Silk

The average per capita dietary intake of the main soy isoflavone, genistein, in the United States is only 1–3 milligrams per day. Some health experts recommend keeping total soy isoflavone intake to no more than 40–80 milligrams a day. Unless you have cancer or have been advised otherwise by your own physician, I believe that this is a prudent recommendation for most healthy adults.

Native Japanese, who enjoy some of the lowest rates of breast and prostate cancer in the world, consume about 40–80 milligrams of isoflavones each day, almost entirely derived from soy. When investigators in a recent study gave a daily dose of 60 grams of soy protein (which contained between 45–70 milligrams of isoflavones) to premenopausal women, it significantly decreased levels of follicle-stimulating hormone and luteinizing hormone and increased menstrual cycle length. Cancer experts believe that translates into a reduced risk of breast, ovarian, and endometrial cancers.

Soy also protects against colon cancer by blocking the carcinogenic effect of secondary bile acids. Primary bile acids are made in the liver and stored in the gallbladder to aid in fat digestion. Secondary bile acids (primary bile acids transformed by normal bacteria in the gut) have been implicated as colon tumor promoters. High-fat diets promote colon cancer by increasing the amount of secondary bile acids in the colon, whereas the phytonutrients in soy foods protect against colon cancer by reducing high levels of secondary bile acids.

It is important to remember that while most research studies have looked at the isolated effects of genistein, there are distinct advantages to consuming soy foods, such as tofu, rather than individual phytonutrients. First, enjoying soy foods and beverages eliminates toxicity concerns because there is no reason to believe that consuming several servings of soy foods and beverages daily is harmful to most people. Second, soy foods and beverages contain a spectrum of cancer-fighting phytonutrients. For example, certain sugars (called *fruto-oligosaccharides*—easier to eat than pronounce) in soybeans promote the growth of friendly bacteria in the colon called *bifidobacteria*. High levels of bifidobacteria have been associated with a lower risk of colon cancer. The level of these sugars is higher in soybeans than in any other food. There are also some provocative studies on the cancer-inhibiting potential of phytic acid, saponins, and protease inhibitors, all of which are found in soy. All of these phytonutrients protect against cancer at several stages in the initiation and promotion of tumors and therefore offer much broader disease protection than the isolated phytonutrients used in many clinical studies.

Soy Mimics Estrogen

Estrogen-related compounds increase cancer risk by binding to breast cells and stimulating unchecked growth that leads to tumor formation. Soy and other plant isoflavones are similar in structure to human estrogen, so they can also attach to the hormone receptors, effectively blocking the cancer-causing effects of estrogen-related compounds. Since isoflavones are very weak estrogen-like compounds, they don't have the deadly effect that human estrogens do. The most widely used drug in breast-cancer treatment, tamoxifen, works in a similar way.

Soy foods are among the richest sources of isoflavones. In a recent clinical study testing the effect of soy against cancer, researchers demonstrated that ordinary soy foods contain enough isoflavones to exert a marked and favorable influence on reproductive hormone levels. Researchers fed a group of women 60 grams of textured vegetable protein (the soy-based meat analogue used in many brands of soy burgers) daily and observed what happened to their menstrual cycles. After 4 weeks, the time between their cycles increased by 2–5 days. Longer menstrual cycles mean a lower lifelong exposure to estrogen and its more potent sister hormone, estradiol, which in turn lowers cancer risk. Oriental-style fermented soy foods, such as miso and tempeh, seem to have the same estrogen-blunting effect, although the safety of fermented soy foods has been called into question by recent research.

Isoflavones and other phytoestrogens are abundant in soybeans and soy products, peanuts, dried beans, split peas, lentils, green beans, and garbanzo beans.

Epidemiological studies (studies of the factors leading to the occurrence of disease among free-living populations) reinforce these findings and suggest soy may help reduce rates of other cancers in addition to those of the breast. And these studies suggest that soy is an important factor in the healthfulness of traditional Asian diets.

Soy Protease Inhibitors Block Tumor Growth

Protease inhibitors are compounds found in soy and other legumes that block the action of certain enzymes that promote tumor growth. Proteases are considered essential for cancer cells during invasion and metastatic growth. They are also capable of inhibiting the activity of the body's digestive enzymes (proteases, amylases, and lipases); however, much of their activity is inactivated by cooking. Pro-

FIGURE 4.1

How Genistein Fights Cancer

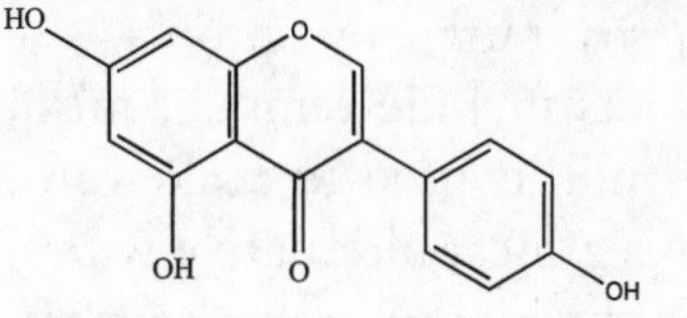

Genistein

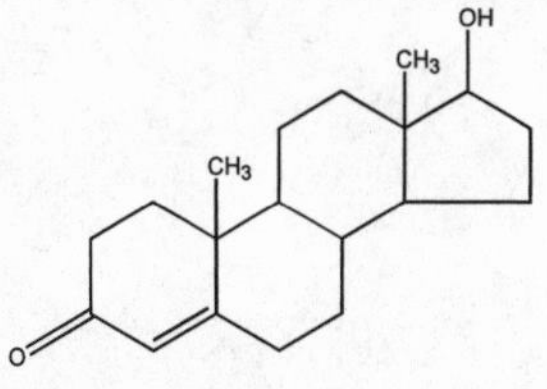

Testosterone

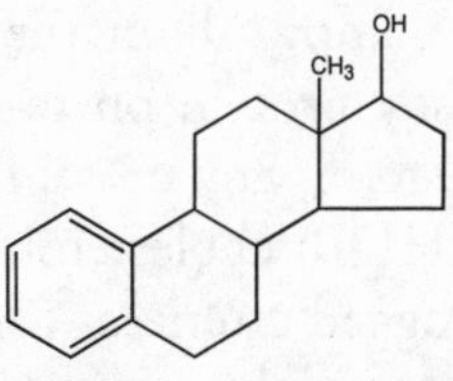

Estradiol

Tricking the Body: Genistein is a phytonutrient found only in soybeans, soy foods, and soy beverages. Its unique molecular structure is similar to the male and female sex hormones, testosterone and estradiol, respectively.

Blocking Hormones: Genistein can block the growth-stimulating effects of testosterone and estradiol by binding to the hormone receptors found in breast, prostate, and other tissues. Since genistein is only about $1/1,000$ as powerful as these sex hormones, it does not possess their cancer-promoting effects.

Stopping Cell Growth: Genistein can block the enzyme tyrosine kinase, a chemical that triggers growth in tumor cells.

Inhibition of Angiogenesis: Tumor cells must develop their own blood supply to grow and spread to other parts of the body. This process of new blood vessel growth is called angiogenesis. Genistein is an inhibitor of angiogenesis and thus can slow down or prevent the growth and metastasis of cancer cells.

tease inhibitors are found in bananas, barley, all kinds of nuts, white and sweet potatoes, wheat, oats, rye, rice, sweet corn, eggplant, sorghum, and pineapple. Fifty percent of the protein in an unripe tomato is in the form of protease inhibitors; ripening decreases that content but does not eliminate it.

The most well known protease inhibitor in soy, called the Bowman-Birk inhibitor (BBI), suppresses cancer induced by a variety of carcinogens. Early studies in rats revealed that the BBI significantly increased their life span and reduced the incidence of chemically induced liver and colon tumors in hamsters. Protease inhibitors suppressed early stages of tumor promotion in mouse skin as well as tumor formation in the bladder, breast, colon, liver, and lung. Pumpkin and squash seeds contain, in addition to soy, protease inhibitors that can block chemically induced carcinogenesis in the intestinal tracts of laboratory animals.

Types of Soy Foods

Soy foods are separated in nonfermented and fermented products. Nonfermented products include soybeans, soy nuts, soy sprouts, soy flour, soy milk, and tofu. Fermented products include tempeh, miso, soy sauces, natto, and fermented tofu. Soy milk is used to make tofu, soy yogurt, and soy-based cheeses. Tempeh is a meat alternative with a unique flavor and texture. Miso is a fermented white to brown soybean paste and is often used in combination with wheat, barley, or rice as a soup base.

Taking Soy to Heart

Most people today are aware of the connection between dietary cholesterol and fat to heart disease. But many don't know about the mounting evidence showing the positive effects of soy protein on reducing harmful low-density lipoprotein (LDL)-cholesterol. Soy protein can also raise beneficial high-density lipoprotein (HDL)-cholesterol, which helps remove cholesterol-filled plaque from clogged arteries.

The amount of soy protein you consume influences the amount of cholesterol reduction. In a recent study, a diet of 25 grams of soy protein per day—equivalent to about ⅔ cup of firm tofu, 1 cup of White Wave's Silk soy milk, or one-half serving of Twinlab's MaxiLIFE Soy Cocktail—caused an average cholesterol drop of 8.9 points, while 50 grams per day resulted in a 17-point reduction.

Dozens of studies have confirmed that when soy protein replaces animal protein in the diet, blood cholesterol levels tend to drop. Impressive cholesterol reductions are now commonly reported in medical studies. For example, a recent soy study demonstrated that one participant with an astronomical cholesterol level of 675 reduced it to 250 in a matter of weeks. The study also showed that people with cholesterol levels greater than 335 milligrams per deciliter could lower cholesterol by 20% by eating a daily average of 47 grams of soy protein. The effect for people with lower cholesterol levels showed a more moderate but nonetheless significant reduction.

The phytonutrients in soy, including amino acids, fiber, and isoflavones, all contribute to soy's powerful cholesterol-lowering effects. Some of these compounds bind with bile acids, which help wash out cholesterol from the body. These same phytonutrients also tend to raise the level of the hormone *thyroxin* in people on soy diets. Thyroxin helps regulate metabolism and body temperature. Some researchers believe thyroxin could be a principal reason for soy's cholesterol-lowering ability.

The connection between eating soy foods and lowering serum cholesterol was first made in the 1960s, quite by accident. A team of researchers investigating the effects of starches and sugars on cholesterol noticed that specially formulated foods made of soy protein caused cholesterol levels to plummet. Dietitians paid little attention to the discovery because they did not consider soy to be much of a food in those days. The research article, published in the June 1968 issue of *The Journal of the American Dietetic Association,* mentioned its cholesterol-lowering effects only in passing. It would be 10 years before anyone set out to systematically study the effects of soy on blood cholesterol levels.

In 1977, at the University of Milan's Center for the Study of Metabolic Diseases and Hyperlipidemia, Cesare Sirtori, M.D., studied a group of people with high blood cholesterol levels (average, 353 milligrams per deciliter) who were already on a low-fat diet. Some of the volunteers ate soy protein; a control group remained on the low-fat diet. Within 2 weeks, the blood cholesterol levels of the volunteers eating soy dropped an average of 14%; in 4 weeks, they were down 21%, to an average of 257 milligrams per deciliter. The control subjects experienced no drop in cholesterol levels. Then, Sirtori removed the volunteers from all soy but kept them on the low-fat diet. Their cholesterol levels crept back up an average rate of 20 points in 2 weeks.

Sirtori then gave another group of volunteers a supplement of 500 milligrams of cholesterol per day to see if that would negate the effects of the soy. Despite the added cholesterol, these volunteers experienced the same drop in blood cholesterol as those who were given no cholesterol supplement.

According to Dr. Sirtori, "individuals with a blood cholesterol above 250 who substitute soy for animal protein in their diets can successfully reduce their cholesterol by as much as 25 percent." Sirtori believes soy is so important to a healthy heart that he also recommends that people at high risk of developing heart disease *make soy their only source of protein.* Soy also affects heart disease risk in ways other than reducing blood cholesterol: soy isoflavones prevent and reverse the formation of plaque deposits on artery walls.

Since Sirtori's study was published, more than two dozen clinical studies have clearly demonstrated that substituting soy protein for animal protein or simply adding soy protein to the diet significantly reduces blood cholesterol levels, regardless of the type or amount of fat in the diet. In many of these studies, about 50 grams of soy protein was given to people with moderately high cholesterol levels (around 240 milligrams per deciliter). The most impressive results are consistently seen in people who have elevated cholesterol levels—generally between 240 and 350 milligrams per deciliter. People with levels of 200 or below do not experience such remarkable reductions in blood cholesterol levels.

Soy-cholesterol studies collectively reveal one simple fact: even moderate amounts of soy foods and beverages—as little as two servings a day—can significantly lower elevated blood cholesterol levels and help prevent and even reverse atherosclerosis.

Soy Protects LDL-Cholesterol from Oxidation

A recent study by a team of Japanese researchers at the Hirosaki University School of Medicine in Japan provides an additional explanation for how soy prevents heart attacks and strokes. University researchers discovered that when they fed rabbits soy milk, their LDL-cholesterol oxidation was dramatically suppressed. LDL oxidation enables the cells that line the arteries to take up cholesterol, leading to plaque formation and, ultimately, heart attacks, strokes, and impotence.

Stopping LDL oxidation may be as important in lowering heart disease risk as lowering blood cholesterol levels themselves. Many scientists agree that oxidized LDL-cholesterol can damage the delicate artery lining that leads to blockage.

There is now sufficient evidence to suggest that even if your cholesterol level is high, you can reduce it substantially by eating just two to three servings of soy foods a day (about 25–45 grams of soy protein) or one to two servings of a concentrated soy beverage. The recipes in this book contain ample amounts of soy foods and beverages that can help you consume adequate soy each day. It's easy to work soy into your diet simply by using soy flour in baked items, by replacing cow's milk with nonfat/low-fat soy milk, and by using soy cocktails and soy foods, such as tofu and soy meat replacers.

Soy and Osteoporosis

The health-promoting benefits of soy don't stop at heart disease and cancer. Scientists are also looking at soy as a preventive for osteoporosis. As I pointed out in 1986 in my book, *Eat to Succeed,* vegetable protein is superior to animal protein for preventing and reversing such degenerative diseases as osteoporosis. A diet based on soy protein, vegetables, and fruits can reduce the amount of calcium lost from the body each day by up to 50% when it replaces animal protein in the diet. Soy protein is also easier on the kidneys than is animal protein. This is especially important to people with impaired kidney function and kidney disease. Always check with your physician, however, before modifying your diet if you have these or any other medical conditions.

Soy Milk Versus Cow's Milk

According to the Soyfoods Association of America (SAA), approximately 5 million people in the United States consumed an estimated $150 million of soymilk in 1996. Soy milk is made by grinding soaked and cooked soybeans and pressing dissolved soy milk out of beans. Commercial soy milks have added ingredients, such as sweeteners, oil, flavors, and salt to improve taste.

The *Permanent Remissions* Plan emphasizes soy milk over cow's milk for several important reasons. Soy milk provides far more disease-fighting phytonutrients. Like cow's milk, soy milk contains a healthy dose of calcium. Soy milk is a good source of iron; while cow's milk contains negligible amounts. And unlike cow's milk, soy milk contains no cholesterol. Soy milk also contains slightly more protein than cow's milk and a similar B-vitamin and mineral profile. The nutritional profile of soy milk and the anticancer nutrients it contains (genistein and daidzein) help to account for the life-saving benefits of switching from cow's milk to low-fat or nonfat soy milk.

Soy milk wins over cow's milk in lowering cholesterol levels in the body. In a recent study, people were fed single test meals identical in composition except for protein source: one group was given soy protein and the other was given milk protein (casein). The group that got the soy-protein diet saw a significant drop in their blood cholesterol levels, while the group that got the milk protein saw a significant rise in serum cholesterol. These results, previously seen in laboratory animal studies, reveal that heart-healthy soy milk is a much wiser choice than cow's milk for lowering a major risk factor in heart disease.

When it comes to preventing cancer, switching from cow's milk to soy milk could save your life. Recent laboratory animal studies reveal that soy milk inhibited mammary tumor formation and metastatic growth to the lungs. Other lab-animal studies have shown that after excision of a primary mammary tumor, growth of additional tumors was inhibited when the diet was changed from a cow's milk protein-based diet to a soy protein-based diet. Small amounts of skim milk and very low-fat dairy products are permitted in a number of *Permanent Remissions* recipes. When used in limited amounts, these dairy products can be used as part of a healthy eating plan.

Recently, the SAA filed a petition with the U.S. Food and Drug Administration (FDA) requesting that the agency develop a "common and usual name" regulation for the term *soy milk*. Up to this point in time, soy milk manufacturers have been prohibited by the FDA from using the term *soy milk* and have instead been labeling soy milk products as "soy drinks" or "soy beverages."

Proof of Soy's Cancer-Stopping Power from Around the World

Population studies on soy intake and its relation to disease have shown that soy foods lower the risk for colon cancer, stomach cancer, lung cancer, gallbladder and bile duct cancer, liver cancer, heart disease, and adult-onset diabetes. Studies that have examined the dietary habits of various countries and religious sects clearly reveal that soy foods make a positive difference in health:

- Native Japanese who consume soy foods and beverages enjoy much lower rates of cancer, heart disease, adult-onset diabetes, osteoporosis, and kidney disease than people in the United States who do not eat soy foods. Soy foods comprise about 10% of the total per capita protein intake in some Asian societies, far more than in Western countries, where soy is rarely eaten. Consumption of nonfermented soy products, such as soy milk and tofu, seem to reduce overall cancer risk, while consumption of fermented soy products, such as miso (a fermented soy paste) and soy sauce tend to show either no protective effect or an increased cancer risk.

- Seventh-Day Adventist women who are vegetarians with a high soy intake and a relatively low incidence of breast cancer have high levels of serum DHEA (dehydroepiandrosterone). DHEA is a hormone related to testosterone that declines with age in men and women and may be related to aging and risk of developing breast and prostate cancer, heart disease, and other degenerative diseases. It is much healthier and more natural to boost DHEA levels with soy foods and beverages than to take DHEA supplements, which can create a hormonal imbalance in the body and possibly fuel the growth of certain cancers.

- A 1989 study of 8,000 Hawaiian men with Japanese ancestry found that men who ate the most tofu had the lowest rates of prostate cancer. A Shanghai study found that premenopausal women who rarely ate soy foods had twice the risk of developing breast cancer than those who ate soy frequently. In both these cases, it was the amount of soy that made the difference, not the amount of fat in the diet.

5

BEATING BREAST CANCER*

Breast cancer is a relatively new disease.

The wives of the Founding Fathers didn't have to worry much about getting breast cancer because it was rare in those days. Why? One reason is that woman's lifetime exposure to estrogen, which usually begins at menarche, is much longer today than it was 200 years ago, when menarche began around 17 years of age. Another reason is that back in Martha Washington's day, less than 30% of women lived to reach menopause. In the United States, the age of menarche has steadily declined over the last 200 years, increasing the lifetime exposure of women to estrogen. Today, about 90% of women reach menopause.

At the time of the American Revolution, women usually bore their first child when they were in their teens and early twenties and often had large numbers of children. Pregnancy lowers cancer risk by reducing the number of epithelial cells in the breast. Women who never have children or who delay childbearing until their late twenties, thirties, or forties may accumulate more epithelial breast cells and increase their lifetime exposure to estrogen, thereby elevating their risk for breast cancer.

Today, the majority of U.S. women give birth much later in life and have just one or two children. The average life span of a woman in the late 1700s was about 40. Today, many women live well into the seventh and eighth decade of life, reaching menopause at about age 52. Thus, the uninterrupted period during which breast cells are exposed

---

*In general, the nutritional principles that prevent and fight breast cancer apply to ovarian and uterine cancer as well.

to their own reproductive hormones and xenoestrogens may now be as long as 30 years instead of 10.

Breast cancer is the second most common cancer among women in the United States, currently accounting for an estimated 207,000 new cases and 46,000 deaths each year. (Lung cancer has become the leading cancer, owing to an increase in cigarette smoking.) About one in nine American women can expect to develop breast cancer at some time during their lifetime. Statistics reveal, however, that the majority of breast cancer occurs in postmenopausal women, with less than 25% of breast cancers occurring in premenopausal women.

Unlike survival rates for many other cancers that tend to level off after 5 years, survival after a diagnosis of breast cancer continues to decline beyond 5 years. According to data published by the American Cancer Society (ACS), 63% of women diagnosed with breast cancer will survive 10 years; 56% will survive 15 years. Overall, survival for patients with metastatic breast cancer *has not significantly improved during the past 30 years.*

Will *You* Get Breast Cancer?

It's a diagnosis that nearly every adult woman lives in dread of hearing from her doctor: "The biopsy came back positive. You have breast cancer."

Are such fears warranted? Perhaps. One of every 2,500 women will get breast cancer while in their thirties. The risk then soars to one in 200 by age 40, one in 50 by age 50, one in 25 by age 60, and one in 11 for a woman in her seventies. If you're an American black woman, you face *twice the risk of dying* from this disease that an American white woman faces. Overall, the risk of getting breast cancer is five times higher in American women than in native Japanese women.

Should you be worried about getting breast cancer? Answer the questions in Table 5.1 to find out.

The increased risk of developing breast cancer associated with each factor varies, roughly from 1.5 to four times the average risk. The more of the risk factors shown in Table 5.1 that apply to you, the higher your risk of getting the disease.

In the United States, a woman's lifetime risk of developing breast cancer is about 12%, if she lives to the ripe old age of 86 (which isn't

---

TABLE 5.1

Assessing Your Risk of Breast Cancer

1. Are you female?
2. Are you fat?
3. Are you 50?
4. Did you start to menstruate before age 12?
5. Did you have your first child after age 30?
6. Have you never carried a pregnancy to term?
7. If premenopausal, do you regularly consume alcoholic beverages?
8. Did you enter menopause after age 55?
9. Have you taken estrogen in any form?
10. Are you a Jew of Eastern European descent?
11. Have you been exposed to high levels of pesticides?
12. Are you tall (5'10" or over)?
13. Did your mother and/or sister have breast cancer?
14. Do you eat few fruits and vegetables?
15. Have you omitted soy milk and soy foods from your diet?
16. Are you sedentary?
17. Are you constantly losing and gaining weight (yo-yo dieting)?
18. Did you bottle-feed instead of breast-feed your baby?

---

that old if you accept that humans following the *Permanent Remissions* Plan can live to blow out 120 candles). In some families, where a genetic tendency for breast cancer is inherited, the risk can be much higher. Scientists now suspect that about 5%–10% of women with breast cancer have a hereditary form of the disease, and these women have a higher risk of developing breast cancer at a younger age than most—usually before menopause.

Most of the known risk factors for breast cancer are linked in one way or another with total lifetime exposure to insulin and reproductive hormones. Dietary fat, percent body fat, obesity, yo-yo dieting, pregnancy, estrogen-replacement therapy, birth-control pills, and estrogen-like pesticides all contribute to the degree of hormone exposure of breast tissue. Exposure to high levels of estrogen begins at menarche.

The average age of menarche in the United States is 12.8, as compared to 17 for China, where breast cancer rates are one fourth those seen in the United States. Studies have shown that many women who begin menstruating at an early age tend to have higher levels of body fat or tend to be overweight or obese, which is a separate risk factor later in life. Since estrogen is produced in fat cells, fat women tend to have higher circulating levels of estrogens. Obesity also affects the metabolism of estrogen unfavorably, raising the risk of breast cancer even higher. Recent studies suggest that apple-shaped women, who carry most of their excess adipose tissue around their middle, tend to have higher breast cancer rates than pear-shaped women, who carry their excess fat around the hips and thighs. Insulin resistance contributes to this unfavorable type of obesity.

THREE IMPORTANT RISK FACTORS FOR BREAST CANCER

Most authors of medical textbooks and published studies on breast cancer agonize over the "fact" that the majority of U.S. women who get breast cancer have no known risk factors for the disease. This is a short-sighted view, given the wealth of research that has been published on the subject. The majority of women who get breast cancer have three important risk factors that caused their breast cancer:

1. A high-calorie, phytonutrient-poor diet (the standard American diet)
2. High insulin levels in the blood (hyperinsulinemia)
3. An unfavorable ratio of unfriendly to friendly dietary fat

Here are the essential dietary strategies that all women should embrace to prevent breast cancer.

EAT A PHYTONUTRIENT-RICH, LOW-CALORIE DIET

Phytonutrients found in soy milk, tofu, and other soy products; tomato-based sauces; and vegetables, such as cabbage and broccoli, can help mitigate the cancer-causing effects of estrogen and estrogen-like chemicals on breast tissue. One of the purposes of *Permanent Remissions* is to educate the medical establishment about the important role phytonutrients play not only in reducing the exposure of breast tissue to estrogen but also in reducing the level of stored body fat—a breeding ground for estrogen.

Studies of people who migrate to the United States from countries with typically low breast cancer rates, such as China and Japan, reveal that dietary factors, rather than genetics, account for changes in breast cancer rates. Once Japanese women who move to Hawaii change their diet, which apparently involves abandoning traditional soy foods in favor of the higher-fat Hawaiian diet, their incidence of breast cancer rises dramatically compared with that of women living in Japan.

Native Japanese women have a much lower breast cancer rate than their siblings living in the United States. The typical Japanese diet, rich in soy-based foods and food products, contains 25% fewer calories than the ordinary diet followed by women in the United States. These two nutritional factors—a phytonutrient-rich diet (low in omega-6 fatty acids) and a reduced caloric intake—are the primary reasons for the lower risk of breast cancer enjoyed by native Japanese women.

Use the *Permanent Remissions* Phytonutrient Guide Pyramid to select foods that can help you prevent breast cancer or, if you already have it, beat the odds by making your conventional therapy safer and more effective.

MAINTAIN MODERATE BLOOD INSULIN LEVELS

Women with diabetes share a common attribute with many breast cancer victims and all women who eat an ordinary American diet: *insulin resistance.*

Insulin resistance occurs when the body becomes desensitized to the actions of the hormone insulin, which is released from the pancreas in response to protein and carbohydrate consumption. Insulin's primary role is to get sugar out of the blood and into muscles, where it can be burned for energy or stored as glycogen for later use.

A woman's entire reproductive tract is sensitive to the growth-promoting effects of insulin. Breast and ovarian tissue, for example, possess special docking sites for the insulin molecule and other insulin-like growth factors (known as IGF-I and -II) that can stimulate cancer cell formation. When cells become resistant to insulin, the pancreas responds by pumping out more of the hormone. And that's the last thing anyone needs if they want to avoid cancer.

Insulin resistance results from overconsumption of fats, sugars, and calories (as evidenced by weight gain), especially after the age of 30. Hyperinsulinemia (high blood levels of insulin) and abdominal obesity are two of the early warning signs that breast cancer could be lurking just around the corner.

The body's resistance to insulin, a hallmark of type 2 diabetes, is also a risk factor for pancreatic cancer. Diabetics have a high rate of pancreatic cancer, and those with the disease generally have more advanced tumors and shortened survival compared to nondiabetic patients with pancreatic cancer. Elevated blood insulin levels are the reason why.

Sadly, the drug tamoxifen, given to many patients with breast cancer, increases levels of insulin-like growth factors, which may increase the risk for endometrial and ovarian cancer cell growth. Several recent studies have reported a significant increase in endometrial cancer incidence in tamoxifen-treated patients with breast cancer. Estrogens are the major growth stimulators of endometrial tumors, but paradoxically, tamoxifen—a drug known to block estrogen—also stimulates their growth through its effect on insulin-like growth factors.

Hyperinsulinemia also promotes colon cancer. Insulin is an important growth factor for colon cells. Indirect evidence supporting the insulin–colon cancer hypothesis comes from observations about the similarity of factors that produce elevated insulin levels to those related to colon cancer risk. A diet high in refined carbohydrates (sugars) and low in phytonutrients and fiber, which is associated with an increased risk of colon cancer, causes rapid intestinal absorption of glucose into the blood, leading to postmeal hyperinsulinemia. Most Americans become hyperinsulinemic after each meal they consume. Is it any wonder that diabetes is on the rise and cancer is the second leading killer in the United States?

TOO MANY UNFRIENDLY FATS AND TOO FEW FRIENDLY ONES

A diet high in unfriendly omega-6 fatty acids, such as those found in safflower, corn, and sunflower oils, raises circulating levels of estrogens. The body can be "persuaded" to make beneficial and harmful estrogens by the type of fats you consume. Unfriendly fats tell the body to make the type of estrogens that promote breast cancer. Saturated fats—those that come primarily from animal foods—promote insulin resistance and the diseases it promotes: cancer, heart disease, and diabetes.

Monounsaturated fatty acids from olive oil and omega-3 fatty acids from seafood, such as salmon, mackerel, and tuna, can help reduce the risk of breast cancer. If you are going to use a vegetable oil, choose olive oil, for it is the friendliest fat in the human diet. As long as you keep total fat intake to 15% of your total daily calories, olive oil and omega-3 fats will help reduce the disease risks associated with consumption of a diet high in omega-6 fatty acids and saturated fats.

PHYTONUTRIENTS, ESTROGENS, AND BREAST CANCER

Reproductive hormones have been linked to the development of cancers of the breast, ovary, uterus, and endometrium because they stimulate cellular growth and proliferation. *Estrogen-related cancers account for more than 50% of all newly diagnosed cancers in women in the United States.*

Women are exposed to estrogen in two ways: *endogenous* estrogen, which is made within the body, and *exogenous* estrogen, which comes from oral contraceptives, postmenopausal hormone-replacement therapy, and environmental toxins. Estrogen-stimulating compounds—such as pesticides; hormones fed to cattle, pigs, chickens, and turkeys; and industrial pollutants that imitate estrogen's cancer-promoting ability—are known as *xenoestrogens* (literally: foreign estrogens). See Figure 5.1 for foods that fight breast cancer.

ESTROGEN'S TWO PATHS: WHICH ONE WILL YOU TAKE?

It's not just the length of a woman's exposure to her own estrogen that puts her at risk but also the chemical form of the circulating estrogens in her body and how much gets into breast cells.

The way the body processes *estradiol*—the biologically active form of estrogen—directly affects the risk of breast cancer. Estradiol can take one of two metabolic paths in the body (Figure 5.2). Pathway 1 leads to a form of estradiol called *2-hydroxyestrone,* which is a much weaker form of the hormone. Pathway 2 leads to a cancer-promoting form of estrogen called *16-alpha-hydroxyestrone.*

Studies that have compared breast tissue of women undergoing mastectomy for breast cancer with tissue from healthy women undergoing breast-reduction surgery found that levels of 16-alpha-hydroxyestrone were almost *eight times higher* in the women with breast cancer. High levels of 16-alpha-hydroxyestrone have also been found in obese women and other women with elevated risk factors for breast cancer. Obese postmenopausal women may have higher risks of breast cancer owing to the ability of body fat to enhance production of estrogens, especially if the fat is distributed in the so-called apple-shaped obesity pattern in which fat is stored in around the center of the torso. Phytonutrients found in soy foods, broccoli, cabbage, and whole grains and cereals can help reverse the high levels of cancer-promoting estrogen associated with this type of obesity. Weight loss and physical exercise help to augment the cancer-protective effects of phytonutrients.

XENOESTROGENS: ENVIRONMENTAL CARCINOGENS

Every two of three cases of breast cancer in the United States puzzle physicians because they simply have no idea what caused the

PHYTOFOODS THAT FIGHT BREAST CANCER

Omega-3 fats from salmon reduce breast cancer inflammation, block the formation of cancer-stimulating reproductive hormones, and inhibit the growth of blood vessels that can feed breast tumors

Olive oil reduces the risk of breast cancer when it replaces other vegetable oils and saturated fats in the diet

Such foods as tomato sauce and watermelon contain lycopene, a potent phytonutrient that can fight breast cancer

Soy foods, soy milk, and soy cocktails block the cancer-causing effects of estradiol in the breast and reproductive organs

Cruciferous vegetables, such as broccoli and cabbage, contain phytonutrients that detoxify cancer-causing chemicals linked to breast cancer

Grapes, grape skins and seeds contain phytonutrients that protect breast tissue against free radical damage

FIGURE 5.2

Estradiol Metabolism: Two Pathways

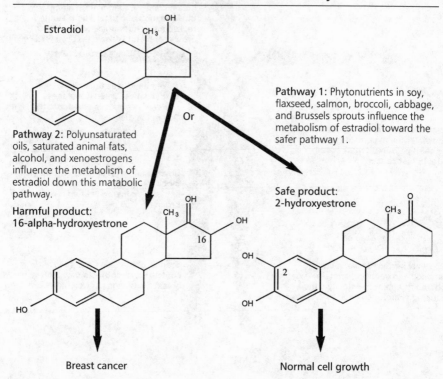

Pathway 1: Phytonutrients in soy, flaxseed, salmon, broccoli, cabbage, and Brussels sprouts influence the metabolism of estradiol toward the safer pathway 1.

Pathway 2: Polyunsaturated oils, saturated animal fats, alcohol, and xenoestrogens influence the metabolism of estradiol down this matabolic pathway.

Harmful product: 16-alpha-hydroxyestrone

Safe product: 2-hydroxyestrone

Breast cancer

Normal cell growth

Estradiol can be converted to two products that differ structurally. Pathway 1 converts estradiol to a relatively safe form of estrogen called 2-hydroxyestrone. Pathway 2 metabolizes estradiol to a form of estrogen, 16-alpha-hydroxyestrone, that promotes the unchecked cellular growth that leads to breast cancer. Cancerous breast tissue from women contains much more 16-alpha-hydroxyestrone than does normal breast tissue. Several xenoestrogens may increase the risk of breast cancer by elevating levels of 16-alpha-hydroxyestrone in breast tissue.

disease. The known breast cancer genes, including the recently discovered BRAC1 and BRAC2 genes, account for perhaps only 5%–10% of all cases. What, then, accounts for the steady rise in the number of women with breast cancer over the years?

A number of cancer researchers believe that environmental toxins (xenoestrogens) mimic the action of estrogen produced in the body or at least alter the hormone's activity. Xenoestrogens found in pesticides, fuels, drugs, and plastics may promote breast and other reproductive disorders, including those that occur in men, such as lowered sperm counts and testicular cancer. Unlike the estrogen-mimicking healthy phytonutrients that are degraded rapidly in the body, many types of xenoestrogens can persist for decades in the fatty tissue in breasts and around other organs, accumulating to high levels. Animal foods high on the food chain, such as meat derived from animals that eat smaller animals or contaminated grain, grass, or water, probably cause more estrogen exposure than vegetables carrying residues of estrogenic pesticides. Safflower, corn, and other vegetable oils also possess estrogenic effects. People who live in areas of high air or water pollution may take in estrogenic chemicals simply by breathing air or drinking contaminated water.

The risk of breast cancer due to pesticides and other environmental carcinogens can be greatly reduced by eating a low-fat diet rich in phytonutrients. From the data I've seen, environmental carcinogens do not pose as high a risk as some researchers believe. The vast majority of breast cancers are due to the factors mentioned above: high-calorie, phytonutrient-poor diets; chronically high levels of insulin; chronically high intake of saturated and polyunsaturated fats; and lack of regular exercise. The *Permanent Remissions* Plan automatically reduces your intake of pesticides and environmental contaminants because the foods that it recommends fall low on the food chain. Since the Plan eliminates most of the foods in the ordinary American diet that are high on the food chain, such as meat, milk, cheese, egg yolks, and fowl, you'll reduce your exposure to pesticides, antibiotics, or other environmental contaminants.

PLASTIC FOOD AND BEVERAGE CONTAINERS

Evidence that ordinary plastic bottles used in food and beverage packaging can be estrogenic has emerged only since the early 1990s, although many scientists long ago suspected that the plastic used in these containers, called *polycarbonate,* was unhealthy. These containers may leach out toxic chemicals and raise cancer risks for those who consume the foods and beverages packaged in them.

In the 1970s, researchers at Stanford University found that an estrogenic chemical, *bisphenol-A,* could leach out of polycarbonate bottles. The ability of bisphenol-A to produce estrogenic effects was discovered when some men in the plastics industry developed prominent breasts after inhaling the chemical in dust. No one has yet figured out exactly how much of this chemical actually seeps into foods and beverages or whether it causes breast cancer in humans when ingested. Another chemical found in household detergents and used to make plastic more flexible, *nonylphenol,* also mimics the effects of estrogen on breast tissue.

YO-YO DIETING, XENOESTROGENS, AND BREAST CANCER

I would like to take this opportunity to cast doubt on the conventional medical wisdom regarding weight cycling, also known as yo-yo dieting. Many health authorities believe that the vicious cycle of repeatedly losing and regaining weight poses no health risks to long-time dieters. I respectfully submit that these authorities are mistaken. Here's why:

There is at least one xenobiotic lurking in your adipose tissue right now, as you read this sentence. It's called beta-HCH *(beta-hexachlorocyclohexane).* This is a chemical related to the insecticide *lindane,* widely used in agriculture and in a medication used to kill head lice in children. If you've eaten animal foods (animals' bodies tend to concentrate this chemical more than plants do), you've got a nice supply of beta-HCH in your body.

Researchers at the Indiana University School of Medicine have conducted laboratory animal research on the effects of beta-HCH, which is released from the body's fat cells during weight loss, exercise, or fasting. When beta-HCH is released, it stimulates uterine growth—a hallmark of estrogen's stimulating effect—even in lab animals that have had their ovaries (the primary estrogen-manufacturing organ) removed.

The Indiana University research team also found that beta-HCH spurs the growth of breast cancer cells but not in the usual way seen with the body's own estrogen. "It didn't do the normal thing that estrogens do," notes physiologist Rosemary Steinmetz, who led the study.

I know I told you that the *Permanent Remissions* Plan can protect breast and ovarian tissue from xenoestrogens, but beta-HCH and bisphenol-A do not bind to estrogen receptors in breast tissue. Devra Lee

Davis, Ph.D., of the World Resources Institute in Washington, D.C., and Michael Osborne, Ph.D., of the Strang Cancer Prevention Center in New York believe that not all xenoestrogens work through the estrogen receptor to increase breast cancer risk—and therein lies the problem. This is one xenoestrogen that may be able to elude the protective effect of phytonutrients.

Helena Mussalo-Rauhamaa, Ph.D., of the Helsinki University Hospital believes that cancer researchers should begin studying yo-yo dieting whenever they probe cancer links to environmental pollution. She found that patients with breast cancer have more beta-HCH in their fat cells than do women without cancer.

So what do these findings mean for those women who want to lose weight to reduce their risk of breast cancer?

My advice is to embrace the *Permanent Remissions* Plan as your lifelong way of eating. Enjoy regular physical activity that burns an additional 1,500–2,000 calories each week. Exercise is one of the easiest ways I know to significantly reduce your risk of reproductive cancers. If you live a *Permanent Remissions*–type lifestyle, your body fat will settle at a healthy level and you won't have to worry about yo-yo dieting and the threat of increasing your risk of breast cancer.

VITAMIN D AND BREAST CANCER

Vitamin D_3 retards the growth of breast cancer cells and activates *apoptosis*—cell death—which eliminates cells that have taken a step toward cancer.

Vitamin D_3 can be toxic in doses required to slow down the spread of breast cancer, so scientists have formulated vitamin-D derivatives that inhibit the proliferation of breast cancer cells and cause regression of experimental mammary tumors. Taken together, these facts suggest that vitamin D and its derivatives may play a role in regulating the expression of genes and protein products that prevent and inhibit breast cancer. The cancer-stopping power of vitamin D has been documented in osteosarcoma (bone cancer), melanoma, colon cancer, and breast cancer. These cancer cells contain vitamin-D receptors that make them susceptible to the anticancer effects of this vitamin-hormone made by the skin when it is exposed to sunlight. Vitamin D–rich foods include salmon, tuna, fish oils, and vitamin D–fortified milk and breakfast cereals. **Caution:** Since vitamin D can be toxic in high doses, people with breast cancer should use vitamin-D supplements only with the permission and supervision of a physician or should ask their doctors about the new synthetic vitamin-D derivatives that do not possess the toxic side effects of ordinary vitamin D_3.

BLACK AND WHITE BIOLOGICAL DIFFERENCES AFFECT BREAST CANCER SURVIVAL

Race and ethnicity can profoundly affect a woman's chances of dying from breast cancer (Table 5.2).

American black women with breast cancer are generally diagnosed at more advanced stages of the disease. The National Cancer Institute's (NCI's) Black/White Cancer Survival Study followed 612 black and 518 white women aged 20–79 years in the Atlanta, New Orleans, and San Francisco–Oakland metropolitan areas. Women in the study were diagnosed with breast cancer in 1985 or 1986, as identified by population-based cancer registries in the three areas, and were followed through 1991.

Researchers found that American black women had a risk 2.1 times greater of dying from breast cancer than did American white women during the study period. Approximately 40% of the difference in survival was due to the fact that disease stage was more advanced at diagnosis for blacks. Fifteen percent of the black–white survival difference was due to histologic differences (appearance of tumor cells under

---

TABLE 5.2

Biological Differences in Breast Cancer in Blacks and Whites

- American black women tend to have more actively dividing tumors. Actively dividing tumors tend to aggressively invade other tissues and metastasize.
- American black women have tumors with cells that appear less differentiated from normal breast cells than those found in whites. Less differentiated tumor cells (meaning they appear more like normal cells) are more likely to respond poorly to some conventional therapies.
- Breast tumors in American black women tend to lack estrogen receptors. These tumor cells are resistant to antiestrogen-type chemotherapeutic drugs.
- American black women tend to have a higher body mass index (BMI—a measure of degree of fatness based on a ratio of height to weight—body weight in kilograms divided by height in square meters). Fat cells manufacture estrogen and help convert it to a form that promotes breast cancer.

microscopic analysis). Some of these differences may reflect underlying biological differences between black and white women. The NCI's Black/White Cancer Survival Study supports the conclusion that socio-economic factors, differences in treatment received, and biological factors are involved.

What are the reasons for the increased aggressiveness of breast cancer in American black women? Scientists are just beginning to unravel some of the mysteries behind this phenomenon:

- Breast tumors in American black women contain genetic mutations in the p53 tumor suppressor gene, believed to control a key step in the breast cancer process. Researchers have found that these genes appear significantly different from those observed in tumors from whites.
- Researchers found that American black women were more likely than American white women to be categorized as overweight based on body mass index (BMI), a measure of body fatness. Women with a high BMI are more likely to die from breast cancer. The amount of body fat a woman carries exposes her to higher levels of the metabolically active form of estrogen, estradiol, which is responsible for stimulating breast cancer.
- Almost half of American black women are overweight, as opposed to a third of white women. Health experts have attributed this disparity to differences in eating, exercise habits, and cultural differences in attitudes toward body weight. But the truth is that higher rates of obesity among black women are partly determined by biology.
- American black women burn nearly 100 fewer calories than American white women do when their bodies are at rest. Even accounting for differences in body weight and muscle mass does not change this observation, borne out by clinical studies at the University of Pennsylvania.

Losing weight is not a hopeless task for people with lower metabolic rates, but it does mean that they may have to be more vigilant in their commitment to follow a healthy diet and exercise regimen. American black women should engage in regular aerobic exercise and strength training to increase muscle mass, which can raise the resting metabolic rate.

Black women have made substantial gains in breast cancer survival in recent decades, from a 5-year survival rate of 46% of women whose disease was diagnosed between 1960 and 1963 to 62% of women whose disease was diagnosed between 1983 and 1988. But American blacks' rates have continued to lag behind those of whites, whose 5-year survival rate was 79% for women whose disease was diagnosed during the same time period. The *Permanent Remissions* Plan is designed to help reduce the known dietary risk factors linked to breast cancer for American black women.

Natural Foods That Fight Breast Cancer

Soy foods and beverages, tomato products, cruciferous vegetables, friendly fats, and certain fruits contain the world's most powerful breast cancer–fighting phytonutrients (Table 5.3).

TABLE 5.3

Phytofood Products That Fight Breast and Ovarian Cancer

The following formula foods (also known as functional foods or biodesigned foods) contain anticancer phytonutrients, vitamins, minerals, and nonvitamin nutrients now being tested by the National Cancer Institute (NCI) and other health research organizations. These formula foods are sold nationwide in health-food stores and some pharmacies and supermarkets. Appendix IV (pages 365–68) contains the names, addresses, and telephone numbers of product manufacturers.

Have one serving of any one of the following products each day.

MaxiLIFE Soy Cocktail: Sold in health-food stores, manufactured by Twin Laboratories. Drink this or any soy cocktail made with a highly concentrated soy protein isolate. This formula contains the phytonutrients that have been shown to be effective against prostate, breast, and reproductive cancers.

MaxiLIFE Phytonutrient Cocktail: Sold in health-food stores, manufactured by Twin Laboratories. This formula contains phytonutrients and other antioxidants shown by clinical and laboratory research to be effective in the prevention and management of prostate, breast, and other reproductive cancers.

Pecta-Sol: Modified citrus pectin (MCP), sold by mail order and manufactured by eco-Nugenics. MCP is currently being tested to determine its clinical effectiveness in blocking cancer-cell metastasis. Use this product only if you have been diagnosed with breast or ovarian cancer. Use only under a doctor's supervision.

Haelan 851: Made by Haelan Products Inc. This not-so-pleasant-tasting fermented soy cocktail contains a rich supply of isoflavones derived from specially grown soybeans.

SOY FOODS AND BEVERAGES

Soy foods and beverages block the cancer-stimulating effects of estradiol, estrogen's powerful sister hormone; it also contains a protease inhibitor that can inhibit the growth of cancer cells. I'd like you to set a goal of consuming enough soy products, including soy meat replacers, soy foods such as tofu, soy milk, and soy cocktails to obtain between 40 and 80 milligrams of soy isoflavones. This level of isoflavone intake should provide for optimum breast cancer protection. Use Table 5.4 to reach this goal each day.

CITRUS FRUITS

Two citrus flavonoids—hesperidin and naringenin, found in oranges and grapefruit, respectively—and four noncitrus flavonoids—baicalein, galangin, genistein (found only in soy), and quercetin—inhibit the proliferation and growth of human breast-cancer cells. Naringenin is present in grapefruit mainly as naringin. These compounds, as well as grapefruit and orange juice concentrates, have been shown in studies to inhibit development of mammary tumors induced by cancer-causing chemicals in laboratory rodents. Rats fed a high-fat diet developed more tumors than rats fed a low-fat diet, but tumor development was delayed in the groups given orange or grapefruit juice. Rats given orange juice had fewer total tumors than did control subjects. Orange and grapefruits are effective inhibitors of human breast-cancer cell proliferation, especially in the presence of quercetin, which is widely distributed in many other foods. Have one to two servings of citrus fruits each day.

TABLE 5.4

Soy Protein Sources

Soy Source	Protein (Grams)	Isoflavones (Milligrams)
Soy cocktail (1 serving)	40	30–40
Soy flour (1 ounce)	10–14	30–40
Soy meat replacer (3.5 ounces)*	17	0–15
Soy milk (1 cup)	4–10	10–30
Tofu (4 ounces)	8–13	30–40

*Many manufacturers of soy meat replacers (e.g., soy ground beef, bacon, sausage, chicken, turkey, pastrami, and ham) use an alcohol extraction process that removes disease-fighting isoflavones from their products. For this reason, I recommend that you use a soy cocktail or increase your intake of tofu and soy milk, both of which contain ample isoflavones and other health-promoting phytonutrients.

TOMATO SAUCES

Tomato sauces (including ketchup, tomato soup, and tomato-based barbecue sauces) contain the richest sources of lycopene, a powerful cancer-bashing phytonutrient. These products, when consumed with a small amount of olive oil in the same meal, provide the body with a concentrated source of lycopene in a biologically available form. Research reveals that five to ten servings per week of tomato sauce (½ cup is a serving) provide protection against cancer.

CRUCIFEROUS VEGETABLES

Broccoli, Brussels sprouts, cauliflower, rutabagas, turnips, and cabbage contain powerful phytonutrients *(indole-3-carbinol* and *sulphorafane)* that prevent breast cancer by inactivating cancer-causing chemicals so that they cannot do damage to breast tissue. Have at least one serving each day (½ cup is a serving) of one of these cruciferous vegetables.

OLIVE OIL

Eating olive oil reduces the risk of breast cancer. Dimitrios Trichopoulos, Ph.D., of the Harvard School of Public Health and his colleagues found that women who eat olive oil only once a day face a 25% higher risk of developing breast cancer than do women who consume it twice or more daily. Olive oil is important, but so is keeping total fat intake and daily calories to low levels. Use olive oil sparingly (1–2 teaspoons a day) in place of other oils and use it in recipes to replace other types of vegetable oils.

OMEGA-3 FATTY ACIDS

Omega-3 fatty acids from salmon, sardines, mackerel, menhaden, and tuna fight breast cancer by reducing inflammation (blocking eicosanoid biosynthesis), blocking the growth-enhancing effects of sex hormones, inhibiting metastasis, blocking blood vessel growth in cancer cells, and helping premalignant cells revert to the normal state. Omega-3 helps sensitize cancer cells to radiotherapy and chemotherapeutic drugs. One serving of salmon (4 ounces) or three servings of tuna fish each week contains a clinically effective dose of omega-3 fatty acids.

Kay Jacobs's Story

The year 1984 marked the beginning of an Orwellian-like nightmare for Kay Jacobs. That was the year she found a lump on the left side of her neck. Despite the fact that she had previously had two benign lumps removed from her breast, her doctor diagnosed the lump in her neck as cancer originating in her thyroid gland.

When Kay sought a second opinion, the doctor told her that her primary tumor probably was in her lung, ovary, or breast. Understandably, she was confused. But not for long. Literally overnight, Kay discovered a marble-size lump in her armpit. A subsequent biopsy revealed that 29 lymph nodes were positive for cancer cells that probably originated in her breast.

Kay's oncologist wanted to irradiate her breasts, but Kay decided to seek yet another medical opinion. After all, her doctor had been wrong before.

Kay went to see Ann Moore, M.D., an oncologist at New York University. Dr. Moore found that Kay had an exorbitantly high level of a blood marker for ovarian cancer, called CA-125. The normal range for CA-125 levels in the blood is 0–35. Kay's level was 1,800. Two more physicians, called in for consultation discovered that Kay's body was riddled with cancer. She remembers their words, uttered during a conference call: "The cancer is everywhere in your body." Her living nightmare just got worse.

After more research, Kay sought the help of Charles Vogel, M.D., a world-renowned breast cancer specialist at the University of Miami School of Medicine. He strongly recommended a chemotherapeutic cocktail called CAP (an acronym for three cancer drugs, cytoxin, adriamycin, and cisplatin). Kay took the treatment, which caused her to lose her hair, hearing, balance, and 35 pounds. The treatment also produced sores in her mouth and vagina and bleeding from her uterus. After 18 weeks of treatment, Kay's CA-125 level was still elevated.

Since chemotherapy failed to control Kay's cancer, she tried the next option: surgery. Kay's doctor recommended a hysterectomy to remove any cancer cells lurking in her ovaries. Kay agreed to the procedure, but her surgeon found no evidence of ovarian cancer. As a result of the operation, Kay was thrown into immediate menopause, suffering night sweats and loss of libido. What did her doctor recommend now? More radiotherapy and chemotherapy.

♦

At that point, most people would have given up and given in, but not Kay Jacobs. This time, Kay decided to play a part in her own cure instead of leaving it in the hands of the medical establishment.

Kay began reading about her disease, nutrition, and new treatments that were outside the bounds of conventional therapy. She devoured everything she could get her hands on about diet and alternative therapies. She resolved to take charge of her own health and visited an "alternative" cancer clinic in San Diego where she received treatments that included megavitamins, BCG vaccine (bacillus Calmette-Guérin, a drug used to treat tuberculosis that is also used against certain types of cancer), and a phytonutrient-rich vegetarian diet. She continued researching the role of nutrients in helping the body heal from cancer. Slowly but surely, she discovered how the body uses the power locked inside phytofoods and vitamins to heal itself (Table 5.5).

Today, 13 years after her initial diagnosis of cancer, Kay, at age 54, remains cancer-free. Despite all the medical misdiagnoses, chemotherapy, radiotherapy, and surgery, Kay stumbled upon the secret to achieving a permanent remission from her cancer. Through trial and error, she discovered how to use nutrition to defeat her cancer. Phyto-

---

TABLE 5.5

Kay Jacobs's Regimen

In 1985, Kay Jacobs began playing an active role in a cure for her breast cancer. In addition to undergoing conventional therapy, Jacobs embraced a phytonutrient rich diet and began taking nutritional supplements. Here is an overview of the regimen she believes saved her life and left her cancer free:

Phytofoods	*Nutritional Supplements*
• Soy milk (non-fat or low-fat) and soy cheese	• High-potency multivitamin-mineral supplement
• Low-fat cottage cheese with tablespoon flaxseed oil	• Vitamin A complex (5,000 international units vitamin A; 1 milligram alpha-carotene; 5 milligrams lycopene; 6 milligram lutein; 0.3 milligram zeaxanthin)
• Fresh vegetables such as broccoli, cabbage, cauliflower, Brussels sprouts	• Vitamin B-complex (high-potency formula)
• Fresh fruit and carrot juice	• Vitamin C (500 milligrams)
• Nuts and seeds	• Vitamin E complex (natural isomers, 400 international units)
• Olive oil	• Coenzyme Q_{10} (200 micrograms)
• Salmon and mackerel	• Pancreatic digestive enzyme complex
• Whole grains and cereals	
• Licorice	

nutrients, vitamins, and conventional medical treatment gave Kay the winning strategy for success.

Today, Kay Jacobs is a cancer lecturer, addressing groups of cancer victims who desperately want a second chance at life. Kay Jacobs took charge of her treatment and her life—and you can, too.

Evelyn Schneider: A Work in Progress

Traditional breast-cancer therapy is designed to kill cancer cells. The problem is that destroying breast cancer cells with drugs and radiation cripples the immune system and ravages healthy cells.

Food, on the other hand, can create such an inhospitable environment for cancer that it eventually gives up. This is partly due to the fact that foods such as legumes, tomatoes, salmon, and broccoli contain powerful anticancer compounds and immune-system stimulants that change the biochemistry of the entire body, not just one part. This ensures that the cancer cannot simply move to another area of the body. But to defeat a formidable foe like cancer sometimes requires a strategy that combines traditional treatments, such as surgery or chemotherapy, with nutrition. And that is exactly how Evelyn Schneider beat her breast cancer into remission.

In 1989, Evelyn Schneider underwent a mastectomy to remove a cancerous tumor in her right breast. Her doctor also prescribed the drug tamoxifen. Doctors don't know which women are likely candidates for a tumor recurrence, so they usually treat breast cancer victims with the drug, which works like phytonutrients in soy foods, to prevent cancer from returning. But tamoxifen causes serious side effects, such as vaginal infections, bleeding, and even uterine cancer years later. Those unpleasant side effects caused Evelyn such severe discomfort that she had to discontinue her tamoxifen therapy.

Almost seven years later a mammogram revealed cancer in Evelyn's left breast. This was a different type of breast cancer, a fast-growing type called ductal carcinoma in situ, comedo type. Evelyn refused further treatment—in this case radiation—and turned to a New York City cancer specialist, Nicholas Gonzalez, M.D., who had been treating her for two years for another medical condition. Dr. Gonzalez recommended a demanding therapeutic regimen that included massive doses of pancreatic enzymes, megadoses of vitamins and minerals, and various types of "cleansing" routines for her liver and intestines. Evelyn's husband, Morton, came under Dr. Gonzalez's care for cancer in 1991 to treat metastases in his pancreas, adrenal glands and liver. (See pages 35–36 for Morton's story.)

Evelyn's dietary protocol contains phytonutrient-rich vegetables and she supplements her diet with vitamins and minerals prescribed by her doctor. Will her new diet beat back her cancer as it did for her husband? Only time will tell, but if her results are similar to those of Dr. Gonzalez's other cancer patients who have used diet and supplements to beat the odds, she stands the chance of sending her breast cancer into permanent remission. (See page 117 for a description of the Gonzalez anticancer regimen.)

Experimental Breast and Ovarian Cancer Diet and Protocol

DIET

The experimental protocol in Table 5.7 contains the phytonutrient-rich foods and nutrients that hold promise for being effective against breast and ovarian cancer. Phytonutrient-rich foods form the foundation of this protocol and should be eaten every day in the amounts listed. Supplementary nutrients should be used only with the permission and under the supervision of a physician. Table 5.8 is a 3-day eating plan to use as a guide for constructing meals based on the experimental breast and ovarian cancer protocol. *Permanent Remission*'s recipes are indicated in bold print.

FOODS TO AVOID

You don't have to completely eliminate any food from your new way of eating, but you should drastically reduce your intake of the following foods in order to achieve optimal reproductive health and a long-term or permanent remission from breast cancer if you have it.

METHIONINE-RICH FOODS

Most animal foods, such as red meats, eggs, milk, cheese, and fowl, contain high amounts of the amino acid methionine. Breast cancer tumors depend on methionine to grow and thrive. Low-methionine

TABLE 5.6

The Gonzalez Regimen

Nicholas Gonzalez, M.D., is a New York City cancer specialist who earned his medical degree from Cornell University and completed an internship at Vanderbilt University Medical Hospital. Gonzalez claims to have helped hundreds of people defeat their cancer—even those whose own doctors gave them merely months to live.

Gonzalez's regimen is exceptionally demanding. It involves a phytonutrient-rich diet, including raw vegetables, vegetable juices, pancreatic enzymes, fiber laxatives, juice fasting, and coffee enemas. This regimen, based on the work of a dentist named William Kelly, who claims to have used it to send his own cancer (pancreatic) into a long-term remission, has met with skepticism and derision by many conventional cancer specialists. Gonzalez staunchly defends the efficacy of his protocol and has recently submitted his research data to the National Cancer Institute for scientific scrutiny. Here is an overview of the Gonzalez anti-cancer regimen:

Phytofoods: Organic raw vegetables, fruits and fruit juices play a major role in the regimen. Gonzalez believes that fresh fruits and vegetables contain important enzymes to help defeat cancer. He also recommends liberal amounts of fresh carrot juice each day. Gonzalez discourages consumption of red meat, but does prescribe it for a small number of patients who have an acid-base imbalance in their blood, as determined by blood chemistry tests.

Pancreatic enzymes: Gonzalez believes that pancreatic enzymes help digest tumor cells and therefore recommends large doses of pancreatic enzymes, usually obtained from overseas suppliers. His patients must take these enzymes throughout the day and evening. Gonzalez often recommends that patients set an alarm to take the enzymes in the middle of the night.

Purgings: Gonzalez advocates four types of body cleansings or purgings: the liver flush, the clean sweep, a two-day juice fast, and coffee enemas.

The liver flush is a five-day course of ingesting olive oil, apple juice, Epsom salts, and phosphoric acid—designed to cleanse the liver and gallbladder.

The clean sweep is a five-day plan ingesting a solution that contains fiber and bentonite (clay minerals) designed to cleanse the intestines.

The juice fast consists of a two-day regimen in which 6 grapefruits, 6 lemons, and 12 oranges are consumed daily, preceded by 3 tablespoons of Epsom salts. Gonzalez believes that this regimen helps draw tumor breakdown waste products out of the body.

The coffee enema is the most notorious of Gonzalez's purging therapies and the one that draws the most criticism from conventional cancer specialists. Gonzalez insists that his patients use organic coffee, a pint at a time, often a dozen times each day (Gonzalez self-administers 4 coffee enemas to himself even though he does not have cancer). He maintains that as a cancerous tumor is digested by pancreatic enzymes, the debris from the tumor can be just as toxic as the cancer itself. The coffee enema, he says, helps flush these toxins out of the body. This allows the immune system and organs such as the liver and kidneys to function at peak levels, thereby accelerating the remission process.

Nutritional supplements: Gonzalez recommends large doses of antioxidant vitamins and minerals, such as the B-complex vitamins, vitamins C, E, A, and minerals such as selenium, magnesium, and calcium.

TABLE 5.7

Experimental Breast and Ovarian Cancer Protocol*

Eat These Phytofoods Each Day	In These Amounts
• Soy meat replacers: soy burgers, hot dogs, bacon, bacon, sausage, turkey, chicken, ground beef, tofu†	• 1–2 servings (as indicated on package) each day or 2½ ounces of tofu in place of all meat, chicken, most fish
• Soy milk (nonfat or low-fat) or soy cocktail‡	• 1 8-ounce serving each day
• Broccoli, cabbage, kale, cauliflower, turnips, Brussels sprouts	• 1 cup raw or ½ cup steamed
• Fresh fruit such as watermelon or guava	• 1 medium slice or 1 small fruit
• Tomato sauce	• ½ cup over pasta or in recipes, or 1 cup of tomato-based soup (3–5 times each week)
• Olive oil, as a replacement for other vegetable oils, butter, and margarine	• 1–2 teaspoons
• Salmon or tuna	• Up to 2 4-ounce servings of salmon each week, or 3 4-ounce servings of tuna
• Citrus fruits: oranges, grapefruits	• 1 medium orange or ½ grapefruit

Vitamins and Minerals

- Vitamin A complex (5,000 international units vitamin A; 1 milligram alpha-carotene; 5 milligrams lycopene; 6 milligrams lutein; 0.3 milligrams zeaxanthin)

- Vitamin B complex (high-potency formula)[§]
- Vitamin C (1,000 milligrams)
- Vitamin D_3 (400 international units)
- Vitamin E complex (natural isomers, 400 international units)

- Calcium citrate (500 milligrams)
- Magnesium citrate (250 milligrams)
- Selenomax (200 micrograms)[‖]
- Zinc gluconate (20 milligrams)
- Chromium picolinate (200 micrograms)

Nonvitamin Nutrients

- Phytonutrient Cocktail (Twin Laboratories)[‡]

- Propolis (caffeic acid esters: 500 milligrams)
- Wine and tea polyphenols (50/250 milligrams)
- Strict vegetarians: flaxseed (1–2 tablespoons, ground and defatted)
- Bioflavonoid complex (500 milligrams citrus bioflavonoids; 30 milligrams grape-skin polyphenols; 200 milligrams quercetin; 50 milligrams rutin; 300 milligrams green tea extract; anthocyanins; 5 milligrams Pycnogenol; 100 milligrams anthocyanins)
- L-glutathione (200 milligrams)
- Coenzyme Q_{10} (90 milligrams)
- N-acetyl-cysteine (500 milligrams)
- Modified citrus pectin (1 teaspoon 3 times each day)
- Conjugated linoleic acid (1,200 milligrams)

*A number of products, such as soy cocktails, phytonutrient cocktails, and choline cocktails, contain most or all of the nutrients listed in this table.
†See brand-name soy-food meat replacers listed in Table 4.7, page 86.
‡See recommended soy cocktails listed in Table 4.4, page 82.
§Use any brand of high-potency B-complex vitamin such as Twinlab, GNC, or Solgar.
‖Selenomax is the trade name for the organic form of selenium manufactured and licensed by Nutrition 21.

TABLE 5.8

Three-Day Sample Breast and Ovarian Cancer Diet

MEAL	DAY 1	DAY 2	DAY 3
Breakfast	• 2 Morningstar Farms Breakfast Strips • **Apple Cinnamon Oatmeal** • 6 ounces fresh orange juice	• **Pigs in the Blanket** • 1 cup soy milk (such as White Wave Silk Soy Beverage)	• **Buttermilk Pancakes with Banana** • 1 cup soy milk • 6 ounces fresh orange juice
Midmorning snacks	• ½ grapefruit	• Apple	• Orange
Lunch	• **Hearty Lasagna** • 1 large wedge of watermelon	• **Tuna Dijon Salad** on whole-grain bread, with lettuce and tomato • Apple	• Green Giant Harvest Burger on whole-grain bun, with lettuce, tomato, ketchup • ½ cup **Cajun Coleslaw**
Midafternoon snacks	• **Super Soy Power Shake**	• **Super Soy Power Shake**	• **Super Soy Power Shake**
Dinners	• **Horseradish-Encrusted Salmon** • ½ cup steamed broccoli with lemon juice • Mixed green salad, olive-oil-and-vinegar dressing • ½ grapefruit	• **Broccoli and Tofu Lo Mein with "Chicken"** • ½ cup fresh berries	• **Rigatoni with Garlic, Tomatoes, and Basil** • 1 slice **Chocolate Bundt Cake with Fruit Ribbon and Mocha Frosting**
Evening snacks	• 1 cup **Fruit Yogurt Crunch**	• 1 cup **Strawberries and "Cream"**	• 1 cup **Pink Citrus Ice**

See pages 227–338 for *Permanent Remissions* recipes listed in this table (boldfaced items).

foods deplete methionine levels in tumor cells, which in turn, lower tumor cells' antioxidant defenses against chemotherapy and radiotherapy. Methionine depletion strongly increases the amount of the drug cisplatin taken up by human breast-tumor cells implanted in laboratory animals. Breast-tumor cells resistant to both methionine depletion and cisplatin alone are very sensitive to the combination of methionine starvation and cisplatin because the intratumoral platinum concentration is higher in combination with methionine starvation than when cisplatin alone is used.

VEGETABLE OILS, EXCEPT OLIVE OIL, CANOLA OIL, AND OMEGA-3 MARINE OILS

Linoleic acid, found in large amounts in most vegetable oils, increases the potential of such environmental toxins as pesticides and chemical waste to stimulate breast-cancer growth. Growth of metastasis to the lung of human breast-cancer cells is increased in laboratory animals fed a diet high in linoleic acid. Linoleic acid increases the progression of breast cancer at several stages of the metastatic process and may stimulate the growth of blood vessels that allow breast tumor cells to metastasize.

ALCOHOL

Recent studies show that as little as one alcoholic drink a day can significantly increase the risk of breast cancer in women. Alcohol increases the amount of estradiol manufactured in the body, which promotes the growth of breast cancer. Women with breast cancer should abstain from consuming alcoholic beverages.

WHOLE MILK, BUTTER, CHEESE, ICE CREAM, MAYONNAISE, AND EGG YOLKS

Milk, butter, and eggs and foods made from them contain too much saturated fat and cholesterol for optimal breast health. If you *must* use these foods, choose skim milk, light butter (contains half the fat of regular butter), soy-based parmesan cheese (available in well-stocked health-food stores), and egg whites or egg substitutes. Egg yolks and red meat contain arachidonic acid, which has been linked to cancer formation and heart disease.

EXERCISE

Regular exercise can also play an important role in reducing the risk of recurrence of cancer. Exercise helps to reduce the circulating levels of estrogens that may contribute to cancer growth. Your goal should be to burn 1,500 calories a week through regular aerobic exercise, such as walking. If you do not currently exercise, obtain your doctor's permission and begin slowly, working up to a 45-minute walk at least 5 days each week.

6

BEATING
PROSTATE CANCER

Gentlemen, start your engines.

The race for your life has begun. Prostate cancer is now the most frequently diagnosed cancer in men in the United States, Canada, and Great Britain, and the second most common cause of cancer-related deaths in men in the United States.

When it comes to cancer, men have not yet begun to fear for their prostates to the extent that women fear for their breasts, but signs of a heightened prostate-cancer awareness among American men looms on the horizon:

- Retired General Norman Schwarzkopf, National Football League Hall of Famer Len Dawson, golfer Arnold Palmer, actors Eddie Albert and Jerry Lewis, Washington, D.C. Mayor Marion Barry, and singer Harry Belafonte have gone public and now speak openly about their battles with prostate cancer.
- The untimely deaths of celebrities such as musician Frank Zappa, Time-Warner President Steve Ross, and actors Don Ameche, Bill Bixby, Telly Savalas, and Dick Sargent have helped publicize the seriousness of prostate cancer.
- Michael Milken, the notorious junk-bond wunderkind of Wall Street and a prostate cancer victim, spent millions of dollars of his own money to found CaP CURE, an organization dedicated to finding a cure for prostate cancer.
- A national TV ad depicting a man at the baseball ballpark urgently leaving to use the bathroom in the middle of an inning has alerted male viewers to an early symptom of prostate disease.

- Urologists report a record number of men have made appointments to be probed, poked, and pricked to find out if they have prostate cancer.
- Men now talk freely and familiarly about formerly obscure medical tests and procedures such as DRE (digital rectal exam), *PSA* (prostate-specific antigen), and TURP (transurethral resection of the prostate).

As with breast cancer, *early detection* has become the catch-phrase for prostate cancer, and it is heavily promoted by the medical and pharmaceutical communities. But does early detection really make a difference in surviving the disease?

Lots of Treatments and Tests but No *Prevention*

American doctors are almost totally absorbed with detection and treatment of prostate cancer. Yet the death rate from prostate cancer has not changed since the 1960s. And no degenerative disease has ever been eliminated by detection and treatment alone. Why has the U.S. medical establishment shown so little interest in finding the cause of prostate cancer and so much enthusiasm for employing and researching painful procedures in treating this disease?

Many doctors are simply not aware of the published data on the role of phytonutrients in preventing and reversing prostate cancer. And why should they be? Doctors are not trained in nutrition *or* the prevention of diet-related diseases. Their professors never taught them the value of nutrition during medical school. While the medical establishment claims to support prevention, it has repeatedly described dietary measures as ineffective and rejected preventive programs well within our reach. A cursory examination of cancer-related medical journals reveals that drug treatments and surgical techniques command the full attention of most physicians who research and treat prostate cancer.

Early detection is important but clearly does nothing to prevent prostate cancer or death from the disease. Prostate cancer occurs in men as young as 30, and *at least 30% of men over the age of 50 have detectable evidence of prostate cancer.* The American Cancer Society (ACS) predicts that more than 240,000 new cases of prostate cancer will be diagnosed this year, resulting in more than 40,000 deaths.

Ironically, prostate cancer may be the most preventable cancer. Medical research has clearly shown that prostate cancer is the most responsive and sensitive of all cancers to the body's sex hormones, to hormonelike drugs, *and* to hormonelike phytonutrients found in soy foods and beverages, whole grains, and vegetables.

Hormones Are the Cause; Phytonutrients Are the "Cure"

Almost all men who reach old age probably have histologic (microscopically verifiable) evidence of prostate cancer; the prevalence of prostate cancer is similar worldwide. But the *risk of dying* from invasive prostate cancer is five times higher among men who eat high-fat, phytonutrient-poor diets.

Whether prostate cancer remains "silent" or rears its ugly head depends on what you eat *and* what you don't eat. Without exception, the vast majority of scientific studies show that phytonutrient-rich diets, low in fat and cholesterol, prevent latent prostate tumors from growing and spreading to other organs. Conversely, studies reveal that diets high in saturated fats from animal foods promote the deadliest form of prostate cancer.

Animal fats, cholesterol, and lack of phytonutrients cause a chronic imbalance between testosterone and estrogen. The idea that men have estrogen at all surprises many people, yet that's just the beginning of the story. Recent research has shown that *male estrogen levels rise and fall with diet* and that this in turn helps determine the risk of developing invasive prostate cancer.

The testosterone–estrogen ratio is one of the most important risk factors for dying from prostate cancer. Men who keep this ratio low during their lifetime seem to avoid getting metastatic prostate cancer. Phytonutrients help reduce the risk of dying from prostate cancer by blocking the cancer-promoting actions of testosterone and its metabolic by-products and by acting like weak estrogens, tipping the testosterone-estrogen ratio in favor of keeping prostate cancer silent.

Changing your diet to favorably influence your own testosterone–estrogen ratio will not diminish your masculinity, libido, or maleness in any way. In fact, recent research has shown that phytonutrient-rich soy foods, rich in estrogen-like compounds, possess all the muscle-building power of traditional high-protein foods favored by bodybuilders, such as fish, fowl, and egg whites. Most animal foods contain amino-acid profiles that can raise serum cholesterol levels and increase the risk of developing cancer and heart disease. Soy protein lowers blood cholesterol levels by as much as 25% and reduces the risk of cancer and heart disease. Sorry, bodybuilders: meat, milk, and eggs are out and soy is in—if you want to live to play with your children's children's children.

Clues from Around the World

Chinese men living in Shanghai enjoy the lowest incidence of prostate cancer in the world: just one in 100,000 men gets the disease. Native Japanese have the next lowest rate, at four in every 100,000 men. Black men living in West Africa (where the traditional diet has little meat or fat) have very low rates, from four to 10 per 100,000. But relocating to the United States exacts a deadly toll on all three groups. The rates rise to 13 in 100,000 for Japanese-Americans, and 19 in 100,000 for Chinese-Americans living in San Francisco. But the group most at risk for prostate cancer is American black men, whose rate approaches 100 per 100,000.

Various migration studies have followed the Taiwanese when they relocated to the United States, the Yemenites and Ethiopians to Israel, and the Asian Russians migrating to European Russian republics. In every one of these studies, *without exception,* people who adopted a higher-fat and lower-fiber diet of the new country they migrated to acquired the elevated cancer rates of that country. Arguments for "genetic protection" from prostate cancer evaporate with these observations. There is one important racial difference between Asians and whites: native Japanese and Chinese men have a substantially lower level of an enzyme, *5-alpha-reductase,* that converts testosterone to its more potent form, dihydrotestosterone (DHT). DHT has been linked to benign prostatic hyperplasia (BPH) and prostate cancer. But I suspect that if men in the United States followed the *Permanent Remissions* plan from childhood, there would be little difference in enzyme levels between the groups.

In Japan, mortality from prostatic cancer is low, *despite the fact that Japanese men have the same rate of prostate cancer as men in the*

United States. The phytonutrient-rich Japanese diet, which contains soy foods and much less animal protein and fat than the ordinary U.S. diet, protects Japanese men from the deadly form of prostate cancer. The death rate from prostate cancer is five times lower in Japan than in the United States. Once Japanese men migrate to Hawaii or the U.S. mainland and adopt the national diet, their risk of the disease approaches that seen in U.S. men.

Intrigued by such findings, U.S. researchers devised the Health Professionals Follow-Up Study (a systematic tracking of the eating habits of 47,855 men between 40 and 75 years old) to examine the role of fat in prostate cancer. They found that men whose diets contained the most fat had a 79% greater risk of developing advanced prostate cancer than those whose diets were lowest in fat.

What were the foods most responsible for the increased risk? Beef, pork, lamb, mayonnaise, cream, salad dressings, and butter. Red meat had the strongest effect, increasing the incidence of advanced prostate cancer risk by 164%. (Other studies have found that a saturated-fat intake of 35 grams a day doubled the risk of developing prostate cancer.) Fish and other seafood were found not to elevate prostate cancer risk.

The most important finding from this study was that the higher the intake of dietary fat, especially fat from red meat (and thus saturated fat and the accompanying cholesterol), *the greater the risk that prostate cancer will progress from a latent disease to a life-threatening disease.* High-fat diets appear to be associated only with advanced prostate cancer, not with the localized, slow-growing form that often remains dormant for many years. Researchers have since found that there is as much as a 120-fold difference in the incidence of more advanced, clinically evident prostate cancer among countries with different fat intake levels.

The Two Important Phytofood Groups for Prostate Health

What types of foods and nutrients provide the most protection from prostate cancer? Worldwide studies have shown that the following two classes of foods help prevent the disease and coax it into remission.

PHYTOESTROGEN-RICH FOODS

Soy foods, such as tofu and miso, soy milk, and soy cocktails (highly concentrated drink mixes of cancer-stopping phytoestrogens sold in health-food stores); soy milk; and legumes, such as garbanzo beans and lima beans, contain hormonelike compounds called phytoestrogens, which protect against invasive prostate cancer. These phytonutrients work by enhancing the body's protective natural estrogen activity and thwarting cancer cells from growing and spreading. One class of phytoestrogens, isoflavones, are abundant in soybeans and other legumes and are especially effective at keeping prostate tumors in check (Table 6.1). Recent studies also show that isoflavones help protect against BPH, a disease in which the prostate enlarges, giving rise to feelings of urinary urgency. Rats fed a soy-free diet develop inflammation of the prostate gland (prostatitis), while none of those fed a special high-soy diet develop the condition.

TABLE 6.1

Phytofood Products That Fight Prostate Cancer

The following formula foods (also known as functional foods or biodesigned foods) contain anticancer phytonutrients, vitamins, minerals, and nonvitamin nutrients now being tested by the National Cancer Institute (NCI) and other health research organizations. These formula foods are sold nationwide in health-food stores and some pharmacies and supermarkets. Appendix IV (pages 365–68) contains the names, addresses, and telephone numbers of product manufacturers. Have one serving of any one of the following products each day.

MaxiLIFE Soy Cocktail: Sold in health-food stores, manufactured by Twin Laboratories. Drink this or any soy cocktail made with a highly concentrated soy protein isolate. This formula contains the phytonutrients that have been shown to be effective against prostate, breast, and reproductive cancers.

MaxiLIFE Phytonutrient Cocktail: Sold in health-food stores, manufactured by Twin Laboratories. This formula contains phytonutrients and other antioxidants shown by clinical and laboratory research to be effective in the prevention and management of prostate, breast, and other reproductive cancers.

Pecta-Sol: Modified citrus pectin (MCP), sold by mail order and manufactured by Eco-Nugenics. MCP is currently being tested to determine its clinical effectiveness in blocking cancer-cell metastasis. Use this product only if you have been diagnosed with prostate cancer. Use only under a doctor's supervision.

Haelan 851: Made by Haelan Products Inc. This not-so-pleasant-tasting fermented soy cocktail contains a rich supply of isoflavones derived from specially grown soybeans.

TOMATO-CONCENTRATE PRODUCTS

Tomato sauce, tomato ketchup, and tomato paste—three staples of the American diet—reduce the risk for developing prostate, digestive tract, and other cancers. One phytonutrient, *lycopene,* found most abundantly in tomato products, watermelon, and guava, provides exceptionally strong protection against prostate cancer.

Increased attention was directed to lycopene in 1995 following the publication of an epidemiological study by Edward Giovannucci, M.D., of the Harvard School of Public Health, that identified a relationship between consumption of processed tomato products and a reduction in the risk of prostate cancer.

Recent studies have confirmed that the intake of lycopene is associated with a reduced risk of developing prostate cancer. The human body does not produce lycopene, so the beneficial effects of this carotenoid can be obtained only through the diet. Processed tomato products provide the most abundant source of lycopene, but the amount of lycopene consumed is not as important to disease prevention as is the amount actually absorbed by the body. In fact, of 46 foods containing fruits and vegetables, only four were associated with reduction in prostate cancer risk: tomato sauce (which had the strongest association), tomatoes, pizza, and strawberries (strawberries are not a source of lycopene).

Lycopene is best absorbed by the body when consumed as tomatoes that have been heat-processed and when a small amount of oil is present, such as in tomato sauce made with olive oil. Lycopene is more efficiently absorbed from tomato sauce, paste, or ketchup than it is from raw tomatoes. Processing concentrates the amount of lycopene present, but combining it with olive oil increases the amount of lycopene your body will absorb. The blood levels of lycopene, unlike those of its cousin beta-carotene, don't seem to be affected by such unhealthy habits as smoking tobacco and drinking alcohol.

The Health Professionals Follow-Up Study, which uncovered a strong link between fat intake and prostate cancer, also found that men who ate 10 or more servings (one serving = ½ cup) of tomato-based foods per week had the lowest risk of developing prostate cancer. However, even those who ate between 1.5 and 10 servings seemed to derive some benefits. Tomatoes contain a variety of cancer-fighting nutrients and carotenoids, in addition to lycopene, which may also play an active role in fighting prostate cancer.

Other Nutrients That Help Fight Prostate Cancer

The following vitamins, minerals, and natural products play a vital role in protecting the prostate from cancer.

CITRIC ACID

Citric acid in citrus fruits blocks the cancer-causing effects of environmental carcinogens. Have at least one serving of citrus fruit each day to prevent prostate cancer, and two servings if you have the disease.

OMEGA-3 FATTY ACIDS

Omega-3 fatty acids, found in such seafoods as salmon, tuna, and mackerel and in flaxseed, inhibit the development of tumors in animals and suppress cell proliferation, cell transformation, and the promotion, growth, progression, and metastasis of a variety of human and rodent cancer-cell lines in the laboratory. They also inhibit blood-vessel formation necessary for cancer cells to metastasize and they sensitize cancer cells to radiotherapy and chemotherapeutic drugs. Have at least one serving of salmon or three servings of tuna each week to obtain a clinically effective dose of omega-3 fatty acids. If you don't enjoy fish, use 1–2 tablespoons of ground flaxseed in salads, soups, or other recipes.

SAW PALMETTO

Saw palmetto berries contain a unique class of fatty acids that can inhibit the enzyme *5-alpha reductase,* which converts testosterone to the more potent DHT in the prostate. DHT is the compound responsible for prostate enlargement and may be involved in the cancer process. Saw palmetto is widely used in Europe to treat BPH. In addition to its cellular growth-inhibiting action on prostate epithelial cells, saw palmetto acts as an anti-inflammatory. Saw-palmetto extract, standardized to contain 85%–95% fatty acids and sterols, is effective in the majority of patients with BPH at a dosage of 160 mg twice daily. BPH develops with increasing age. It occurs in about 8% of men in their thirties, in more than 40% at 50–60 years of age, in more than 70% at 61–70 years of age, and in over 80% in men older than 80 years of age. Anyone experiencing symptoms of BPH should first see a physician to be tested for prostate cancer. Unlike finasteride, a prescription drug used to treat BPH, saw palmetto also blocks the binding of DHT to sites on prostate epithelial cells. As a result, clinical studies of saw palmetto have demonstrated its superiority to finasteride in the treatment of BPH. More research is needed to determine the clinical effectiveness of saw palmetto extract.

VITAMIN D

Prostate cancer death rates are lower in regions that receive more ultraviolet (UV) light, which is required for the synthesis of provitamin D in the skin. Vitamin D (1,25-dihydroxyvitamin D_3) affects the function and growth of healthy and cancerous prostate cells. Men who develop prostate cancer are more likely to be deficient in vitamin D. In men older than 57 years of age, decreased blood levels of 1,25-dihydroxyvitamin D_3 are an important predictor of risk for prostatic tumors. It's becoming increasingly clear that vitamin D can inhibit the growth of tumor cells. Several animal studies have demonstrated that even moderate amounts of vitamin D can slow the growth of prostate cancer cells. Milk is a major source of dietary vitamin D for many people in the United States, but the vitamin D content of fortified milk and milk products is inconsistent; you can't be certain you're getting enough vitamin D from them. A study by researchers at the Boston University School of Medicine found that 80% of milk samples taken in the United States contained either 20% less or 20% more vitamin D than the labels claimed. Fourteen percent of the samples had undetectable amounts of the vitamin. The dosage of vitamin D required to inhibit the growth of prostate cancer may be much higher than the recommended daily allowance (RDA) of 400 international units per day. Since vitamin D can be toxic in doses that greatly exceed this value, researchers have developed synthetic analogues of vitamin D that retain the ability to inhibit cancer cell growth without the toxicity associated with high doses. These analogs have been successfully used in animal models of leukemia and breast cancer. Vitamin D may be related to other cancers. One study found that women who get low levels of sunlight experience high rates of breast cancer, suggesting that low vitamin D levels may play a preventive role in the disease. Low blood levels of vitamin D have been found in people with colon cancer. Vitamin D–rich foods include salmon, tuna, fish oils, milk, and vitamin-fortified cereals.

VITAMIN E

Vitamin E taken at 50 milligrams per day significantly decreased the incidence of prostate cancer in a large study of Finnish smokers. At least three other published studies have found a protective effect for vitamin E in prostate cancer. Always choose natural vitamin E instead of the D-alpha form (synthetic vitamin E) because natural E contains a spectrum of isomers (related chemical forms) of vitamin E that are necessary for optimal disease protection. Since an ordinary diet cannot supply anywhere near the daily doses of vitamin E shown to be clinically effective (200–400 international units), you must supplement your new way of eating with this vitamin.

ZINC

The prostate contains more zinc than any other human organ. This implies that zinc might be associated with the prostate's housekeeping and manufacturing functions. Studies show that there appears to be a strong correlation between zinc concentrations in prostatic secretions and prostate diseases. In patients who have died of cancer, prostatic zinc levels are usually low. Foods high in zinc include pumpkin seeds, oysters, and legumes.

MODIFIED CITRUS PECTIN

A special form of citrus pectin has been shown to interfere with cancer-cell metastasis by inhibiting the ability of cancer cells to adhere to other cells in the body. Modified citrus pectin (MCP) combats galectin-3, a protein that helps cancer cells bind to normal tissue and makes metastasis possible. Laboratory studies show that the MCP acts as an antiadhesive agent, a type of cellular Teflon that inhibits the metastatic process. In addition, it enhances the activity of immune cells involved in destroying migrating cancer cells in the bloodstream. Research on MCP is still inconclusive; however, preliminary results suggest that it is safe and should be considered for use by cancer patients who can afford it. Ordinary pectin, found in fruits such as grapefruit and oranges, does not possess the metastasis-stopping power of MCP.

MCP interferes with cell-to-cell interactions. Such interactions are important in the metastatic process because they are a necessary step in the formation of a new cancerous colony of tumor cells. MCP is a phytochemical product manufactured by modifying the carbohydrate chain length of commercial citrus pectin, the type used in jellies and jams.

To date, preliminary studies have demonstrated that MCP can inhibit the spread of prostate cancer in laboratory animals. An Italian research team established specifications and standards for clinically effective MCP. The cancer-stopping power of MCP seems to depend on whether it can be absorbed by the digestive tract into the bloodstream. It is within the bloodstream that the binding action on the migrating cancer cells takes place. Pecta-Sol (manufactured by EcoNugenics) is the first commercially available MCP, and it is manufactured to the specifications established by an Italian research team that conducted the first study to document the cancer-stopping power of MCP.

MCP can be used daily if you have prostate cancer. One tablespoon mixed with 1 cup of juice or soy milk taken twice each day provides a clinically effective dose that has been shown to be effective against the disease.

Further research is required before scientists can determine if MCP is truly effective at blocking the spread of prostate or other types of cancer in the human body. Pecta-Sol is now being studied in human trials to determine if it can inhibit the spread of metastatic prostate cancer in humans. Discuss the possibility of using MCP with your physician. *Do not use this product without medical supervision.*

Howard Fuerst, M.D.: A Taste of His Own Phytomedicine

The stomach pain started simply enough. An invisible power drill began boring into the lower abdomen of Howard Fuerst, M.D. It wasn't really a sharp pain at first; it was more of a deep, dull ache, and it didn't become bothersome until it felt like it was chewing a hole through to his spine. It made itself felt in an authoritative way, as if to say, "This is no passing pang, pal; you're going to remember me."

As a board-certified internist with 35 years of clinical practice under his belt, Dr. Fuerst, now 66, knew the difference between ordinary pain and what he calls "oops" pain. With ordinary pain, such as a muscle pull, you will hurt, but it's not significant and you work through it with a couple of aspirin or ibuprofen tablets. With "oops" pain, you'd better stop and do something about it. This was full-blown "oops" pain, no question about it. But since doctors are their own worst patients, Howard Fuerst ignored the sage advice he had dispensed to patients for over 3 decades and worked through a week's worth of serious pain until it subsided by itself. That pain, Dr. Fuerst believes, was an early signal of his disease.

Dr. Fuerst recalls: "I was diagnosed with a highly aggressive form of prostate cancer *and* heart disease six years ago. Talk about a double whammy! What was especially disconcerting was that my PSA level was 4,000. Typically, patients with prostate cancer have PSA values between 5 and 15. I had never seen a value approaching my own, let alone heard or read of one. So I had my doctor repeat the test. Back came that ridiculous number—4,000! I called the company that manufactures the test and talked to their chief scientist. He told me that a PSA of 11,000 was indeed possible and that the test was very accurate. I sank into a deep depression.

"My daughter, who is a book publicist, gave me a number of diet and alternative-medicine books to read. My strategy for beating cancer and heart disease included a little of everything: surgery, drugs, meditation, a macrobiotic diet, Ayurevedic medicine, motivational and visualization tapes, and even traditional psychotherapy," reflects Dr. Fuerst. "But timely medical treatment and my phytonutrient diet formed the foundation of my remarkable remission."

Dr. Fuerst bases his diet around phytonutrient-rich vegetables, soups, a small amount of salmon (for omega-3 fats), whole grains and cereals, and fruits. He likes to get his soy isoflavones the old-fashioned way—by drinking soy milk and eating steamed soybeans, tofu, and miso, a fermented soy paste used in soups and salad dressings. Dr. Fuerst's phytonutrient-rich diet contains all of the nutrients known shown to be effective against prostate cancer in clinical and laboratory studies.

Today, Dr. Fuerst's PSA level is normal and his heart disease (diagnosed shortly after he learned about his prostate cancer) appears to be in remission. He is thoroughly enjoying his retirement with his wife Sheila, his children, and grandchildren.

A 1-day sample of the diet that Dr. Fuerst first used to keep his prostate cancer in remission is shown in Table 6.2.

TABLE 6.2

Sample Day in Dr. Fuerst's Diet

Meal	Foods
Breakfast	• Oatmeal made with soy milk • One slice sourdough bread with unsweetened apple butter
Midmorning snack	• One-half grapefruit
Lunch	• One cup miso soup • Hummus on pita bread with vegetables and miso dressing • One cup green tea
Midafternoon snack	• One medium apple
Dinner	• Six-ounce poached salmon fillet • Steamed broccoli with lemon juice • Mixed green salad with miso dressing • One serving fresh fruit
Evening snack	• One cup chamomile tea • Brown rice cakes with unsweetened apple butter

Hal Pritchard: Shaken but Not Stirred

Hal Pritchard, 73, is on a mission to save the world—or at least the men in it—from prostate cancer. And he is as passionate about his ambitious quest as he is about the soy cocktail that he credits with saving his life.

Hal is a consummate proselytizer. He hands out printed information on the life-saving powers of soy in shopping malls and restaurants and talks to anyone interested in what he has to tell them about diet and cancer.

Hal's one-man mission to alert others to the life-saving benefits of soy began in 1991. It was in that year that Hal began experiencing symptoms of urinary urgency that prompted him to visit his doctor for a prostate examination. Hal's PSA test results came back abnormally high. A subsequent biopsy confirmed his doctor's suspicion: Hal had an aggressive prostate cancer.

Hal's physician believed that the cancer was advanced enough to recommend external-beam radiation, in which the prostate is irradiated from an external source, as opposed to brachytherapy, in which radioactive pellets are premanently inserted into the prostate and radiate the gland from within. Radiation oncologists regard brachytherapy as a precise way of zapping the prostate and not the surrounding vital structures, thereby avoiding damage to the nerves feeding the prostate gland. This can help avoid unpleasant side effects associated with irradiation of the prostate, such as urinary incontinence, impotency, and severe infections. But brachytherapy may be used only when the cancer is clearly confined to the prostate. Doctors use external-beam radiation when the tumor is too large for brachytherapy or has spread beyond the prostate.

According to Hal's doctor, without external-beam radiation, the cancer would continue growing. But to Hal, the possible side effects of impotence or urinary incontinence were as unacceptable as dying prematurely from cancer.

Hal's physician was critical of his decision to forgo radiotherapy, but Hal decided, nevertheless, to pursue a nutritional remedy for his disease.

Hal decided to play a role in his own cure by trying an alternative approach to radiotherapy. He had read that phytonutrients in soybeans could help slow down or stop the progression of certain types of prostate cancer; he opted for a natural-foods approach to healing his cancer. Hal became a pioneer, trailblazing a new path toward healing his disease.

Hal read everything he could get his hands on about soy and prostate cancer. He discovered a soy cocktail that contained a large amount of cancer-fighting isoflavones and other phytonutrients that were active against cancer.

Soy contains a number of phytonutrients that attack prostate cancer at several levels, such as cutting off the blood supply to tumor cells and preventing the growth-stimulating effects of testosterone-related compounds. Hal knew from his research that soy could keep prostate tumor cells from growing, keeping them silent even though they remained in the prostate. After all, Japanese men get prostate cancer as frequently as men in the United States, but soy phytonutrients keep their prostate tumors from growing and spreading, allowing them to live a normal life and life span. Hal wondered if soy could do the same for him.

Hal devised his own treatment regimen, drinking a soy cocktail twice each day to obtain a clinically effective dose of soy isoflavones, protease inhibitors, and antiangiogenesis compounds that would stop his tumor from getting into his bloodstream and spreading to other organs. (A soy cocktail is a beverage mix that contains a clinically effective dose of soy isoflavones in addition to other phytonutrients, antioxidants, vitamins, and minerals. People who don't eat soy foods can use any commercially prepared soy cocktail—sold in most health-food stores and natural-food markets—to obtain genistein, the powerful disease-fighting phytonutrient available only in soybeans.) Within a month, Hal's symptoms—pain, urinary urgency, lethargy—and the worry and anxiety that accompanies them—began to disappear. His energy levels improved by leaps and bounds. During the next year, Hal's symptoms disappeared entirely—without surgery, without drugs, without radiotherapy. Five years later, Hal remains symptom free. He doesn't care if he still has cancer in his body. He believes that he can peacefully coexist with his disease, without the disastrous side effects of radiotherapy, surgery or drugs.

Hal Pritchard credits his soy drink with allowing him to take a kinder and gentler approach to beating his prostate cancer. "Today, my soy cocktail is a morning ritual: I drink 1 1/2 glasses each morning on an empty stomach and then sit down to enjoy my morning coffee and start my day. I am now 73 years old, but the drink has made me feel like I'm in my fifties. Something else that has happened is that my skin looks like the skin of a man in his fifties."

Hal cannot prove that his soy cocktail was the reason his prostate cancer no longer poses a threat to his life, but he believes that every man should be using it on a daily basis to head off cancer. A large body of scientific research backs up his belief in the healing power of soy.

Although Hal Pritchard was able to send his prostate cancer into remission without the medical intervention, most men should consider the variety of options available for the medical treatment of the disease. Consult your physician and seek additional opinions before deciding on the treatment strategy that's right for you. I recommend that you read Michael Korda's informative account of his own battle with prostate cancer, *Man to Man* (Random House, 1996). His success story makes clear the importance of getting more than one medical opinion before beginning treatment for prostate cancer.

American Black Men and Prostate Cancer

American black men have the highest incidence of prostate cancer in the world. Being older than 55, regardless of race, is also a risk factor for the disease. This suggests a common rate of prostate cancer initiation between blacks and whites but differences in tumor promotion. American black men have higher PSA levels (owing to a larger tumor volume), higher prostate cancer rates, more severe disease at the time of diagnosis, and higher mortality rates than Chinese and Japanese men, who have a *30-fold lower* prostate cancer rate. But native Africans have a markedly decreased risk of prostate cancer when compared to Americans of all races. The incidence of prostate cancer in American black men is 50% higher than in American white men.

Why do native African men have a significantly lower prostate cancer rate, whereas American black men have the highest rate in the world? Current research indicates that diet and biological differences play vital roles. Here is what I believe contributes to these differences:

- Young adult American blacks have a higher circulating testosterone level than American white men. Testosterone and its metabolites promote cancer cell growth.
- American black women have higher first-trimester testosterone levels than American white women, which may predispose their sons to prostate cancer later in life.
- The high dietary fat intake of many American blacks increases production of testosterone, which raises the risk of prostate cancer.

American black men have higher levels of a particular fatty acid (stearic acid) stored in their body fat than white American men. This may be significant, but further research is needed to confirm that this poses a risk of developing prostate cancer.

The *Permanent Remissions* Plan contains the foods and food products (e.g., soy cocktails and meat analogs) that can help reduce the cancer-promoting effects of testosterone and its metabolites. If you are an American black, you can use the plan now to reduce or eliminate the future risk of prostate cancer for you and your children.

Experimental Prostate Cancer Diet and Protocol

The experimental protocol shown in Table 6.3 contains the phytonutrient-rich foods and nutrients that hold promise for being effective against prostate cancer. Phytonutrient-rich foods form the foundation of this protocol and should be eaten every day in the amounts listed. Supplementary nutrients should be used only with the permission and under the supervision of a physician. Table 6.4 is a 3-day eating plan

TABLE 6.3

Experimental Prostate Cancer Protocol*

Eat These Phytofoods Each Day	In These Amounts
Soy meat replacers: soy burgers, hot dogs, bacon, sausage, turkey, chicken, ground beef, tofu†	2 servings (as indicated on package) each day or 2½ ounces of tofu in place of all meat, chicken, most fish
Soy milk (nonfat or low-fat)	1 8-ounce serving each day
Citrus fruits: oranges, grapefruits	1 medium orange or ½ grapefruit
Watermelon or guava	1 medium slice or 1 small fruit
Tomato sauce	½ cup over pasta or in recipes, or 1 cup of tomato-based soup
Olive oil, as a replacement for other vegetable oils, butter, and margarine	1–2 teaspoons
Salmon or tuna	1 4-ounce serving of salmon each week or 3 4-ounce servings of tuna

Dietary Supplements	Vitamins and Minerals
Soy-protein cocktail (40–80 milligrams total isoflavones per serving‡)	Vitamin A complex (includes 5,000 international units vitamin A; 1 milligram alpha-carotene; 5 milligrams lycopene; 6 milligrams lutein; 0.3 milligram zeaxanthin)
Grape seed extract (50 milligrams)	Vitamin B complex (high-potency formula)§
Wine and tea polyphenols (50/250 milligrams)	Vitamin C (1,000 milligrams)
Flaxseed (1–2 tablespoons, ground and defatted)	Vitamin D₃ (400 international units)
Propolis (caffeic acid esters: 500 milligrams)	Vitamin E complex (natural isomers: 400 international units)
L-glutathione (250 milligrams)	Calcium citrate (500 milligrams)
Coenzyme Q₁₀ (90 milligrams)	Magnesium citrate (250 milligrams)
N-acetyl-cysteine (500 milligrams)	Selenomax (200 micrograms)‖
Modified citrus pectin (1 teaspoon 3 times each day)	Zinc gluconate (20 milligrams)

*A number of products, such as soy cocktails, phytonutrient cocktails, and choline cocktails, contain most or all of the vitamins, minerals, and other nutrients listed in this table.
†See brand-name soy-food meat replacers listed in Table 4.7, page 86.
‡See brand-name soy cocktails listed in Table 4.4, page 82.
§Use any brand of high-potency B-complex vitamin such as those made by Twinlab, GNC, or Solgar.
‖Selenomax is the trade name for the organic form of selenium manufactured and licensed by Nutrition 21.

PHYTOFOODS THAT FIGHT PROSTATE CANCER

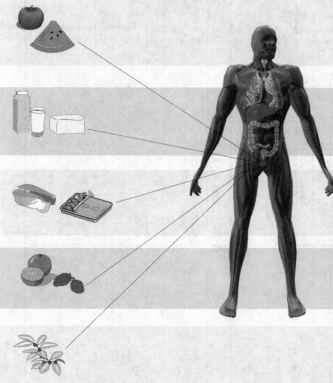

Processed tomato products and watermelon contain lycopene, a phytonutrient that can reduce the risk of prostate cancer.

Soy foods, soy milk, and soy cocktails enhance the body's protective natural estrogen activity to stop prostate cancer cells from growing and spreading.

Omega-3 fatty acids found in salmon, sardines, tuna, and mackerel inhibit prostate tumor growth and metastasis.

Citrus fruit and strawberries reduce the risk of prostate cancer and inhibit the growth of prostate tumors.

Saw palmetto berries prevent the conversion of testosterone to a compound that promotes prostate inflammation and prostate cancer.

TABLE 6.4

Three-Day Sample Prostate Cancer Diet Guide

MEAL	DAY 1	DAY 2	DAY 3
Breakfast	• **Apple Cinnamon Oatmeal** • 2 Morningstar Farms Breakfast Patties	• **Super Soy Shake** • 1 **Mandarin Orange Muffin**	• **Biscuits 'n' Sausage** • 6 ounces fresh grapefruit juice
Midmorning snacks	• ½ grapefruit	• Apple	• Orange
Lunch	• Green Giant Harvest Burger on whole-grain bun, with lettuce, tomato, and ketchup • ½ cup grapes	• **Egg "Fu" Salad Sandwich** on whole-grain bread, with lettuce and tomato • Apple	• **"Meatball" Oven Grinder Sub** • ½ cup **Cajun Coleslaw**
Midafternoon snacks	• **Super Soy Shake**	• **Super Soy Shake**	• **Super Soy Shake**
Dinners	• **Tricolor Pasta with Salmon** • ½ cup steamed broccoli with lemon juice • Mixed green salad with olive-oil-and-vinegar dressing • ½ grapefruit	• **"Beefy" Bean Burrito** • Large mixed salad with **Creamy Garlic Dressing** • 1 cup **Pink Citrus Ice**	• **Rigatoni with Garlic, Tomatoes, and Basil** • 1 slice **Tuscan Garlic Bread** • 1 cup **Strawberries and "Cream"**
Evening snacks	• 1 cup **Fruit Yogurt Crunch**	• 1 cup **Strawberries and "Cream"**	• 2 **Chewy Oatmeal Chocolate Chip Cookies** • 1 cup White Wave Chocolate Silk Soy Beverage

See pages 227–338 for *Permanent Remissions* recipes listed in this table (boldfaced items).

to use as a guide for constructing meals based on the experimental prostate cancer protocol. *Permanent Remissions* recipes are indicated in bold print.

FOODS TO AVOID

You don't have to completely eliminate any food from your new way of eating, but you should drastically reduce your intake of the following foods in order to achieve optimal prostate health and a long-term or permanent remission from prostate cancer if you have it.

RED MEAT

Red meats, including beef, lamb, and pork, contain saturated fats and are often contaminated by hormones and other toxic chemicals put there not by nature but by agribusiness. One large human study found an association between beef consumption and elevated risk for prostate cancer. These risks were stronger in men diagnosed before age 72.5. This study provides further evidence that animal fat and perhaps other compounds, such as arachidonic acid, contained in animal flesh, promote prostate cancer and it indicates that fat may act by shortening the latency period of the disease.

VEGETABLE OILS, EXCEPT OLIVE OIL, CANOLA OIL, AND OMEGA-3 MARINE OILS

Israelis consume one of the highest dietary polyunsaturated–saturated fat ratios in the world; the consumption of vegetable oils is about 8% higher than in the United States and 10%–12% higher than in most European countries. In fact, Israeli Jews may be regarded as a population-based dietary experiment on the effect of a high–vegetable oil diet, a diet that has been widely recommended by some physicians and health faddists. In Israel, there is a very high cancer rate, cancer mortality (especially among women), and high rates of cardiovascular disease, hypertension, type 2 diabetes mellitus, and obesity, compared with Western countries. The trend in many countries of increasing polyunsaturated fat intake is associated with an increasing frequency of prostate cancer. Studies suggest that excessive vegetable oil consumption might account for the high incidence and mortality of this disease.

ALCOHOL

You may have heard of the "French paradox," in which it is claimed that wine and other alcoholic beverages somehow protect the

French from heart disease. Alcohol may lower the risk of heart disease in some people, but it can raise the risk of prostate, breast, liver, pancreatic, and gastrointestinal cancers. If you have any of these cancers, *do not drink any type of alcohol.* It's like pouring gasoline on a fire.

WHOLE MILK, BUTTER, CHEESE, ICE CREAM, MAYONNAISE, AND EGG YOLKS

Milk, butter, and eggs and foods made from them contain too much saturated fat and cholesterol for optimal prostate health. If you *must* use these foods, choose skim milk, light butter (contains half the fat of regular butter), soy-based parmesan cheese (available in well-stocked health-food stores), and egg whites or egg substitutes. Egg yolks and red meat contain arachidonic acid, which has been linked to cancer formation and heart disease.

EXERCISE

Regular exercise can also play an important role in reducing the risk of recurrence of cancer. Exercise helps to reduce the circulating levels of testosterone that may contribute to cancer growth. Your goal should be to burn 1,500 calories a week through regular aerobic exercise, such as walking. If you do not currently exercise, obtain your doctor's permission and begin slowly, working up to a 45-minute walk at least 5 days each week.

7

BEATING DIABETES MELLITUS

Evelyn Potter has discovered how to have her cake and eat it, too.

Evelyn's "death-by-chocolate" cake is to *die* for, but Evelyn plans on being around for a quite a while. She's not going to let diabetes get in the way of enjoying her favorite recipe. And she doesn't have to. Evelyn has learned how to enjoy delicious desserts without jeopardizing her health.

Sugar is sweet, but not when you're one of 16 million Americans who have diabetes, up from 11 million in 1983. Evelyn has the adult form (type 2) of *diabetes mellitus,* Latin for "sweet that passes through" (so named for the sweet taste of urine in diabetics, and to distinguish it from an unrelated disease, *diabetes insipidus*). High blood sugar glucose levels, the hallmark of diabetes mellitus, can blind, cripple, and kill. There's nothing sweet about that.

The number of Americans with diabetes has risen almost 50% since 1983 and the disease rate has tripled since 1958, primarily because Americans are getting older and fatter. About half of people with diabetes don't know it because they don't recognize the meaning of symptoms, such as excessive thirst and urination.

Annually, diabetes causes an estimated 39,000 cases of blindness, 13,000 new cases of end-stage kidney disease, 54,000 amputations, and 90,000 cases of heart disease and stroke-related deaths. The risk of leg amputation is 30 times greater for a person who has diabetes than for those without the disease.

All who develop type 1 diabetes, the so-called juvenile type, know they have the disease because they must take daily insulin injections (a blood sugar–lowering hormone made in the pancreas) to survive. This will soon change with the advent of newer oral medications that control blood sugar equally as well as do insulin injections. But at least half the people with adult (type 2) diabetes in the United States—about 8 million, according to recent estimates—don't know they have this insidious disease. Many will find out only after serious complications develop. Yet there is growing evidence that almost all of these complications can be prevented or forestalled by using phytonutrient-rich low-fat foods, dietary supplements, and exercise to normalize blood sugar and the body's need for insulin.

Many Americans Become Temporary Diabetics Each Day

The high fat, high sugar, and high animal protein content of the American diet causes blood sugar levels to soar after meals. This dietary onslaught forces the beta-cells of the pancreas to pour out more and more insulin in a futile attempt to get sugar out of the blood and into the cells where it can be properly metabolized. What most of us consider ordinary American fare—typically high in fat, animal protein (saturated fat), and sugar, causes muscle cells to become insensitive to the sugar-lowering effects of insulin. So sugar accumulates in the blood, creating a host of health hazards, including diabetes, cancer, and heart disease.

After eating a typical American dinner, insulin levels can be three to five times higher than normal in response to abnormally high blood-sugar levels, essentially making many Americans *temporary diabetics*. After years of such chronic abuse, pancreatic cells give up the ghost, creating an insulin shortage while the body becomes progressively more insensitive to the hormone. This is the vicious circle that eventually makes so many people diabetics.

Type 2 diabetes disproportionately afflicts nonwhites, with rates about two times as high in American blacks, two to three times as high in American Hispanics, and five to six times as high in American Indians as it is in American whites.

Insulin Insensitivity

Diabetes works silently and relentlessly to damage almost every organ in the body. Even though doctors refer to type 2 diabetes as "insulin-independent" diabetes, many adult diabetics have to rely on insulin because they can't control their blood sugar effectively without the hormone. In fact, most type 2 diabetics shouldn't be on insulin, because this form of the disease can be controlled by using a phytonutrient-rich diet, dietary supplements, and regular exercise. Some doctors, however, don't have the time or nutritional training to properly counsel patients, so they place them on oral medications or insulin injections instead.

Like those with high blood pressure, many people with diabetes may not even know they have the disease, making it all the more insidious. In diabetes, sugar remains trapped in the blood. After a while, it oxidizes, becomes toxic, and damages delicate proteins in the eye, kidney cells, heart muscle, blood vessels, nerves, and other organs.

Diabetes leads to the diseases we associate with aging: retinopathy (degeneration of the retina, which can cause blindness), cataracts, kidney failure, stroke and heart attacks, arm and leg amputations, and nerve damage. Slowly, and with juggernaut-like tenacity, diabetes prematurely ages it victims, killing them slowly but surely.

About 80 million Americans are insensitive to their own insulin but have not yet developed overt diabetes. About a quarter of them will probably become ill later in life with symptoms of diabetes, which include fatigue, nerve damage, obesity, stroke and heart disease, and blindness. Insulin is produced in the pancreas and circulates to virtually every tissue in the human body. It is taken into cells through an insulin receptor that sits in cell membranes. Once insulin docks with a receptor, like a lock and key, the receptor triggers enzymes inside the cell that promote growth. For this reason, overproduction of insulin has been linked to promoting the unchecked cellular growth that can lead to cancer.

The Incidence of Type 2 Diabetes Is on the Rise

The incidence of type 2 diabetes has risen sharply in recent decades. It now afflicts more than 3% of Americans, up from less than 1%

in 1958, with no sign that the rise will slow. Three percent of all pregnant women develop gestational diabetes, which can complicate pregnancy and increase the risk of later developing adult diabetes.

People of minority ethnic groups tend to get the disease earlier in life, and because they have it longer, they tend to develop complications sooner than do American whites. All together, about 25%–30% of Americans carry a gene that predisposes them to developing type 2 diabetes.

Before Evelyn Potter came to me for counseling, she had had little luck with controlling her diabetes. Her doctor had prescribed an oral medication, called a *sulfonylurea,* but it did not work, so he placed her on daily insulin injections. Insulin cannot be taken orally because it is digested in the stomach. And insulin is *not* a cure for diabetes. Even worse, too much of the hormone can foster premature heart disease, obesity, high blood pressure, and eye damage and can stimulate the growth of latent cancer cells.

I have taught all my diabetic patients how to use phytonutrient-rich foods, dietary supplements, and regular exercise (walking is excellent) to lower their blood sugar into the normal range. With this new way of eating, many diabetics become so sensitive to their body's own insulin that they can, with their doctor's permission, gradually discontinue their insulin injections or oral medications. Evelyn no longer required insulin injections or other medications after just 6 weeks of following her new diet. To this day, she remains in what apparently will be a permanent remission from her disease.

How Do You Know If You Have Diabetes?

The routine testing of urine for the presence of glucose is useless in diagnosing most cases of adult type 2 diabetes *before* it causes serious harm to the body. By the time significant amounts of glucose spill into the urine, the disease is fairly well advanced. There is about a 7-year gap between the onset of diabetes and its diagnosis. Symptoms that should prompt you to visit your doctor for a thorough check of your body's ability to handle glucose include urinary frequency, unusual thirst, blurred vision, and unexplained weight loss.

Your doctor will give you diagnostic tests that include measurements of the amount of sugar in blood after an all-night fast and, if this level is unduly high, a glucose tolerance test, which involves drinking a concentrated sugar solution after a 3-day diet high in carbohydrates and an all-night fast. Blood glucose levels are then checked periodically for 3–5 hours.

A simple and routine screening test for blood glucose can help your doctor decide if you should be tested more thoroughly. The test can be done on a drop of blood from a finger prick. The blood is taken after a fast or 2 hours after a meal. Most pharmacies now sell digital blood glucose monitors that allow you to perform this simple test at home.

OBESITY: A PRIMARY RISK FACTOR

During World War II, adult type 2 diabetes virtually disappeared because of food and gasoline shortages—testimony of the efficacy of caloric restriction and regular exercise in preventing and reversing the disease. A recent study (the Nurses' Health Study), which followed the health profiles of about 120,000 middle-aged female nurses, found that a weight loss of 11–44 pounds can reduce the risk of diabetes by 30%.

Obesity is a leading risk factor for developing type 2 diabetes, especially abdominal obesity, which often results in insulin resistance. Americans who are overweight are nearly three times more likely to develop diabetes as people of normal weight. Obesity is the most important lifestyle determinant of diabetes. The recent rise in diabetes is directly linked to the rise in obesity, a result of increasing inactivity without a compensating decrease in caloric intake.

Weight loss and regular exercise remain the cornerstone for controlling blood sugar adequately, but phytofoods and certain vitamins and minerals may be required to bring blood sugar into the normal range.

DIABETES: A DISEASE THAT GETS ON YOUR NERVES

From 10% to 15% of all diabetic patients develop painful nerve disorders, called neuropathies, usually after having the disease for many years. "Early on, neuropathy can cause excruciating pain," notes Douglas Ishii, Ph.D., a biochemist at Colorado State University who studies nerve growth factors, natural substances that nourish and maintain nerves in the brain, spinal cord, skin and muscle.

"People [with diabetes] can't stand the weight of a bedsheet on their bodies. In time, the nervous system is lost. People can no longer feel things. They step on objects and get wounds that don't heal," notes Ishii. In 1996, over 50,000 amputations of feet or parts of feet were performed on diabetics. Thousands of others suffered bladder problems, sexual dysfunction, and abdominal complaints, all stemming from diabetic neuropathy.

Metabolic abnormalities and demyelination in nerves (loss of insulating material that surrounds most nerves) of diabetic patients may be due to the direct exposure of nerve tissue or nearby blood vessels to high concentrations of glucose. Glucose and fat undergo auto-oxidation in diabetic patients, forming free radicals that damage nerves and blood vessels. Powerful hormonelike chemicals, made by the body in response to a high-fat, high-sugar diet, can also cause inflammation and damage to these tissues.

Nutrients That Fight Diabetes

You can beat diabetes, with your doctor's help, by using the *Permanent Remissions* Plan. In addition, there are several nutrients that can make you body more sensitive to its own insulin. You must work with your doctor to do this, because you will need to regularly monitor your blood sugar levels and adjust the dosage of any medication you might be taking.

Even though the nutrients in the list below have been used in clinical studies with relative safety and efficacy, only your doctor can properly monitor your response to these supplements and adjust your medication according to ever-changing needs. *Use these dietary supplements only with your doctor's approval and supervision.*

ALPHA-LIPOIC ACID

Alpha-lipoic acid (ALA) is a multifunctional compound made by the body that helps control carbohydrate and fat metabolism. It prevents destruction of insulin-producing cells in the pancreas that leads to type 1 diabetes, enhances glucose uptake in type 2 diabetes, prevents toxic sugar-protein reactions, helps maintain normal intracellular levels of vitamin C, and slows the diabetic development of nerve and retina damage while preventing cataracts. These beneficial effects will not normally be apparent until weeks to months of treatment. ALA has been used with success in Germany to control diabetic neuropathy. ALA improves nerve blood flow, reduces oxidative stress, and improves distal nerve conduction in experimental diabetic neuropathy. Clinical studies have used daily doses between 300 and 600 mg. A 1995 German study of 13 diabetic patients was the first clinical study to demonstrate ALA's effectiveness at clearing glucose from the blood and to show that ALA increases insulin-stimulated glucose disposal in type 2 diabetes. ALA is also a therapeutic metal-chelating antioxidant.

ACETYL-L-CARNITINE

Acetyl-L-carnitine (ALC) is a compound based on the body's own fat transport molecule, L-carnitine. ALC is sold as a dietary supplement. It has been used in clinical studies in the United States and Europe (dosage: 1,000–3,000 milligrams each day) with success to prevent and mitigate the effects of diabetic neuropathy, neuromuscular disorders, and cardiovascular disease. Diabetes disrupts normal fat metabolism, but ALC helps restore it to normal, especially in the heart, retina, and nerves in the hands and feet.

CARNOSINE

Carnosine is an antioxidant found in muscle tissue that can help protect damage to the body's vital protein-containing tissues in diabetes. Carnosine blocks blood sugar from oxidizing and combining with the body's proteins while it protects fats from oxidizing and causing cellular damage. Carnosine has also been used to protect against radiation damage and may be useful in those people undergoing radiotherapy for cancer. At present, carnosine supplements are not widely available; however, dietary supplement manufacturers may begin to formulate products containing carnosine in the near future because of its many suspected health benefits. At present, only one product marketed in the United States (MaxiLIFE Phytonutrient Cocktail, manufactured by Twin Laboratories) contains a clinically useful dose of carnosine.

CHROMIUM PICOLINATE

Chromium picolinate is a form of the mineral chromium that has been reported to increase the sensitivity of tissues to insulin. The observed moderate reductions in serum glucose achieved with 200 micrograms per day of chromium picolinate imply an effect on insulin receptors. Diabetes leads to changes in the brain typically seen in normal aging. Conversely, promoting brain insulin activity with chromium picolinate may help to maintain the brain in a more functionally youthful state. The pineal gland (which helps control wake–sleep cycles through the release of the hormone melatonin) and thymus (involved in regulating the immune system) are dependent on insulin activity, and chromium may aid their function as well.

L-GLUTATHIONE

L-glutathione is an antioxidant that can protect cells against free-radical damage caused by high blood sugar levels. L-glutathione can be manufactured in small amounts in the body from amino acids. A typical supplementary dose of L-gluthathione is 500 milligrams.

L-GLUTAMINE

L-glutamine is an amino acid that has been shown to be effective in preventing diabetes in laboratory animals. Duke University researchers found that L-glutamine, which increases the body's stores of the antioxidant glutathione, protected laboratory animals from experimentally induced diabetes. When they added L-glutamine to the diets of diabetic mice in a follow-up study, the diabetes disappeared altogether. L-glutamine also protected the mice from becoming obese. A typical supplementary dose of L-glutamine is 500 milligrams.

N-ACETYL-CYSTEINE

N-acetyl-cysteine (NAC) is an antioxidant that protects vital organs from free-radical damage resulting from elevated blood glucose levels. NAC is effective at raising the level of L-glutathione in the body, another powerful antioxidant. A typical dose of NAC is 500 milligrams.

VITAMIN B$_6$

Vitamin B$_6$ deficiency may contribute to diabetic retinopathy. A 1991 study of 18 patients with diabetes mellitus, some of whom had retinopathy, were treated with steroids and vitamin B$_6$. Investigators followed these people for periods of 8 months to 28 years. The investigators found a total absence of retinopathy in vitamin B_6–treated diabetic patients over the study period. Since many B vitamins work in tandem, use a B-complex vitamin supplement. Vitamin B_6 can be toxic in large doses. *Never supplement your diet with a single B vitamin unless advised to do so by a physician.*

VANADYL SULFATE

Studies have shown that vanadyl sulfate and bis (maltolato) oxovanadium (BMOV), a trace mineral, promote sugar metabolism that helps lower blood glucose levels. Vanadyl sulfate and BMOV may activate insulin receptors and reduce the amount of fatty acids carried in the blood (triglycerides). Small oral doses of vanadyl sulfate and BMOV do not alter insulin sensitivity in nondiabetic people, but it does improve insulin sensitivity in liver and muscle cells in people with type 2 diabetes. Two recent studies showed that after just 3–4 weeks of treatment with vanadyl sulfate (50 milligrams twice daily), people with insulin-resistant type 2 diabetes experienced improved insulin sensitivity. Vanadyl sulfate at the dose used was well tolerated and resulted in modest reductions of fasting plasma glucose. More research is needed to determine the usefulness of this mineral in controlling carbohydrate metabolism and insulin sensitivity.

VITAMIN C

Human beings, and perhaps other species requiring vitamin C, need insulin for the transportation of the vitamin into the cells of certain tissues. The impairment of insulin function that occurs with diabetes disrupts the transportation of vitamin C into cells. Certain insulin-sensitive tissues, lacking vitamin C, tend to develop a type of scurvy that leads to the formation of faulty connective tissue, fragile blood-vessel walls, hemorrhage, and thickening of cell blood-vessel basement membranes. Vitamin C and glucose share the same transportation mechanism. If elevated blood sugar levels disrupt the transportation of vitamin C into cells, this may lead to nerve damage. Supplementary vitamin C may help overcome this effect of high blood sugar levels. Experimental dosages of vitamin C usually range between 200 and 2,000 milligrams.

VITAMIN D₃

Vitamin D_3 is a hormonelike vitamin essential for insulin secretion. It also lowers fasting blood glucose concentrations and serum triglycerides and controls the absorption of calcium from the gastrointestinal tract. Daily intakes of vitamin D_3 should not exceed 400 international units (unless advised otherwise by your physician), because of potential toxicity.

VITAMIN E (NATURAL FORM)

In its natural form, vitamin E is a fat-soluble antioxidant that improves the body's sensitivity to insulin. Natural vitamin E contains a complex of disease-fighting isomers not found in synthetic vitamin E. Clinical studies typically use 400 international units per day.

WHAT ABOUT DHEA?

The adrenal-gland hormone dihydroepiandrosterone (DHEA) is currently sold as a nonprescription dietary supplement in the United States and has been shown to improve insulin sensitivity and reduce blood glucose levels. The ratio of DHEA to testosterone in the body is an important regulator of insulin sensitivity and glucose tolerance.

At this time, the safety and efficacy of long-term use of the hormone remains unknown. DHEA, if improperly used, can cause unwanted side effects, such as facial hair growth in women, and may accelerate the growth of preexisting cancer. If you decide to use DHEA, I strongly advise you to use it only with your doctor's permission and under his or her strict medical supervision.

Sugar in Your Foods

Carbohydrate foods are broken down in the digestive tract and absorbed into the blood as glucose. Insulin is released by the pancreas in response to carbohydrate and protein in foods, facilitating the entry of glucose into cells. Glucose, a simple carbohydrate, rapidly increases blood glucose levels. Complex carbohydrates, such as found in vegetables, oatmeal, brown rice, and legumes, are digested more slowly and provide a more constant supply of glucose into the blood.

Scientists have measured the blood glucose–raising effects of a number of individual foods and rated them in what is known as the glycemic index (Table 7.1). This index indicates the speed at which carbohydrates are digested and release their glucose into the blood.

TABLE 7.1

Glycemic Index Values*

Food	Mean Value	Food	Mean Value
Breads		**Fruit (continued)**	
Rye (crispbread)	95	Orange juice	71
Rye (whole grain; i.e.,		Raisins	93
pumpernickel)	68	Yam	74
Wheat (white)	100		
Wheat (whole grain)	100	**Legumes**	
		Baked beans (canned)	70
Breakfast cereals		Butter beans	46
All Bran	74	Chickpeas (canned)	60
Cornflakes	121	Green peas (canned)	50
Muesli	96	Garden peas (frozen)	65
Oatmeal	89	Kidney beans (canned)	74
Puffed rice	132	Kidney beans (dried)	43
Puffed wheat	110		
Shredded wheat	97	**Lentils**	
		Lentils (green, canned)	74
Cereal grains		Lentils (green, dried)	36
Barley (pearled)	36	Lentils (red, dried)	38
Buckwheat	78	Pinto beans (canned)	64
Bulgur	65	Pinto beans (dried)	60
Millet	103	Peanuts	15
Rice (brown)	81	Soybeans (canned)	22
Rice (instant, boiled 1 minute)	65	Soybeans (dried)	20
Rice (polished, boiled 10–25			
minutes)	81	**Pasta**	
Rice (parboiled, boiled		Macaroni (white, boiled	
5 minutes)	54	5 minutes)	64
Rye kernels	47	Spaghetti (white, boiled	
Sweet corn	80	15 minutes)	67
Cookies		**Root vegetables**	
Oatmeal	78	Potato (instant)	120
Shortbread cookies	88	Potato (mashed)	98
		Potato (russet, baked)	116
Dairy products		Potato (sweet)	70
Ice cream	69		
Skim milk	46	**Snack foods**	
Whole milk	44	Corn chips	99
Yogurt	52	Potato chips	77
Fruit		**Sugars**	
Apple	52	Fructose	26
Apple juice	45	Glucose	138
Banana	84	Honey	126
Orange	59	Lactose	57
		Sucrose	83

*All foods listed are compared to the glycemic index of white bread, which has been arbitrarily set at 100 for comparison purposes.

One way to slow down the release of glucose from consuming foods high on the glycemic index is to consume them with more slowly digested foods such as soy foods, legumes, whole fruits, and vegetables.

This list of commonly eaten foods reveals some surprises: a baked potato, eaten alone and without topping, actually raises blood sugar more than a Snickers candy bar (the fat in the candy bar slows down sugar absorption from the stomach). A plain baked potato raises blood sugar because it contains almost no fat to delay sugar release into the blood. Fructose (fruit sugar) is five times less powerful at raising blood sugar than glucose, a sugar added to many processed beverages and foods. One caution about fructose: this sugar stimulates fat synthesis in the body, even in someone with diabetes, because the enzyme fructokinase, which catalyzes the first step in fructose metabolism, is not regulated by diet or hormones.

The glycemic index of foods is useful for gauging the rise in blood sugar after consuming foods individually on a relatively empty stomach. The glycemic potential of these foods is drastically reduced when they are consumed as part of a mixed meal.

Weight Loss and Fat Intake

Weight reduction improves the body's ability to handle blood sugar because it helps sensitize muscle cells to sugar-lowering actions of insulin. Studies have shown that people who eat a phytonutrient-based diet enjoy lower morbidity and mortality from type 2 diabetes in part because they are not as fat as compared to people who eat an animal protein-based diet.

Regular aerobic exercise, such as brisk walking, increases the body's sensitivity to insulin and increases the burning of sugar by muscle tissue. One study has shown that men considered to be at high risk of developing type 2 diabetes who engaged in intense exercise of moderate duration reduced their risk of the disease by well over 80% compared to men who did not exercise. Aerobic exercise should be carried out only in diabetics with good metabolic control of blood glucose, which means that they are able to keep their blood sugar to near normal levels. *Always consult with your physician before beginning an exercise program.*

Minority Groups and Diabetes Risk

Diabetes mellitus is more prevalent in American blacks than in American whites. The incidence of the disease is steadily increasing in blacks, and there is evidence that it is accompanied by a greater severity of diabetic complications. In addition, death rates are higher in blacks, and black women are more seriously affected than black men. Reasons for these differences include obesity, socioeconomic status, and genetics.

Obesity is a growing problem among American blacks, particularly in women. Both the amount and the distribution of fat contribute to the high rate of diabetes in blacks. Although the prevalence of obesity is higher in the poor economic groups, poverty cannot explain all of the excess obesity that occurs in U.S. blacks. Recent studies have shown that on average, American black women burn about 100 calories less each day than American white women. That can translate into a 10-pound weight gain over the period of just 1 year. More research is needed into a possible genetic predisposition of blacks to obesity and diabetes on the ordinary American diet and into the interrelationship between the two conditions.

Diabetes increases the chance of dying from heart disease by nine to 10 times for women but by only two to three times for men. American black women run a much higher risk of dying from diabetes-induced heart disease than white women (blacks, 39%; whites, 27%); American black men run a higher risk than American white males (blacks, 19%; whites, 14%).

Numerous studies have shown that the occurrence of insulin resistance in black men is related to *where* they tended to store body fat rather than if they were obese. Researchers have found that it is the proportion of fat stored in the abdominal area that determines diabetes risk and severity—the so-called apple body type. Studies with black men have shown that blood sugar levels and diabetes risk seem to be unrelated to the amount of total muscle tissue or total body fat.

American blacks suffer diabetic retinopathy, a leading cause of blindness, earlier than do other minority groups. One study found that American blacks are diagnosed with retinopathy 5 years earlier than are American Hispanics (58 years versus 53 years, respectively). The high percentage of patients in both groups with severe diabetic retinopathy at the time of initial diagnosis suggests that earlier patient referral from primary-care physicians and better patient education about the need for earlier eye examinations should be encouraged in these two groups.

Experimental Diabetic Diet and Protocol

DIET

The experimental protocol in Table 7.2 contains the phytonutrient-rich foods and nutrients that hold promise for being effective against type 2 diabetes mellitus. Supplementary nutrients should be used only with the permission of and under the supervision of a physician. Table 7.3 is a 3-day eating plan to use as a guide for constructing meals based on the experimental diabetic protocol. *Permanent Remissions* recipes are indicated in bold print.

EXERCISE

Regular exercise can also play an important role in normalizing blood sugar levels by making the body more sensitive to its own insulin. Your goal should be to burn 1,500 calories a week through regular aerobic exercise, such as walking. If you do not currently exercise, obtain your doctor's permission and begin slowly, working up to a 45-minute walk at least 5 days each week.

Diabetics' Food Exchange Guide

Diabetics who use exchange lists to help control blood glucose levels may use the following list for determining portion sizes. Each serving can be exchanged for another within the same group. One serving of any food on the list can be exchanged for one serving of any other food in the same group. Each food provides about the same calorie count and the same number of carbohydrate, protein, and fat grams as other foods within the same group:

Proteins (legumes, seafood): about 200 calories per serving
- 4 ounces soy ground "beef"
- 1 cup beans

- 1 ½ cup peas
- 1 cup lentils
- 5 ounces salmon
- 7 ounces lobster
- 2 ½ cups nonfat soy milk
- 5 ounces tuna

Starches (cereals, grains, and breads): about 80 calories per serving
- ½ cup cooked corn
- ½ cup cooked pasta
- ½ cup shredded wheat
- ¼ cup yam
- ¼ cup sweet potato
- ⅓ cup cooked brown rice
- 1 slice whole wheat bread
- 1 small baked potato

Fruits: about 60 calories per serving
- ½ medium red grapefruit
- 1 cup berries
- ½ cup fresh fruit salad
- 1 cup melon
- ½ small banana
- 1 medium apple, orange, peach, or pear
- ½ cup fruit juice
- 2 tangerines

Vegetables: about 25 calories per serving
- ½ cup cooked vegetables
- ½ cup vegetable juice
- 1 cup raw vegetables

TABLE 7.2

Experimental Diabetes Protocol*

Take These Vitamins and Minerals

- Vitamin A complex (5,000 international units vitamin A; 1 milligram alpha-carotene; 5 milligrams lycopene; 6 milligrams lutein; 0.3 milligram zeaxanthin)
- Vitamin B complex (high-potency formula)[†]
- Vitamin C (1,000 milligrams)
- Vitamin D₃ (400 international units)
- Vitamin E complex (natural isomers: 400 international units)
- Calcium (500 milligrams)
- Chromium picolinate (200 micrograms)
- Magnesium (250 milligrams)
- Selenomax (200 micrograms)[§]
- Vanadium (5 milligrams)
- Zinc gluconate (30 milligrams)

Take These Nutrients

- Alpha-lipoic acid (100 milligrams)
- Acetyl-L-carnitine (500 milligrams)
- Carnosine (500 milligrams)[‡]
- Coenzyme Q₁₀ (50 milligrams)
- Choline (1,500 milligrams)
- Gingko biloba (60 milligrams)
- L-carnitine (500 milligrams)
- L-glutamine (500 milligrams)
- L-glutathione (250 milligrams)
- N-acetylcysteine (500 milligrams)
- L-taurine (500 milligrams)

Note: A number of products, such as soy cocktails, phytonutrient cocktails, and choline cocktails contain most or all of the nutrients listed in this table.

*This experimental diabetes protocol may augment the blood glucose–lowering effects of oral hypoglycemic medications, including sulfonylureas and injectable insulin.

†Use any brand of high potency B-complex vitamin such as those made by Twinlab, GNC, or Solgar.

‡Carnosine can be found in MaxiLIFE Phytonutrient Cocktail (Twin Laboratories).

§Selenomax is the trade name for the organic form of selenium manufactured and licensed by Nutrition 21.

TABLE 7.3

Three-Day Sample Diabetic Diet

MEAL	DAY 1	DAY 2	DAY 3
Breakfast	• **Biscuits 'n' Sausage** • ¾ cup oatmeal with ½ banana • 4 ounces apple juice	• **Pigs in the Blanket** • 1 cup soy milk (such as White Wave Silk Soy Beverage)	• **Buttermilk Pancakes with Banana** • 1 cup soy milk • 4 ounces apple juice
Midmorning snacks	• ½ grapefruit	• Apple	• ½ grapefruit
Lunch	• **Hearty Lasagna** • **Spinach Salad with Warm "Bacon" Dressing** • 1 large wedge of watermelon	• **Shrimp Wrapped in "Bacon"** • **Southwestern Corn Chowder** • Apple	• Green Giant Harvest Burger on whole-grain bun, with lettuce, tomato, and ketchup • ½ cup **Cajun Coleslaw** • **Tomato Rice Soup**
Midafternoon snacks	• **Super Soy Shake**	• **Super Soy Shake**	• **Super Soy Shake**
Dinners	• **Horseradish-Encrusted Salmon** • ½ cup steamed broccoli with lemon juice • Mixed green salad with olive-oil-and-vinegar dressing • ½ grapefruit	• **"Meatball" Oven Grinder Sub** • ½ cup brown rice	• **Lobster Malabar** • ½ honeydew melon
Evening snacks	• **Fruit Yogurt Crunch**	• **Strawberries and "Cream"**	• Ambrosia

See pages 227–338 for *Permanent Remissions* recipes listed in this table (boldfaced items).

8

BEATING
CARDIOVASCULAR DISEASE

It just doesn't make sense.

Any cardiologist worth his or her salt (substitute) will tell you that the Masai of Kenya and Tanzania eat *all wrong*. The African herders consume enough meat and milk to give every man, woman, and child in the tribe a massive heart attack. Make that two massive heart attacks. Yet the Masai, whose cholesterol levels are a third lower than the U.S. average, enjoy much lower rates of heart disease than do Americans.

Ah, you say, these lactocarnivores must be genetically endowed with a cast-iron constitution. Such is not the case. Other groups with very low rates of heart disease, such as the Japanese and Chinese, lose any putative "genetic" protection when they migrate to the United States. Once they abandon their traditional cuisine in favor of Big Macs, Whoppers, Dunkin' Donuts, and Ben & Jerry's, their disease rates soar, approaching our own. Who can blame them? No one ever claimed that tofu and rice packs the palate-pleasing power of Häagen-Dazs mint chocolate chip ice cream.

So how on earth do the Masai gorge on cholesterol-laden fare yet remain so heart healthy?

The Masai consume a soup laced with powerful disease-bashing phytonutrients. The soup is made from a bitter bark and roots rich in *saponins*—the same type of compounds found in soy foods and other legumes and vegetables that confer disease protection on native Japanese and Chinese who eat them daily. If you're still not convinced, consider this: Masai who do not consume the soup develop heart disease.

Please don't get the idea that you can live off the fat of the land like the Masai just by washing down a 16-ounce filet mignon with a cup of herbal soup. It's not *that* simple. There are other factors involved. The Masai lead a radically different lifestyle than most Americans. They get much more exercise, often walking 25 miles a day as they tend their herds. The meat they eat has a healthier fat profile than American beef. And they eat far less sugar and trans fatty acids (TFA)—cholesterol-raising fats found in margarines, processed foods, and fast-food french fries—than we do.

The important lesson to be learned from the Masai and other cultures who enjoy even lower rates of heart disease is that phytonutrients play a key role in helping to prevent or forestall the appearance of heart disease and other serious health problems. The Masai diet is not a healthy diet, but the phytonutrients they eat and the exercise they get each day do provide a degree of protection against heart disease. And that's the important message about the Masai.

Fad weight-loss diets that promote a high intake of protein from animal foods contradict the latest scientific knowledge on disease prevention and treatment. Such diets are clearly linked to cancer, cardiovascular disease, and osteoporosis and are the polar opposite of the *Permanent Remissions* Plan. Phytonutrient-rich foods, not animal protein, are the key to life extension and a healthy heart.

The Doctor Is In

Twenty-one years ago, Jaswant Singh Pannu, M.D., felt a shortness of breath during exercise. He didn't think much about it because after all, he had just played a hard game of tennis. He took a few deep breaths, but the shortness of breath was still there. He began to sweat profusely—but it was a cold sweat. And even though all the doors in his house were open and a cool breeze was blowing, it seemed very stuffy in the room.

On that Thanksgiving afternoon in 1976, Dr. Pannu suffered a heart attack. "Until that day, I was a practicing physician, working in Fort Lauderdale, enjoying perfect health for a man of 42, exercising regularly and showing no signs of any serious physical problems.

"The doctor read my ECG and told me that I had suffered a heart attack. I opted for coronary bypass surgery at the Miami Heart Institute. I read the statistics on bypass operations and knew that I might die on the operating table. I also knew that there was a good chance the bypass would close up within the first year."

Dr. Pannu recalls craving a fast-food hamburger following his surgery. He distinctly remembers the hospital food as "unappetizing." That started him thinking, for the first time, about his diet. As a confessed junk-food junkie, Dr. Pannu instinctively knew he would probably have a hard time giving up his favorite fast foods. But he also knew that if he wanted to beat the odds, he'd have to make a few adjustments in his diet.

"After my surgery, my doctor's job was done. But what I needed was to make sure it didn't happen again. And most doctors know next to nothing about nutrition."

On the day he came to my clinic—his newly replaced coronary arteries stitched firmly in place—Dr. Pannu's blood cholesterol level was 328 milligrams per deciliter. With that much cholesterol in his blood, he would have surely had another heart attack with 1 or 2 years. Within 4 weeks, I was able to reduce Dr. Pannu's cholesterol level by 100 points.

"In my own heart, I believe that diet is the one cause of heart disease that can be controlled. You can't do too much about heredity," Dr. Pannu observes. "I've always wanted healthy food that tastes like fast-food hamburgers, hot dogs, and the like. Now, with the new soy products on the market, I can enjoy 'hamburgers' and 'fried chicken' to my heart's content. Soy meat substitutes that are appetizing to children and adults are as important as proper nutritional education. But diet education alone isn't going to help children learn to eat properly. Children must have foods that taste good because the child does not see that what he eats today may affect him 40 years later."

Since Dr. Pannu began following my dietary recommendations (see Table 8-11, Experimental Atherosclerosis Reversal Protocol, page 200), he says his wife, Debbie, has also been following the plan (Table 8.1). It is the dieter who has to diet alone who runs into problems, he says.

"Diets cannot be followed alone. That's the reason why most people go off their healthy diets. It helps tremendously to have your spouse or boyfriend or girlfriend or children to also go on the diet," Pannu observes. "Perhaps I would not have been successful were it not for my wife's help."

Today, Dr. Pannu has no evidence of heart disease. At age 63, he

---

TABLE 8.1

Dr. Pannu's Diet Guidelines

Carbohydrates (2–4 servings per day)
  Oatmeal (¾ cup cooked)
  Brown rice (1 cup cooked)
  Whole-grain breads (1 slice)

Vegetables (3–5 servings per day)
  Tomatoes (½ cup sauce, 1 whole)
  Carrots (½ cup cooked, 1 cup raw)
  Baked potato (1 medium)
  Broccoli (½ cup cooked; 1 cup raw)
  Corn (½ cup)
  Cabbage (½ cup)
  Carrots (½ cup)
  Tomato- and vegetable-based soups
  (1 cup)

Dairy (1 serving per day)
  Low-fat yogurt (1 cup)
  Skim milk (1 cup)

Garlic and Onions (1 serving per day)
  1 garlic/onion supplement capsule
  4 tablespoons chopped onion
  2 cloves garlic

Fruit (2–3 servings per day)
  Apples (1 medium)
  Oranges (1 medium)
  Grapefruit (½ medium)
  Bananas (1 medium)
  Kiwi (½ cup)
  Watermelon (1 medium slice)
  Papaya (½ medium)

Legumes (1 serving per day)
  Lentils
  Beans
  Peas

Seafood (1–2 servings per week)
  Salmon (4 ounces)
  Tuna (7 ounces)
  Shrimp (3 ounces)

Friendly fats (1–2 servings per day)
  Olive oil for cooking (up to 2 teaspoons each day)

---

still enjoys competitive tennis and leads a full and active life. Since his heart attack 21 years ago, Dr. Pannu has pioneered new surgical techniques and devices for use in ophthalmology, established the Pannu Eye Institute in Fort Lauderdale, Florida, and continues to travel throughout the United States and to India, lecturing on the power of dietary change to prevent and reverse heart disease.

Why Cholesterol Matters

In 1983, 1 year before my book, *Eat to Win,* was published, only 3% of Americans knew their blood cholesterol number. Most had no

♦

idea which foods contained cholesterol, how much cholesterol was in those foods, or what cholesterol did in the body.

When *Eat to Win* became the number-one best-selling hardcover self-help book of 1984 and the number-one best-selling softcover in 1985, millions of Americans learned about the importance of knowing their cholesterol and reducing it to safe levels. Following my advice, they began to visit their doctors in record numbers to learn their cholesterol number. Since then, America has become the most cholesterol-conscious nation in the world. Statistics show that:

- Some 70 million to 80 million American adults who in 1983 were unaware of their cholesterol level have now learned their blood cholesterol numbers.
- Forty-nine percent actually know their own cholesterol level, up from 37% in 1990 and 3% in 1983.
- Twenty-two percent of people overall have been told by their doctors that their cholesterol level is too high.
- Sixty-nine percent have read or heard that a desirable cholesterol level is below 200 (a safe cholesterol number is actually below 160).
- Ninety percent of doctors know their own cholesterol number and 67% say they've made dietary changes to lower it.

Cholesterol is an essential element of all the cells in our body, especially in the brain, nerves, and spinal cord. The body makes sex hormones from cholesterol and cholesterol provides a layer of protection in the skin to prevent the loss of water and the absorption of toxic substances. But too much cholesterol can cause serious health problems (Table 8.2). Here's why:

Shortly after a typical meal, cholesterol levels begin to rise in the blood, carried in waterproof packets called *lipoproteins* (the most well-known lipoproteins are low-density lipoproteins [LDL] and high-density lipoproteins [HDL]). Because of its contribution to the formation of arterial plaque, LDL-cholesterol is often called "bad" cholesterol. But LDL isn't bad at all; in fact, it is necessary for life because it transports essential fats and vitamins to all cells. As you will discover, there is nothing inherently harmful about LDL-cholesterol unless it is overwhelmed by free radicals. LDL-cholesterol becomes harmful when the blood does not contain enough antioxidant vitamins and phytonutrients. The HDL lipoprotein is often called "good" cholesterol because it transports excess cholesterol from the artery wall back to the liver for disposal, thus helping to prevent the formation of plaque.

TABLE 8.2

Key Risk Factors for Heart Attack and Stroke

- Low phytofood intake
- High animal-protein/saturated-fat diet
- High blood pressure
- Elevated low-density lipoprotein (LDL) levels
- Decreased high-density lipoprotein (HDL) levels
- Elevated triglyceride (blood fat) levels
- Obesity
- Family history of premature heart attack before the age of 55
- Personal history of heart disease
- Cigarette smoking
- Simultaneous use of oral contraceptives and cigarette smoking
- Being male
- Presence of diabetes mellitus

Antioxidants in the blood (such as vitamin E, vitamin C, lycopene, and other carotenoids) rush to defend LDL-cholesterol against the attack of oxygen and other chemical compounds that can convert it into a toxic form that damages the artery wall. Then, and only then, can LDL-cholesterol be properly called "bad" or harmful.

Perhaps now you understand why it is vital that you consume phytonutrient-rich foods—which are chock full of heart-friendly anti-oxidants—*with each meal.* When you "package" dietary antioxidants with cholesterol and other volatile compounds (including most polyunsaturated vegetable oils) in the LDL carrier molecule, you minimize the level of oxidized cholesterol—the form that damages cell membranes and artery linings—in the blood. Most cardiologists remain unaware of the importance of consuming phytonutrients and antioxidant dietary supplements with every meal.

If the blood contains a sufficient amount of antioxidants and a low level of LDL-cholesterol, a healthy balance is struck and very little toxic cholesterol is formed and arteries remain clean and healthy. Trouble comes when an imbalance occurs and some cholesterol is converted to its artery-damaging oxidized form. Years of chronic damage help establish a tumorlike plaque—a kind of "cancer" of the arterial wall—that can lead to heart attack and stroke.

How much cholesterol do we need to eat each day? *The body requires not a single molecule of cholesterol from foods.* There is controversy over how much dietary cholesterol growing children should eat.* Our liver manufactures all the cholesterol we need–about 1,000 milligrams each day (1000 milligrams = 1 gram). On average, Americans consume about 300 milligrams of cholesterol each day, but many consume in excess of 500 milligrams daily. Our metabolic machinery can safely dispose of perhaps an additional 100 milligrams of cholesterol from the diet each day, beyond what the liver makes, but no more than that. Even a dietary intake of 200 milligrams of cholesterol each day is enough to give many Americans a head start toward heart disease. The American Heart Association (AHA) recommends that you limit your average daily cholesterol intake to less than 300 milligrams. My research shows that this is clearly a far too generous recommendation for optimal protection against heart disease (Table 8.3).

Why Fat Matters

So now we know that the body can safely handle about 1 gram of cholesterol each day made by the liver and that dietary cholesterol in excess of 100 milligrams a day can overwhelm the body. But what about fat? Everyone knows that's bad for your heart, right?

Well, yes and no. Saturated fats found predominantly in foods of animal origin (which are, coincidentally, the only foods in which you'll find cholesterol) raise the body's production of cholesterol. The less you eat, the healthier you'll be. Vegetable oils, with one or two exceptions, can also pose a health risk if overconsumed. Vegetable oils, with the exception of olive oil, can turn on the body's manufacturing system for hormonelike chemicals that promote tumor growth and insulin resistance that leads to type 2 diabetes.

Here is an overview of the ordinary fats and oils found in the American diet and what they do.

POLYUNSATURATED VEGETABLE OILS

Polyunsaturated vegetable oils derived from safflower seeds, peanuts, sesame seeds, and corn, for example, contain unsaturated fatty acids, which can oxidize and help convert cholesterol and fats in cell

---

*Some health experts suspect that a child's nervous system requires a small amount of dietary cholesterol each day to develop properly, but this suspicion remains unproven at present.

TABLE 8.3

Cholesterol Content of Selected Foods

Cholesterol (Milligrams)	Amounts	Foods
482	3.50 ounces	Beef liver, pan-fried
166	3.00 ounces	Steamed shrimp
121	3.50 ounces	Pork spareribs, broiled
105	3.80 ounces	Fried chicken leg with skin
99	3.50 ounces	Ground beef, extra lean, broiled
98	3.50 ounces	Pork, center loin, broiled
96	3.00 ounces	KFC Original Recipe chicken breast
93	3.00 ounces	Steamed oysters
89	3.50 ounces	Turkey, dark meat with skin, roasted
88	3.50 ounces	Chicken, broiler/fryer, w/skin, roasted
83	6.80 ounces	McDonald's Big Mac
76	3.50 ounces	Turkey, light meat with skin, roasted
65	3.00 ounces	Spanish mackerel, raw
63	3.00 ounces	Pacific halibut, broiled
62	3.50 ounces	Ham, cured, canned, roasted
61	3.00 ounces	Lobster, northern, steamed
58	3.00 ounces	Freshwater bass, broiled
57	3.00 ounces	Steamed clams
56	3.00 ounces	Chinook salmon, broiled
35	3.00 ounces	Tuna, white meat, canned in spring water
35	1 cup	Milk, whole, 3.7% fat
33	3.00 ounces	Swordfish, broiled
27	1.00 ounces	American cheese, processed
19	1.00 ounces	Parmesan cheese, hard
18	1 cup	Milk, low-fat (2% fat)
16	1.00 ounces	Mozzarella cheese, part skim
10	1 cup	Milk, low-fat (1% fat)
4	1 cup	Milk, skim

membranes into toxic substances. These oils have also been linked to increased risk of cancer, gallbladder disease, and obesity. So just as with saturated fats, less of these oils is better for everyone.

MONOUNSATURATED OILS

Monounsaturated oils, particularly olive oil, don't seem to cause heart disease or cancer. In fact, several studies suggest that olive oil, when used in place of other added fats and oils in the diet, may actually lower the risk of some types of cancer. This research is still preliminary but is encouraging nonetheless. Olive oil contains over twice the calories of proteins and carbohydrates, so you should limit your intake of this friendly fat to no more than 2 teaspoons each day. The resistance of the fatty acids in olive oil to oxidation may be one important reason why a Mediterranean-type diet, which uses monounsaturated olive oil in place of other vegetable oils, confers protection against heart disease on those who embrace it.

MARINE OILS

Marine oils, as found in such fish as salmon, mackerel, tuna, sardines, and menhaden, contain omega-3 fatty acids (the fatty acids found in vegetable oils are called omega-6). Omega 3 is unique in that it tends to lower serum cholesterol and make the blood less sticky, which helps reduce the risk of developing blood clots that can cause heart attacks and strokes. Omega-3–Rich seafood is permitted on the *Permanent Remissions* Plan, but you should limit your consumption to a 4-ounce portion no more than twice each week. Those who do not care for these fish can use a small amount of flaxseed (about 1–2 tablespoons), which can be ground in a battery-powered coffee grinder and sprinkled on salads or used in recipes (such as the hummus recipe on page 240). Flaxseed is not as beneficial as fish oils, but it is an alternative, cholesterol-free source of omega-3 fatty acids.

There are other types of fats, called *triglycerides,* found in your blood. These fatty molecules (three fatty acids linked to a three-carbon backbone) are manufactured in the intestine and liver in response to the amount of fat, sugar, and alcohol in the diet. Many health experts believe that high levels of triglycerides increase the risk of getting coronary heart disease.

The type of fat you eat each day influences the amount of choles-

terol converted to oxysterols, a toxic form of cholesterol that accumulates in arteries (Table 8.4). The most abundant fatty acid in the LDL-
cholesterol complex is linoleic acid (found in vegetable oils). LDL molecules enriched in linoleic acid are increasingly susceptible to oxidation.
These oxidized vegetable oils (but not olive oil) can lead to the formation of the oxysterols *25-hydroxycholesterol* and *26-hydroxycholesterol*.
Such toxic forms of cholesterol damage smooth muscle cells in the arterial wall, leading to the formation of a tumorlike growth that forms
artery-clogging plaque.

Why Protein Matters

Want to get into the zone of optimal cardiovascular health? Then
get out of the high-protein zone, quickly.

The myth of high-protein eating for health and weight loss resur-
faces every decade or so in diet books, none of which have ever been
written by an author with a graduate degree in nutrition. And it shows.

What's wrong with eating a high-protein diet? After all, didn't our
moms tell us to eat lots of protein to grow up to be big and strong?

Mom, God bless her well-meaning heart, was *wrong*.

Okay, so what's so bad about foods such as meat, eggs, milk,
cheese, and fowl?

When eaten sparingly, none of these foods poses a health risk. The

TABLE 8.4

Effect of Fats and Oils on Lipoprotein Cholesterol Levels

Type of Fat	Selected Food Sources	Effects on LDL and HDL
Saturated	Meat, milk, butter, coconut oil, palm oil	Raises LDL; lowers HDL
Monounsaturated	Olive oil and canola oil	Lowers LDL; maintains HDL
Transfatty acid	Margarine, baked goods, fast-food french fries, snack chips, potato chips, and other processed foods	Raises LDL; lowers HDL
Omega-3	Oils from salmon, mackerel, sardines, tuna, swordfish, menhaden, lobster, and flaxseed	Lowers LDL; raises HDL
Omega-6	Oils from corn, soybeans, cotton, sunflowers, sesame seeds	Decreases LDL; decreases HDL

HDL, high-density lipoprotein; LDL, low-density lipoprotein.

problem is that most Americans don't know how to do that. My research shows that the body can safely handle up to 100 grams of animal
protein each day—that's 3½ ounces for those who are metrically chal-
lenged. A 3½-ounce chicken breast, about the size of deck of playing
cards, contains about 100 milligrams of cholesterol. But most us eat far
more than that—about six to seven times more.

I'm against high-protein diets for the following reasons:

- High-protein animal foods are the only food source of cholesterol in
  the diet and are the primary source of cholesterol-raising saturated
  fats.
- Animal-protein foods contain no disease-fighting fiber.
- Animal-protein foods increase the level of *homocysteine* in blood. This
  compound is toxic to arteries and can damage them in much the same
  way that excess cholesterol does. A high-protein diet increases the
  body's requirement for the nutrients that protect arteries from homocysteine damage—vitamin B_6, vitamin B_{12}, folic acid, vitamin E, and
  vitamin C. Since high-protein animal foods usually contain a poor
  supply of these heart-healthy nutrients (except vitamin B_{12}), homocysteine in the blood increases the risk of heart attack and stroke.
- Protein from animal foods contains an amino-acid profile (individual
  amino acids bonded together form proteins) that can accelerate the
  loss of calcium and other minerals from the skeleton. Many animal-
  protein foods are relatively high in the sulfur-containing amino acids
  methionine and cysteine. Some preliminary research has linked a
  high-methionine diet to cancer in laboratory animals; several studies
  have shown that low-methionine diets may help prevent or reverse
  cancer. Other conflicting studies suggest a role for methionine in protecting against some forms of cancer. What is clear is that methionine
  is also one of the raw materials the body uses to manufacture artery-
  damaging homocysteine. That's why the *Permanent Remissions* plan
  takes most of its protein from soy products and legumes. Vegetable
  protein contains an amino-acid profile consistent with protection
  against cancer, heart disease, diabetes, and osteoporosis.

The graphs in Figure 8.1 compare 100 calories of cooked soybeans
to 100 calories of lean beef. Notice that soy contains an essential
amino-acid pattern similar to that of beef but supplies safer levels of
the amino acids MET (methionine) and CYS (cysteine). That's why
many professional bodybuilders who want to avoid the health risks associated with eating large amounts of animal protein have switched to

FIGURE 8.1

Comparison of the amino-acid profiles of soybeans and beef. Phe, phenylalanine; Tyr, tyrosine; Leu, leucine; Ile, isoleucine; Val, valine; Trp, tryptophan; Met, methionine; Cys, cysteine; Arg, arginine; His, histidine; Thr, threonine; Lys, lysine.

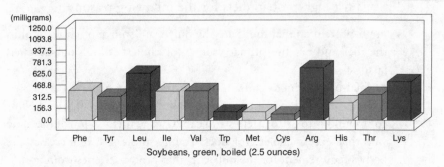

Soybeans, green, boiled (2.5 ounces)

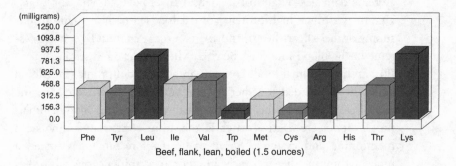

Beef, flank, lean, boiled (1.5 ounces)

soy-based foods and beverages. Twenty-first-century athletes will eat to win with soy protein, not with animal protein.

Homocysteine and Artery Damage

It's a fire you can't feel, but it burns in your arteries every day. That's the scary part of the artery-clogging disease atherosclerosis. Yet, many Americans go about their daily lives oblivious to the fact that their coronary arteries are chronically inflamed. High-protein diets, especially those that do not provide sufficient heart-healthy phytonutrients, vitamins, and minerals, help fuel this coronary conflagration.

People who eat steak, chicken, eggs, and dairy products consume large amounts of the amino acid *methionine*. When methionine is broken down by the body, it forms a compound called *homocysteine* that inflames arteries.

High levels of homocysteine in the blood do, in fact, wreak havoc on blood vessels, raising the risk of heart disease 30 times higher than in people with normal levels of the compound. About 25% of patients who have had heart attacks and 40% of stroke victims carry high levels of homocysteine in their blood. And even in people who don't have this condition, higher levels of homocysteine have been linked to greater heart disease risk.

Homocysteine levels rise when you eat a high-protein diet—even when blood levels of B vitamins such as folic acid, vitamin B_{12}, and vitamin B_6 are in the normal range. Phytofoods, such as soy foods and beverages, green leafy vegetables, and fruits, are naturally lower in methionine than animal foods and they contain a healthy supply of B vitamins that keep homocysteine levels in check. (**Note to strict vegetarians:** vitamin B_{12} is found only in animal products, fortified food products such as breakfast cereals, and vitamin supplements.)

Now, scientists are taking a hard look at homocysteine's involvement in other health problems. Cancer researchers are now wondering if homocysteine is involved in tumor growth. Scientists are also searching for links to diabetes, organ rejection, and some nerve disorders. Homocysteine may even cause problems in pregnancy. And the elderly are especially vulnerable to homocysteine damage because they often have trouble absorbing B vitamins from food.

"With regard to heart disease, high homocysteine is about as dangerous as smoking," says Killian Robinson, M.D., a cardiologist at the Cleveland Clinic. "Each confers a twofold increase in risk." And not just to arteries in the heart: homocysteine seems to damage blood vessels in the brain, too.

For years, scientists have wondered why heart disease rates rise so dramatically as people enter their golden years. Now, it seems, a deficiency of B vitamins may be part of the problem. Researchers from the U.S. Department of Agriculture (USDA) working at Tufts University took blood samples from 1,100 aging men and women in Massachusetts. The researchers found excesses of homocysteine in 29% of the volunteers over age 67 and in 40% of the patients over age 80. The higher the homocysteine readings, said the scientists, the lower the amounts of folic acid and vitamin B_6. Since the elderly may have trouble absorbing adequate vitamin B_{12}, many should take a B-complex vitamin supplement.

Homocysteine damage to arteries may also help explain why estrogen seems to protect women from heart attacks. Estrogen and estrogen-like drugs protect women from heart disease by helping the body get rid of homocysteine. Until menopause, women run a much lower risk of heart disease than men; then their risk rises steadily, even though their cholesterol levels tend to fall. "We know now that homocysteine concentrations rise around the time of menopause," says Peter Berger, M.D., a cardiologist at the Mayo Clinic.

Homocysteine may also be responsible for increasing a woman's chances of having a baby with neural-tube defects, such as spina bifida or anencephaly. Recently, James Mills, Ph.D, an epidemiologist at the National Institutes of Health (NIH) analyzed blood samples from 400 pregnant women in Ireland. Of these, 81 gave birth to babies with neural-tube defects. They had higher homocysteine and lower B_{12} levels than did the mothers of normal children. But almost none of the women actually had a B-vitamin deficiency by current standards. A number of studies have also linked neural-tube defects with a deficiency of another B vitamin, folic acid.

The *Permanent Remissions* Plan reduces blood levels of homocysteine caused by high protein consumption and protects the body against its toxic effects. To insulate yourself against the toxic effects of homocysteine and reduce the risk of heart disease, cancer, and birth defects, avoid high-protein fad diets and enter the zone of optimal health with the *Permanent Remissions* Plan.

The Cancer–Heart Disease Connection

Cancer and heart disease may be kissing cousins. One theory holds that the plaque buildup that eventually blocks the blood flow in an artery arises from a tumor in the arterial wall. The similarities between cancer-tumor initiation and promotion and smooth muscle cell tumors that eventually occlude arteries leading to the heart may explain why the identical antioxidant vitamins and phytonutrients so effective against cancer also help prevent and reverse atherosclerosis.

According to this theory, called the *monoclonal origin of atherosclerosis,* damage to artery walls is initiated by oxidized fat, cholesterol, homocysteine, and other free radicals. This damage gives rise to cellular mutations in arterial smooth muscle cells. A single mutated cell then forms a tumor, which eventually forms the arterial plaque responsible for many heart attacks and strokes.

Heart disease and cancer are linked by this process, but it does not mean they are identical. For example, scientists have found no evidence that heart disease is caused by genetic mutations of the p53 gene that helps prevent normal cells from turning cancerous.

Lowering dietary cholesterol levels has beneficial effects related not only to preventing cardiovascular disease but also to preventing cancer. Dietary cholesterol has been shown to induce pancreatic cancer in laboratory animals exposed to environmental carcinogens. A cholesterol-free diet decreased the level of free radicals in the blood of hamsters given carcinogenic chemicals. A variety of phytonutrients that lower blood cholesterol in rats inhibit the formation of breast cancer caused by environmental carcinogens.

We now know that the same phytonutrients that fight cancer also fight heart disease. Recent studies have clearly shown that heart disease can be reversed by using a phytonutrient-rich diet, regular exercise, and relaxation techniques such as meditation. It remains to be proven that cancer can be reversed through the use of a similar strategy. But the evidence is mounting.

Reversing Heart Disease and the "160" Watch

Late one night in the fall of 1986, I received a telephone call from a legendary motion picture personality (I'll refer to him as Mr. Jones to protect his privacy) who had suffered a heart attack. Calling from his hospital, he asked me to come to see him immediately. He knew from the health literature he had read that nutrition could play an important role in his recovery.

It was 9:30 P.M. "Aren't visiting hours over?" I asked.

"Don't worry. I've taken care of that. A nurse will meet you at the hospital entrance and escort you to my room." Ah, the privileges of celebrity.

So that night, from his hospital bed, we began working on reversing his heart disease.

I have clinical experience in helping heart-attack victims reverse their disease. I also have helped individuals who have been classified by their cardiologists as so-called terminal cases—those sent home from the hospital with inoperable heart disease and little hope of living out the year. In one case, described in the following section, a man with inoperable heart disease was given less than 3 months to live by his cardiologist. But the man's daughter brought him to my clinic, with the hope that her father could beat the odds. One year later, he walked 5 miles from his home to his cardiologist's office just to say hello.

Mr. Jones had every intention of beating the odds and living to a ripe old age. His plan was to combine the best medical care with the best nutritional advice to beat his disease into a permanent remission. And that's exactly what he did. I devised a phytonutrient-rich diet, based on his favorite foods, created special recipes to suit his tastes, and developed a dietary supplement program to help protect his coronary arteries from closing. And of course, I insisted that he begin a regular aerobic exercise program. He chose stationary cycling—a good idea, since he lived in Manhattan, a city not known for its clean air or light traffic.

During the next 8 weeks, Mr. Jones embraced a new way of eating that provided all of the cholesterol-lowering phytonutrients and antioxidant supplements that would protect the delicate lining of his arteries. He exercised 6 days a week, starting slowly and building up to a respectable 45 minutes on his exercise bicycle.

I explained to Mr. Jones at the outset that he would have to bring his elevated cholesterol level (256 milligrams per deciliter) down to 160 milligrams per deciliter or below to help the plaque in his arteries regress and to prevent another heart attack. People with a total cholesterol of 160 or below rarely die of atherosclerosis. Researchers conducting the famous Framingham Heart Study, an ongoing analysis of people living in a small Massachusetts town since 1948, have discovered that Framingham residents with a *blood cholesterol level below 160 do not die from heart disease.* But as their cholesterol numbers rise, so does the death rate from heart attacks.

Eight weeks after I began working with Mr. Jones, he visited his cardiologist for a checkup and his all-important blood cholesterol test. That afternoon, there was a knock at my door. His assistant had come to deliver a package from Mr. Jones. After she left, I opened it. The enclosed note read: "I call this the '160' watch. Thank you." I opened the box to find a gold watch from Cartier jewelers. Mr. Jones didn't know it, but his true gift to me was achieving an impressive recovery from his heart attack and reaching his new heart-safe cholesterol value. To this day, it appears he is in permanent remission from heart disease. And that is a present far more precious than gold.

David Levy's New Heart

As I write this account of David Levy's case, I'm reminded of an old Rodney Dangerfield one-liner: "My doctor gave me 6 months to live, but when I couldn't pay the bill, he gave me another 6 months."

David Levy's cardiologist gave *him* 6 months to live. But when David came to me, I gave him more than another 6 months; I taught him how to send his "terminal" heart disease into a long-term remission. David's seemingly miraculous recovery is testimony to the disease-fighting power locked inside the phytonutrient-rich foods and antioxidant vitamins and minerals that make up the *Permanent Remissions* Plan.

The day that David Levy's daughter brought him to my clinic, he could barely walk more than 100 feet or so without resting. He had such severe coronary artery stenosis (blockage) that almost any physical exertion—even the act of shampooing his own hair—caused him severe chest pain (angina pectoris).

David's blood lipids—his total cholesterol (365 milligrams per deciliter) and triglycerides (258 milligrams per deciliter)—were dangerously high, while his HDL-cholesterol (25 milligrams per deciliter), which helps remove artery-clogging plaque, was extremely low.

Within 8 weeks, I had helped David reduce his blood lipids to much safer levels. His total cholesterol had dropped to 170, his triglycerides fell to 94, and his HDL rose to 35. More importantly, he was walking 15 minutes each day without chest pain. Within 3 months, he was walking 30 pain-free minutes each day. His blood lipid profile continued to improve. His energy levels soared and he regained a vibrancy that had eluded him for the last 20 years of his life. Six months after he began his new diet, he returned to his cardiologist for a checkup. David Levy strode into his doctor's office as living proof that you can defeat "terminal" heart disease. His cardiologist came face-to-face with a patient whom he had thought would be dead by that time. But David Levy beat the odds.

David did something his doctor couldn't help him do: he learned how to save his life with an ordinary knife and fork. He discovered how to extend his life by using the heart-saving nutrients locked in phytofoods.

Table 8.5 is a sample 3-day diet that David Levy used to send his heart disease into a long-term remission. *Permanent Remissions* recipes are indicated in bold print.

TABLE 8.5

David Levy's Atherosclerosis Diet: Three-Day Sample

MEAL	DAY 1	DAY 2	DAY 3
Breakfast	• Oatmeal with ½ banana • 1 cup low-fat soy milk • 2 slices rye toast with unsweetened apple butter • 2 soy-sausage patties • 6 ounces fresh orange juice	• Egg-white omelet made with tomatoes, peppers, and onions • 2 slices rye toast with unsweetened apple butter • 6 ounces fresh orange juice)	• Oatmeal with ½ banana • 1 cup low-fat soy milk • 2 slices rye toast with unsweetened apple butter • 6 ounces fresh orange juice
Midmorning snacks	• ½ grapefruit	• Apple	• ½ grapefruit
Lunch	• 1 bowl tomato-vegetable soup • Soy-turkey sandwich on whole-grain bread, with soy mayonnaise, lettuce, and tomato • Mixed garden salad with fat-free dressing • 1 cup fresh berries	• 1 bowl **Pasta e Fagiole** • Mixed-green salad with nonfat dressing • Veggie burger on whole-grain bun, with ketchup, lettuce, tomato • Apple	• Baked potato with nonfat sour cream and chives • Mixed garden salad with fat-free dressing • 1 cup fresh strawberries
Midafternoon snacks	• **Super Soy Shake**	• **Super Soy Shake**	• **Super Soy Shake**
Dinners	• Whole-wheat pasta with marinara sauce • Mixed-green salad with olive-oil-and-vinegar dressing • ½ grapefruit	• Vegetarian lasagna made with low-fat mozzarella and ricotta cheeses • ½ cup corn • ½ fresh strawberries	• 4 ounces poached salmon • 1 cup steamed broccoli–carrot medley • ½ cup brown rice • ½ cup frozen low-fat yogurt
Evening snacks	• ½ cup low-fat frozen yogurt	• ½ grapefruit	• ½ cup blueberries topped with nonfat sour cream

See pages 227–338 for *Permanent Remissions* recipes listed in this table (boldfaced items).

Nutrients That Fight Heart Disease

The following are the heart healthy nutrients and phytonutrients that can protect your cardiovascular system from damage.

SOY PHYTONUTRIENTS

The world may have marveled at the Russians when they launched the first artificial satellite to orbit the earth, but in my opinion, their finest scientific contribution to the world was the discovery that soy protein protects against heart disease. It wasn't an earth-shaking discovery back in 1909, because in those days, heart disease was far from the number-one killer disease it is today. At the beginning of the twentieth century, Americans ate more disease-fighting phytonutrients in vegetables, less trans fatty acids (found in fast foods, baked goods, and margarine), got more exercise, and were thinner than Americans today. The diet and lifestyle they enjoyed helped prevent premature heart attacks. Heart disease was so rare, in fact, that medical texts devoted little space to it.

The early Russian soy–heart disease discovery assumes much greater significance today, when nearly one of every two Americans dies of the disease or is crippled by it. The cholesterol-lowering action of soy protein as compared to animal protein has been confirmed in numerous laboratory and human studies since then. When researchers replace animal protein with soy protein in the diets of laboratory animals and human volunteers, cholesterol levels and the risk of coronary heart disease plummet. People with elevated blood levels of cholesterol can reduce their cholesterol level by 15%–20% simply by consuming between 30–45 grams of soy protein—about two to three servings of soy products daily (Table 8.6).

Phytonutrients called *saponins* in soybeans lower cholesterol by blocking cholesterol absorption from the intestines, by enhancing cholesterol excretion, and perhaps by influencing thyroid gland metabolism. Soy foods provide enough saponins and other phytonutrients to prevent LDL-cholesterol from forming toxic by-products that damage delicate artery walls and lead to heart disease. Soy isoflavones, particularly genistein (found only in soy), help block the formation of arterial plaque and blood clots.

TABLE 8.6

Soy Protein Sources*

Soy Source	Protein (Grams)	Isoflavones (Milligrams)
Soy cocktail (1 serving)	40	30–40
Soy flour (1 ounce)	10–14	30–40
Soy meat replacer (3.5 ounces)	20	0–15
Soy milk (1 cup)	4–10	10–30
Tofu (4 ounces)	8–13	30–40

*Many manufacturers of soy meat replacers (e.g., soy ground beef, bacon, sausage, chicken, turkey, pastrami, and ham) use an alcohol extraction process that removes disease-fighting isoflavones from their products. For this reason, I recommend that you drink a soy cocktail or increase your intake of tofu and soy milk, both of which contain ample isoflavones and other health-promoting phytonutrients.

CAROTENOIDS

Carotenoids, found in such foods as yams, carrots, spinach, and kale (including alpha- and beta-carotene, lycopene, zeaxanthin, lutein, and cryptoxanthin), provide a degree of protection against coronary heart disease and heart attacks. Dietary carotenoids inhibit the oxidation of LDL-cholesterol and stop the progression of atherosclerosis. Studies have shown that men with the highest amount of carotenoids in their blood enjoy almost a twofold reduced risk of heart disease compared to men with the lowest level of serum carotenoids. For men who have never smoked, the risk is almost four times lower. Carotenoid-rich phytofoods include tomatoes, carrots, yams, yellow squash, spinach, and kale.

CARNOSINE

You've probably never heard of this nutrient, but don't let that throw you. Carnosine presents a new way for doctors to control and regulate the levels of calcium in the heart. Changes in levels of carnosine may play a role in life-threatening irregular heartbeats that can occur during ischemic heart disease and such inflammatory disorders as bacterial infections. Dietary supplementation with carnosine and vitamin E can increase the concentration of both nutrients in the heart and liver. Carnosine can also protect healthy cells against damage caused by radiotherapy. Carnosine is difficult to find, but manufacturers may make it more widely available in the near future. At present, only one product marketed in the United States (MaxiLIFE Phytonutrient Cocktail, manufactured by Twin Laboratories) contains a clinically useful dose of carnosine. Use this nutrient only under a physician's guidance.

FRIENDLY FATS (OLIVE OIL AND OMEGA-3 FATTY ACIDS)

Olive oil and omega-3 fatty acids from seafood reduce the clumping of blood platelets, which reduces the risk of developing coronary heart disease. Eskimos of Greenland and Alaska and native Japanese living in fishing villages enjoy a low death rates from cardiovascular disease, owing, in part, to their large dietary intake of omega-3 fatty acids. Eskimos of Greenland have low concentrations of serum cholesterol and triglycerides. People living in Mediterranean countries (where diets are rich in olive oil) enjoy one of the lowest death rates in the world from coronary heart disease—twice as low as people living in Finland, where consumption of olive oil is much lower.

VITAMINS C AND E

Vitamins C and E interact intimately, often working together to reduce the risk of cardiovascular disease. Vitamin C is a powerful water-soluble free-radical scavenger that protects against atherosclerosis. Some studies have found that artery-cleansing levels of HDL-cholesterol are linked to high levels of vitamin C carried in the blood. Studies also show a relationship between a high supplemental intake of vitamin E and reduction of rates of death from cardiovascular disease. Vitamin E has shown promise in treating existing vascular disease in some but not all clinical studies.

A study of over 87,000 women showed that the risk of coronary heart disease was 41% less in women who took vitamin-E supplements for more than 2 years. Another large study revealed that a relatively small daily intake of vitamin E (60 international units) reduced the incidence of coronary heart disease in 39,000 healthy male health-care professionals.

I believe that most people would do well to take at least 200 international units of natural vitamin E. (The natural form contains all the isomers of vitamin E that help fight cancer, heart disease, and the effects of aging.) Many labels list vitamin E in international units instead of milligrams. For natural vitamin E, 1 milligram equals 1.43 interna-

---

Vitamin E Quinone: A Clot-Busting Compound

Although vitamin E has long been known to have some anticoagulant properties (people with bleeding problems are cautioned against taking supplements of it), its clot-busting ability has largely been ignored by most researchers. While natural vitamin E itself, or *D-alpha-tocopherol*, has almost no ability to retard blood clotting, one of its main metabolites—*vitamin E quinone*—has significant anticlotting effects. Vitamin E quinone inhibits an enzyme that activates clotting factors in the blood and also shuts them down before they get out of control. The process depends on a little-appreciated nutrient, vitamin K (found in dark green leafy vegetables). This vitamin, which can be produced in small amounts by bacteria that live in the intestines, stimulates the release of chemicals that promote clotting and proteins that stop the clot from spreading beyond the site where it is needed. Vitamin E quinone interferes with this process. Vitamin E quinone competes with vitamin K's ability to initiate the clotting process. This is why some people have to be careful about how much vitamin E they take. Each person's metabolism is different, and some people may form more vitamin E quinone than others. The anticoagulant medications doctors now use act indirectly and slowly to inhibit clotting. Vitamin E quinone acts directly and faster, which could save lives, time, and money when someone is in danger of forming life-threatening blood clots. The *Permanent Remissions* plan emphasizes foods rich in vitamins E and K. **Warning:** Do not take vitamin E if you have blood-clotting problems, take anticlotting medications, have retinitis pigmentosa, or have any medical condition that might preclude you use of this vitamin. Always consult with a physician before you take vitamin E or any other dietary supplement.

---

tional units; for synthetic vitamin E, 1 milligram equals 1.1 international unit.

A recent study that examined the vitamin C and vitamin E intake of 11,178 senior citizens revealed that when the effects of these two vitamins were combined, risk of death from all diseases and especially coronary artery disease was reduced by 34% and 63% respectively.

The most telling finding of this recent study was that people who took a low-potency "once a day"–type multiple vitamin supplement fared no better than those taking nothing at all. People who took higher doses of vitamin C and vitamin E derived the health benefits of vitamin supplementation.

Natural vitamin E contains the isomers that protect the LDL-cholesterol molecule from oxidation. Taking natural vitamin E with meals incorporates this antioxidant vitamin into the LDL molecule, thereby reducing atherosclerosis. Vitamin C helps regenerate vitamin E "used up" as it protects the body against free-radical attack.

SELENIUM

The heart and blood vessels can be damaged by free radicals formed by a high-fat, high-cholesterol diet and exercise. Chronic alcoholics have low serum selenium and a high risk of dying from heart disease. Studies have shown that selenium provides greater protection against heart disease in smokers than in nonsmokers. One recent study found that organic selenium clearly reduces the chance of getting several forms of cancer and heart disease. Garlic grown in selenium-rich soil, salmon, tuna, sunflower seeds, and whole grains contain appreciable amounts of selenium.

COENZYME Q_{10}

Coenzyme Q_{10} is not a phytonutrient but rather a compound made by the body in small amounts. Coenzyme Q_{10} inhibits LDL-cholesterol oxidation more efficiently than either lycopene, beta-carotene, or vitamin E. Studies have shown that coenzyme Q_{10}:

- Significantly reduces hospitalization times and the incidence of serious complications in patients with chronic congestive heart failure. Patients with stabilized heart failure who received a daily dose of 50 milligrams of Q_{10} for 4 weeks, in addition to receiving conventional therapy, experienced improved breathing at rest and with exercise and reduced heart palpitations, liver enlargement, pulmonary rales, ankle swelling, heart rate, and systolic and diastolic blood pressure. Overall, Q_{10} led to a decrease in the signs and symptoms of heart failure and in the quality of life.
- Levels are usually much lower in patients with heart failure when compared to levels found in people without heart disease: almost two thirds of a series of 40 patients in severe heart failure treated with 100 milligrams of Q_{10} daily showed subjective and objective improvement. Investigators have concluded that Q_{10} is a safe and effective long-term therapy for chronic cardiomyopathy.
- Can improve the ability to do exercise or work in people with stable angina pectoris. One study, in which participants received Q_{10} (150 milligrams per day in three daily doses) for 4 weeks, showed that Q_{10}

reduced the frequency of angina attacks and nitroglycerin intake (a drug used to alleviate the pain of angina) by 50% for 2 weeks compared with patients receiving a placebo.

Canned white albacore tuna packed in water is a good source of coenzyme Q_{10} *and* omega-3 fatty acids. Small amounts of tuna (up to 12 ounces per week) can be used on the *Permanent Remissions* Plan to reduce the risk of cardiovascular disease.

L-TAURINE

L-taurine (Table 8.7) is a powerful antioxidant amino acid manufactured in small amounts by the body from other amino acids and vitamin B_6. Foods rich in L-taurine include clams, tuna fish, oysters, and human milk. L-taurine increases the calcium availability in heart muscle for contractions while it protects against calcium overload. Like coenzyme Q_{10}, L-taurine has been tested in people with chronic congestive heart failure. One study tested the effects of L-taurine (3 grams per day) in 17 patients with congestive heart failure. L-taurine improved the ability of the heart to pump blood after 6 weeks.

GARLIC

Garlic has been used as a medicinal agent for over 5,000 years. The ancient Egyptians used the bulb to cure two dozen ailments. During the Tang Dynasty of China (618–907 B.C.) garlic was cultivated as a food and used as medicine. The ancient Romans and Greeks used garlic for cooking and medicine. Aristophanes advised athletes to eat garlic in order to maintain their endurance. French priests in the Middle Ages used garlic to protect against the bubonic plague. Louis

TABLE 8.7

Cardiovascular Effects of L-Taurine in the Body

- Improves insulin sensitivity
- Reduces blood stickiness (clotting)
- Improves heart pumping function
- Lowers blood pressure
- Reduces heart arrhythmias
- Improves the efficacy of digitalis (heart medication)

Pasteur discovered that garlic killed bacteria. Soldiers in World Wars I and II used garlic to prevent infection in battle wounds. Studies at the State University of New York at Buffalo and at Brown University Medical School have shown that garlic protects against heart disease in several ways. Four to five cloves a day has been found to lower potentially harmful LDL-cholesterol by 10%. Garlic blocks cholesterol from adhering to artery walls and prevents blood cells from clumping together, which lowers the risk of developing blood clots. There are dozens of sulfur-containing compounds in garlic that individually and in combination contribute to its therapeutic value. One study found that dietary supplementation with one half to one clove of garlic a day decreased total cholesterol levels by 9% in individuals with very high cholesterol levels. Although garlic comes in a variety of forms, each abounds in the same disease-fighting properties. Whole garlic cloves contain *alliin*, the precursor of *allicin*. Allicin is the phytonutrient released from garlic when it is cut or damaged and gives the bulb its signature scent. Encapsulated garlic supplements sold in health-food stores do not usually contain appreciable amounts of allicin (in one recent study, only one of 39 different garlic supplements tested contained the total amount of organosulfur compounds equal to or higher than those found in garlic cloves). The effectiveness of garlic against cardiovascular disease is still being investigated. Aged garlic supplements contain disease-fighting phytonutrients not found in fresh garlic.

CHOLINE

Choline is a key component of lecithin, known chemically as phosphatidylcholine, a member of a family of fatty substances known as phospholipids. Studies have shown that choline plays an important role in brain development and memory and decreases the risk of getting heart disease and cancer. Like folic acid, choline can help lower homocysteine levels in the body. Twinlab's MaxiLIFE Choline Cocktail contains 1,000 milligrams of choline, a clinically effective dose, and heart-protective antioxidant vitamins and minerals. Foods rich in choline (Table 8.8) include wheat germ (1,400 milligrams per 1/4 cup), peanuts (1,111 milligrams per 1/2 cup), whole-wheat flour (613 milligrams per 1/2 cup), and pecans (333 milligrams per 1/2 cup).

L-CARNITINE

L-carnitine is an amino acid made in the body in small amounts that shuttles fatty acids into cellular furnaces called mitochondria. Nor-

TABLE 8.8

Choline-Rich Foods

Food	Milligrams of Choline
Wheat germ (½ cup)	2,820
Peanuts (½ cup)	1,113
Whole-wheat flour (½ cup)	613
White rice (½ cup)	586
Trout (3.5 ounces)	580
White flour (½ cup)	346
Pecans (½ cup)	333

mal heart function requires adequate levels of carnitine; a deficiency of this amino acid is associated with an increased risk of developing angina pectoris. Human studies have used 300-mg L-carnitine three times daily to ameliorate angina. In chronic heart failure, the heart muscle may require additional L-carnitine acid to normalize its metabolism. The L-carnitine level in the heart of patients with chronic heart failure has been shown to be lower than in individuals without heart disease. L-carnitine has been tested in patients with acute myocardial infarction, myocardial ischemia (with beneficial effects on symptoms and stress tolerance), and peripheral vascular disease. Preliminary results in patients with cardiac failure suggest that this nutrient may reduce cardiac arrhythmias and may allow the reduction of digoxin therapy. L-carnitine, which can stabilize the cell membranes of heart muscle cells, can reduce the risk of edema (swelling) that can follow anesthesia and surgical intervention. L-carnitine is found in muscle meats, but since it keeps company with some very unhealthy compounds, such as saturated fats and cholesterol, you may want to use an L-carnitine supplement (250–500 milligrams)—but only if advised to do so by your physician.

PROANTHOCYANIDINS

Peanuts, cranberries, red wines, grape skins and seeds, and citrus peels contain phytonutrients (catechins, flavonols, anthocyanins, proanthocyanidins, and soluble tannins) with powerful antioxidant properties.

The antioxidant activity of proanthocyanidins is much greater than either vitamin C or vitamin E. In addition, proanthocyanidins protect against radical damage in both water soluble and fat soluble components of the cell. Extracts from grape skin and grape seed have been shown to improve blood flow to the brain and heart and have been used to treat varicose veins and atherosclerosis. These substances in wines may help explain, in part, why French men enjoy heart disease rates 60% lower than those of American men. The French consume large amounts of fruits and vegetables in addition to large amounts of red wine. If you want to fortify your diet with red-wine polyphenols but prefer not to drink wine, you can enjoy purple grape juice. But you'll have to drink about three times more grape juice than wine to have the same heart-healthy effects.

NIACIN

Niacin (nicotinic acid) is a form of vitamin B_3 that has been used to lower elevated blood cholesterol. Niacin has been used with the prescription drug colestipol to achieve remission (reversal) of coronary atherosclerosis. Studies have shown that in daily doses of 2–3 grams, niacin can reduce total cholesterol and LDL-cholesterol between 20%–30%. It also lowers triglyceride levels between 35% and 55% and increases HDL-cholesterol levels by 20%–35%. Research indicates that niacin therapy, under medical supervision, can reduce death from heart disease when used to slow or reverse the progression of atherosclerosis, often with the use of bile acid resins.

Even though niacin is technically a vitamin (B_3), I do not approve of its use unless recommended by a physician. Most people can lower cholesterol and triglycerides by using the *Permanent Remissions* Plan and the phytonutrients and other nutrients discussed in this chapter without the use of niacin or cholesterol-lowering drugs (all of which are associated with toxic side effects). Daily doses of more than 100 milligrams of niacin have been associated with toxic side effects. Niacin increases heart rate and workload and reduces peripheral arterial resistance, making it inappropriate for those people who suffer from reduced blood flow to the heart. Niacin is acidic, and individuals with hypersensitivity to niacin or those with gastrointestinal disease, including stomach ulcers, should avoid using niacin. *Never use niacin unless advised to do so by a physician.*

ALPHA-LIPOIC ACID

Alpha-lipoic acid (ALA) is a coenzyme (similar in function to a vitamin) that directs the calories we eat to be burned as energy instead of stored as fat. ALA is synthesized in the body and absorbed from the diet. ALA is a potent antioxidant that can inhibit the oxidation of fat and cholesterol in the blood, arteries, and heart muscle. ALA helps regenerate vitamins E and C and helps protect cholesterol carried in LDL-lipoproteins from oxidation, thereby preventing the artery damage that leads to heart attacks. ALA also prevents blood sugar from combining with proteins in the body—a toxic chemical reaction that accelerates aging. Some evidence exists to recommend the use of ALA to aid recovery from heart attacks. ALA supplementation, at a dose of 100–600 milligrams a day, has been used to treat heart disease and diabetes. Use ALA only under a physician's supervision.

GREEN TEA

Studies suggest that green tea may protect against cardiovascular disease in four ways:

- Reducing total cholesterol and elevating HDL-cholesterol
- Inhibiting abnormal clotting in blood vessels
- Reducing high blood pressure
- Inhibiting the oxidation of LDL-cholesterol

Dietary surveys in Japan reveal that people who consume 4–6 cups of green tea each day have lower rates of breast, pancreatic, stomach, liver, lung, esophageal, and skin cancers. Green tea may prevent cancer by:

- Neutralizing cancer-causing agents
- Protecting cells against mutations from carcinogens
- Protecting against free-radical damage
- Protecting against radiotherapy damage

Green tea has also demonstrated an ability to reduce blood glucose levels, inhibit bacteria and viruses, and act as a general antioxidant.

FIBER

Such phytofoods as carrots, whole grains, oat bran, or citrus fruits and apples contain the type of soluble fiber that lowers blood cholesterol levels. Many bulk laxatives sold in the United States use psyllium husk fiber, which also has a cholesterol-lowering ability. Oatmeal, brown rice, and barley lower plasma total and LDL-cholesterol in people with normal or mildly elevated plasma cholesterol levels. Other phytonutrients that lower cholesterol are garlic and onions. These phytonutrients cost over 100 times less than prescription drugs used for lowering high blood cholesterol levels and don't cause the dangerous side effects. The soluble type of pectin fiber found in apples is a well-known cholesterol-lowering compound, and you can easily lower your blood cholesterol level by eating several apples per day.

ALCOHOL, WOMEN, AND HEART DISEASE

You're damned if you do and damned if you don't. That's the mixed message health experts are sending women who enjoy alcoholic beverages.

Women clearly suffer more of the adverse health effects of alcohol than do men. For example, women have a lower level of *alcohol dehydrogenase,* an enzyme that metabolizes alcohol, so they feel the effects of alcohol faster. Alcohol also disperses in the body water. Since women have less body water compared to men, they are more likely to have a higher alcohol concentration in their system. Monthly hormonal changes associated with the menstrual cycle also affect the way the body handles alcohol. Women suffer from premature death due to cirrhosis of the liver because they are more vulnerable to liver damage than are men. Worst of all, women who drink one or more alcoholic beverage a day are at increased risk of developing breast cancer later in life. Here's why:

Alcohol raises blood levels of the hormone estradiol and other reproductive hormones. Some studies have linked high estrogen levels to an increased risk of developing breast cancer. In one study of more than 3,000 women aged 20–44, women who reported consuming 14 or more alcoholic beverages (beer, wine, or spirits) per week in their thirties were 80% more likely to develop breast cancer than those who were nondrinkers. In another study conducted at the University of California Los Angeles, investigators questioned over 6,000 women with breast cancer and 9,000 healthy women about alcohol intake. *Those women who averaged one drink a day—a can of beer, a glass of wine, or a standard mixed drink—were 39% more likely to develop breast cancer than were women who did not drink. Women who consumed even one alcoholic beverage a day from their teens through their thirties were more likely to develop breast cancer.*

On the other hand, studies show that moderate alcohol consumption apparently lowers a woman's risk of coronary heart disease, which kills twice as many women as does breast cancer. Some researchers think that alcohol protects against heart disease by interfering with blood clotting; others think alcohol may elevate artery-cleansing HDL-cholesterol levels.

Women who drink moderately usually have lower serum insulin concentrations than nondrinkers, suggesting a role for insulin in explaining the relationship between alcohol and coronary heart disease. But for many people, alcohol is addictive, and alcohol consumption has been linked to an increased chance of dying from hypertension, stroke, stomach and throat cancer, cirrhosis of the liver, and fetal alcohol syndrome, which causes birth defects, mental retardation, and low birth weight in babies. Finally, binge drinkers have a high risk of sudden death. Alcohol consumption also hastens the loss of calcium from the body, setting the stage for osteoporosis later in life.

Age, heredity, gender, weight, and amount of body fat all affect the level of alcohol intake considered "moderate" for a given individual. Use this simple guide to determine your own alcohol intake: one or two "standard" drinks daily is considered "moderate." A standard drink contains about the amount in 12 ounces of beer, 5 ounces of wine, or 1½ ounces of 80-proof (40%) hard liquor.

Men, Alcohol, and Heart Disease

Doctors at Harvard University Medical School have good news for men who enjoy drinking alcoholic beverages. They studied 22,071 male doctors over an 11-year period and found that men who had two to four drinks a week had the lowest death rate—22% lower than those who eschewed alcohol. But men who averaged one drink a day lost the heart-saving benefits attributed to alcohol. Those who averaged two drinks or more a day had a death rate 63% higher than that of nondrinkers.

Other studies have shown that men who drink moderately increase their blood level of beneficial HDL-cholesterol and significantly decrease their coronary disease risk. Over 90% of Americans who drink consume less than 30 grams alcohol per day (considered the upper limit for "moderation"). Thirty-three percent of Americans abstain from alcohol.

Doctors who treat prostate disease have long known that any alcohol consumption irritates the urinary tract and promotes an inflammatory condition in the prostate gland (prostatitis). Some health experts believe that chronic prostatitis may be linked to benign prostatic hyperplasia (BPH), which enlarges the prostate, creating symptoms of urinary urgency and prostate cancer.

To Drink or Not to Drink:
What Should You Do?

A Mediterranean-type diet, which is similar in several respects to the *Permanent Remissions* plan (high in fruits, vegetables, and grains; small amounts of seafood and olive oil), also typically includes one or two drinks per day. But it is also high in the very phytonutrients that protect against breast and prostate cancer and cardiovascular disease.

Alcohol consumption seems to reduce the risk of cardiovascular disease in populations throughout the world, especially among the French. However, several studies have linked alcohol consumption (even amounts equivalent to two drinks daily) to increased rates for certain cancers.

Pick your poison carefully: the type of alcohol you drink may be an important factor in cardiovascular-disease risk reduction. A 15-year study of nearly 130,000 people found that wine—red or white—and beer appeared to protect the heart more than did other alcoholic beverages.

"People who drank liquor were protected, but people who drank beer or wine were better protected," notes study investigator Arthur Klatsky, M.D., an epidemiologist and cardiologist at the Kaiser Permanente Medical Care Program in Oakland, California. The study revealed that drinking a glass of wine or beer a day lowered the risk of developing heart disease by 20%. Drinking hard liquor lowered the risk by 10%, compared with those who did not drink any alcoholic beverages. And in a small study of healthy people and monkeys, researchers at the University of Wisconsin Medical School found that drinking three glasses of purple grape juice a day reduced blood stickiness by about 40%, making grape juice about as effective as alcohol for reducing the risk of life-threatening blood clots.

Whether one or two glasses of wine or beer adversely affect heart disease or cancer incidence in people who eat a Mediterranean diet has not been fully investigated. With the evidence currently available, I would expect that alcohol, when consumed responsibly and moderately, can be a component of the *Permanent Remissions* Plan. I would not recommend, however, that those who don't drink alcohol begin: if you don't drink, don't start! You will enjoy better health without using alcohol if you embrace the dietary strategies in this book.

Warren Cromartie

Warren Cromartie, a former member of the Kansas City Athletics and a national baseball hero in Japan, knows how to knock a 95 mile-per-hour fastball out of the ballpark, but he can't seem to keep his blood pressure from soaring out of the normal range.

When Warren sits down to a plate of spaghetti marinara at his favorite *ristorante,* he sets off a chain reaction in his body that raises his blood pressure to dangerous levels. But he loves the salty sauce on his pasta, so he eats it anyway. Sure enough, the next day, his blood pressure ascends into the stratosphere. But as Warren knows, there's nothing heavenly about that.

Why can't Warren enjoy salty foods and dishes without putting himself at risk of developing heart disease, kidney disease, and stroke?

Because Warren is an American black. And, like millions of blacks, his body is not equipped to handle the high salt content of many processed meats, fast foods, and restaurant dishes that he enjoys. And that, by itself, is enough to make eating a salty sauce risky business.

Warren has learned that a phytonutrient-rich diet can help him keep his high blood pressure in check. I've taught him the principles of the *Permanent Remissions* Plan. Does he still get to enjoy his favorite salty dishes? Not as much as he'd like. But for millions of blacks, a high-sodium diet can be a time bomb. So Warren grumbles a bit but passes on the pasta marinara when dining out and enjoys a salmon fillet with steamed broccoli and carrots instead. And to Warren, that's a grand-slam dinner that will keep him in the ballpark for a long time to come.

Blacks and Hypertension

Researchers have observed striking racial differences in hypertension between blacks and whites. American black men suffer hypertension at rates twice as high as those of American white men. Some research suggests that black men seem to respond more unfavorably to the level of sodium in the ordinary American diet than do whites. They may be correct: African blacks, who eat a much lower sodium diet than American blacks, have very low rates of hypertension.

Blacks with high blood pressure have higher rates of stroke and kidney damage but a lower incidence of coronary artery disease than do hypertensive whites. Blacks may also handle sodium differently than other groups: both blacks with normal blood pressure and those with high blood pressure tend to be salt sensitive. Blacks also tend to have lower renin levels (a blood pressure–controlling hormone) than do whites. These differences and others make it mandatory that hypertension among blacks be managed initially with salt restriction.

Sodium is just one cause of hypertension. Excessively high intakes of saturated and polyunsaturated fats, sugar, and animal-protein foods contribute to hypertension in most cases.

If you are an American black, the *Permanent Remissions* Plan can help you reduce the risk of suffering from hypertension and the diseases it causes because it prevents hypertension on all fronts simultaneously. Remember: hypertension is a silent killer. It rarely produces symptoms until the victim has a heart attack or stroke. And then it may be too late.

While most physicians routinely prescribe blood pressure-lowering medications for their patients, there is strong evidence that exercise and diet could eliminate the need for placing many American blacks on medications that cause harmful side effects.

In a recent study, doctors tested the effects of exercise on 46 American black men whose blood pressure was higher than 180/110 without medical treatment. They placed half the men on an exercise program that consisted of riding stationary bikes 45 minutes a day at about 75% of their maximum heart rates.

All the men received standard high-blood-pressure medicines. After 16 weeks, the exercising men's diastolic blood pressure—the lower of the two numbers—fell from 88 to 83. It rose slightly to 90 in the nonexercising comparison group. Men who cycled were able to reduce their doses of blood pressure medicine by 30%–40%. Heart enlargement, a common complication of high blood pressure, also decreased when the men exercised. About 60% of American white men over age 60 have high blood pressure, compared with 71% of black men.

The Role of Exercise

Regular aerobic exercise and physical activity reduce the risk of heart disease and stroke. Dozens of studies have shown a clear reduction in the known risk factors for cardiovascular diseases. For example:

- Nearly 75% of hypertensive people experience a reduction of blood pressure by exercising at just 50% of their maximum pulse rate. (Your maximum pulse rate is 220 minus your age.)
- Couch potatoes who never exercise have a much higher heart disease risk when compared with those who are constantly active. (A reduced heart rate is protective against death from heart disease and stroke: the relative risk in men with heart rates less than 90 beats per minute, in comparison with those with heart rates less than 60 beats per minute, is $2^{1}/_{3}$ times lower for total noncardiovascular death rates and over $1^{1}/_{2}$ times lower for death from cancer.)
- In some individuals with mild hypertension, a physical training program is sufficient to bring blood pressure to within normal limits.
- High levels of physical exercise and low-fat diet have been associated with a reduced prevalence of cardiovascular disease mortality and a reduced progression of cornonary atherosclerosis.
- Physical activity reduces serum lipids, partly because of a reduced serum insulin concentration and decrease in level of body fat.
- Endurance exercise, such as jogging or cycling, elevates HDL-cholesterol and reduces triglyceride levels.
- Increased physical activity in women is associated with higher HDL-cholesterol and a lower LDL-cholesterol and plasma total cholesterol level in both premenopausal and postmenopausal women.

- The fall in blood pressure in physically trained individuals may often be as great as or greater than the fall seen with drug treatment.

Contrary to conventional wisdom, people who are overweight may be able to remain so while they exercise their way to cardiovascular fitness. Excess body weight per se does not prevent the improvements in cardiovascular fitness due to regular aerobic exercise. While excess body fat can increase the risk of developing certain types of cancer, type 2 diabetes, gallbladder disease, and osteoarthritis, studies have shown that individuals who remain overweight may still enjoy good cardiovascular fitness if they burn approximately 1,500 calories each week during exercise beyond normal activities (Table 8.9).

Many people are justifiably worried about heart attacks and strokes brought on by exercise. Strenuous physical exercise is associated with increased rates of sudden cardiac death. The majority of people who have died from sudden cardiac arrest during or immediately following exercise, however, generally have medically documented evidence of prior angina pectoris or autopsy evidence of heart disease. That is why it is mandatory that you obtain a physician's permission before beginning any exercise program, especially if you have been inactive for any length of time. Studies have shown that the risk of heart attack during exercise is about 10-fold greater for those who exercise

TABLE 8.9

Calories Burned During Selected Activities

Activity	Calories per Hour (Approximate)
Running 10 miles per hour (6-minute miles)	1,200
Jogging 5.5 miles per hour (11-minute miles)	700
Cross-country skiing	700
Bicycling 12 miles per hour	400
Bicycling 6 miles per hour	220
Swimming 25 yards per minute	250
Swimming 50 yards per minute	500
Tennis (singles)	400
Walking 2 miles per hour (30-minute miles)	220
Walking 3 miles per hour (20-minute miles)	300
Walking 4.5 miles per hour (13.3-minute miles)	420

◆

less than 20 minutes each week than in those who exercise for more than 140 minutes each week.

I recommend that you embrace the *Permanent Remissions* Plan, visit your physician for a thorough examination, and then, with your doctor's permission, begin a regular exercise program of walking. Start slowly with a 15-minute walk and gradually increase your time (and mileage) every 2 weeks until you can comfortably walk at least 45 minutes at a brisk pace.

Exercise and Die on the American Diet

You gather all the resolve your tired body can muster, don your workout clothes, then pause for a moment, and think, "Do I really have the energy to do this today?" Well, not really, but you do it anyway. After all, this is part of your daily commitment to fitness. So you jog, stair-climb, cycle in place, and step-class your way to better health. Or so you think. Does all that exercise really do any good?

A well-oiled body runs best on a mixture of fuels derived from plant foods rich in antioxidant vitamins, phytonutrients, and soy protein, with small amounts of fats (those found in olive oil and seafood such as salmon). Exercise—whether one is stalking game on the African veldt for dinner or running on a high-tech treadmill in a trendy health club—speeds up the metabolism of dietary fats and carbohydrates. As the gears of the body's metabolic machinery whir ever faster, they pump out pesky free radicals that can damage organs, delicate artery linings, cell membranes, and DNA (deoxyribonucleicacid).

If you follow the *Permanent Remissions* Plan, you can relax: phytofoods contain a wealth of antioxidants that mop up toxic free radicals before they can do real damage. The trouble is, most Americans simply don't eat this way.

What's so bad about eating a "normal" diet and exercising? Physical exercise damages exercising muscle groups, releasing muscular enzymes such as *creatine kinase,* which researchers point to as clear-cut evidence of injured and aching muscles. And strenuous exercise generates lactic acid, which can reduce the effectiveness of cellular antioxidant systems. Even more important, exercise can shake loose artery-clogging plaque, found in the blood vessels of a majority of all Americans beyond the age of 20. Once that happens, the risk of heart attack and stroke soars.

Imagine a jogger running along his neighborhood road. He looks fit and serene, enjoying the scenery as he wends his way back home. If you could look inside his arteries, you might see gelatinous growths (arterial plaque) attached to his blood-vessel walls, bouncing and jiggling with every footstrike. Suddenly, one of these jellylike blisters breaks away from its mooring and is swept along the blood stream until it reaches the heart or brain, leading to a heart attack or stroke. The results can be disastrous: Remember Jim Fixx, the author who helped popularize jogging in the late 1970s? Jim sent me a copy of his cholesterol test results after I met him at a book-signing party. I warned him that his blood cholesterol level was in the danger zone and that he had to eschew his high-fat, high-cholesterol diet before running another step. But Jim laughed off my concern. Within a year, at age 52, Jim died of a massive heart attack while jogging.

Regular exercise is vital to achieving and maintaining optimal health but not when you eat a phytonutrient-poor American diet, which is far too high in fat, cholesterol, unrefined carbohydrates, sodium, and calories. The *Permanent Remissions* Plan provides a fuel mixture that fosters optimal health and promotes peak athletic performance—while lowering the risk of cardiovascular disease and sudden death.

And Last but Not Least . . .

Need I even mention it? Tobacco consumption—smoking cigarettes, cigars, or pipes—can give you heart disease, stroke, lung cancer, and emphysema. Snuff and chewing tobacco are no better, unless you don't mind cancer of the mouth, tongue, lip, or other areas of the mouth and throat. Tobacco products are the *only* consumable products that, when used as directed by the manufacturer, can kill you.

Even if tobacco use doesn't kill you, it can contribute to the damage of some very important body parts: the arteries (atherosclerosis and angina pectoris), the legs (claudication), the eyes (blindness), the ears (hearing loss), the nose (loss of taste and smell), the penis (impotence), and the face (wrinkles). When George Orwell said, "By the age of 50, you have the face you deserve," he might have had smokers in mind.

Cigarette smoking causes more lung damage in women than in men and affects black women worst of all because they generally have

smaller lungs than whites. Women have smaller lungs and air passage-
ways than men, so they have a greater percentage of loss of breathing
capacity for a given amount of smoke. Researchers at Tulane University
Medical School measured the amount of air a person can exhale by
studying 27,000 blue-collar workers. Among smokers, black women
scored lowest, black men scored lower than white men, and overall,
women scored worse than men. Since smaller lungs make it harder to
recover from damage caused by smoking, blacks did not recover as
much lung capacity after quitting smoking.

A more recent study by researchers at the Centers for Disease
Control and Prevention (CDC) revealed that women's lower lung capacity and an increase in smoking rates from the 1950s to the mid-
1980s have taken a deadly toll. From 1979 to 1992, women's deaths
from lung disease rose 108%, while deaths in men declined 2%. This
reflects the fact that men's smoking rates peaked several decades ago,
while women's rates have increased.

I hesitate to mention this, but in fact, the *Permanent Remissions*
Plan can protect you against some of the damage to arteries caused by
tobacco products. But please do not use this as a license to take up
smoking or to continue the habit. Phytonutrients can help put out
some of the fire of cellular damage caused by the thousands of harmful
products created during tobacco combustion, but why start the fire in
the first place?

Experimental Protocol for Angina Pectoris

Angina pectoris—pain in the chest—generally indicates underlying coronary artery disease. The experimental protocol shown in Table
8.10 contains nutrients that may be effective in ameliorating angina
pectoris. Use this experimental protocol only under the supervision of
a physician.

Experimental Atherosclerosis
Diet and Protocol

DIET

The experimental protocol shown in Table 8.11 contains the
phytonutrient-rich foods and nutrients that hold promise for being ef-

TABLE 8.10

Permanent Remissions Experimental Formula for Angina Pectoris

- Acetyl-L-carnitine (500 milligrams)
- L-taurine (500 milligrams)
- Coenzyme Q_{10} (90 milligrams)
- Calcium (500 milligrams)
- Magnesium (250 milligrams)
- Vitamin E (400 international units)
- Vitamin C (500 milligrams)
- Selenium (200 micrograms)

Caution: Do not use these or any other supplements unless you first obtain your physician's approval. These nutrients may help alleviate the pain of angina pectoris. If you have this health problem, discuss this formula with your physician to determine if it is right for you.

fective against atherosclerosis. Phytonutrient-rich foods form the foundation of this protocol and should be eaten every day in the amounts listed. Supplementary nutrients should be used only with the permission of and under the supervision of a physician. Table 8.12 is a 3-day eating plan to use as a guide for constructing meals based on the experimental atherosclerosis protocol. *Permanent Remissions* recipes are indicated in bold print.

EXERCISE

Regular exercise can also play an important role in reducing the risk of recurrence of atherosclerosis. Your goal should be to burn 1,500 calories a week through regular aerobic exercise, such as walking. If you do not currently exercise, obtain your doctor's permission and begin slowly, working up to a 45-minute walk at least 5 days each week.

TABLE 8.11

Experimental Atherosclerosis Protocol*

Eat These Phytofoods Each Day	In These Amounts
Soy meat replacers: soy burgers, hot dogs, bacon, sausage, turkey, chicken, ground beef, tofu†	2 servings (as indicated on package) each day or 2½ ounces of tofu in place of all meat, chicken, most fish
Soy milk (nonfat or low-fat) or soy cocktail‡	1 8-ounce serving each day
Olive oil, as a replacement for other vegetable oils, butter, and margarine	1–2 teaspoons
Salmon or tuna	1 4-ounce serving of salmon each week or 3 4-ounce servings of tuna
Tomato sauce	½ cup over pasta or in recipes, or 1 cup of tomato-based soup
Broccoli, cabbage, kale, cauliflower, turnips, Brussels sprouts	½ cup, 2 servings each day
Skim milk or low-fat yogurt (optional)	1 cup
Apple	1 medium
Banana	1 medium
Citrus fruits: oranges, grapefruits	1 medium orange or ½ grapefruit
Garlic and onion	2 bulbs/2 tablespoons, or use a dietary supplement

Take These Vitamins and Minerals

Vitamin A complex (5,000 international units vitamin A; 1 milligram alpha-carotene; 5 milligrams lycopene; 6 milligrams lutein; 0.3 millgram zeaxanthin)

Vitamin B complex (high-potency formula)[§]

Vitamin C (1000 milligrams)

Vitamin D_3 (400 international units)

Vitamin E complex (natural isomers: 400 international units)

Calcium (500 milligrams)

Chromium picolinate (200 micrograms)

Magnesium (250 milligrams)

Selenomax (200 micrograms)[‖]

Vanadium (5 milligrams)

Zinc gluconate (30 milligrams)

Take These Nonvitamin Nutrients

Alpha-lipoic acid (100 milligrams)

Acetyl-L-carnitine (500 milligrams)

Choline (1,000 milligrams)

Coenzyme Q_{10} (50 milligrams)

DMAE (100 milligrams) Dimethylaminoethanol (DMAE)

Gingko biloba (60 milligrams)

L-carnitine (500 milligrams)

L-glutathione (250 milligrams)

N-acetylcysteine (500 milligrams)

Phosphatidyl serine (500 milligrams)

Wine and tea polyphenols (50/250 milligrams)

*A number of products, such as soy cocktails, phytonutrient cocktails, and choline cocktails contain most or all of the vitamins, minerals, and other nutrients listed in this table.
[†]See brand name soy food-meat replacers listed in Table 4.7, page 86.
[‡]See recommended soy cocktails listed in Table 4.4, page 82.
[§]Use any brand of high-potency B-complex vitamin such as those made by Twinlab, GNC, or Solgar.
[‖]Selenomax is the trade name for the organic form of selenium manufactured and licensed by Nutrition 21.

TABLE 8.12

Three-Day Sample Atherosclerosis Diet

MEAL	DAY 1	DAY 2	DAY 3
Breakfast	• **Apple Cinnamon Oatmeal** • 2 Morningstar Farms Breakfast Patties • 6 ounces fresh orange juice	• **Buttermilk Pancakes with Banana** • 1 cup soy milk (such as White Wave Silk Soy Beverage)	• **2 Mandarin Orange Muffins** • 1 cup soy milk
Midmorning snacks	• ½ grapefruit	• Apple	• ½ grapefruit
Lunch	• **Beefy Bean Burrito** • **Pasta e Fagiole** • 1 large wedge of watermelon	• **Po' Boy ("Chicken Style")** on whole-grain bun, with lettuce and tomato • Mixed-green salad with olive-oil-and-vinegar dressing • Apple	• **Spinach Pita Puffs** • **Sweet Carrot Side** • **Sweet-and-Sour Cabbage with "Beef" Soup**
Midafternoon snacks	• **Super Soy Shake**	• **Super Soy Shake**	• **Super Soy Shake**
Dinners	• **Tricolor Pasta with Salmon** • ½ cup steamed broccoli with lemon juice • Mixed-green salad with olive-oil-and-vinegar dressing • ½ grapefruit	• **Lobster Malabar** • **Festive Kasmati Rice** • 1 slice **Chocolate Bundt Cake with Fruit Ribbon**	• Mexican "Beef" • **Red Beans and Rice** • 1 cup fresh berries
Evening snacks	• 1 cup **Fruit Yogurt Crunch**	• 1 cup **Strawberries and "Cream"**	• **Ambrosia**

See pages 227–338 for *Permanent Remissions* recipes listed in this table (boldfaced items).

9

BEATING OSTEOPOROSIS

It is a silent thief that stealthily robs you of your health, height, and happiness.

It can prevent you from picking up a child, hugging a loved one, or taking a romantic walk on the beach.

It is osteoporosis (*osteo* = bones; *porosis* = porous). And for 25 million people in the United States alone (close to 80% of whom are women), these everyday activities are difficult or impossible because the disease has ravaged their skeletons. Many people believe that osteoporosis affects only women, but such is not the case. Between 5 million and 10 million men in the United States are diagnosed annually with the disease. Most of the risk factors for osteoporosis are the same for men and women.

When someone has osteoporosis, even the slightest injury can cause a broken bone. Most typical are fractures of the hip and wrist and collapsed vertebrae of the spine, which can cause postural deformity and loss of height.

"It is normal to lose bone tissue gradually as you age," says Michele Bellantoni, M.D., codirector of the Osteoporosis Center at the John Hopkins Bayview Medical Center. "But osteoporosis involves much more than gradual loss. It endangers your health. It is so important for people, especially women, to know what to do to reduce bone loss and prevent osteoporosis."

Is it possible to prevent osteoporosis? What if you already have the disease? Can it be reversed?

Stopping Bone Loss

Why is preventing and reversing osteoporosis so important? Because each year, the disease is responsible for more than 1.5 million fractures that run up $10 billion in health-care costs and result in 40,000 deaths, usually within 6 months of the fractures. Fifty percent of all people who suffer hip fractures due to osteoporosis *never regain the ability to walk independently.*

Building strong bones during childhood and early adulthood depends on proper diet and exercise. That's when most of the eating and lifestyle habits that will last for life are established. Physicians recommend three or more daily servings of calcium during young adulthood (five servings during pregnancy and lactation) and weight-bearing exercises to prevent osteoporosis. Many now routinely recommend calcium supplements to their patients. But is that enough?

The answer, quite simply, is no. It takes more than a roll of Tums to beat a disease like osteoporosis. The idea that taking calcium supplements can prevent osteoporosis misses the mark entirely. Yet many physicians and nutritionists have fostered the notion that osteoporosis can be prevented by adding calcium to diet, through liberal use of dairy products and/or taking calcium supplements. This approach will fail for most people who eat an ordinary American diet because it fails to address the cause of the disease. Osteoporosis is as much a disease of calcium *retention* as it is a disease of calcium loss.

No amount of calcium will build a healthy skeleton on its own. Calcium and other minerals provide the raw materials that exercise and a healthy lifestyle can forge into bone. The more you bend or pull bones, the stronger they grow.

Aerobic exercise has long been touted as a way to prevent or slow bone loss, but researchers increasingly emphasize the benefits of strength training, such as weight lifting, to prevent bone loss at any age. A 1994 study published in the *Journal of the American Medical Association* revealed that women as old as 70 who lifted weights twice a week for a year avoided the expected loss of bone and even increased their bone density slightly.

Like skin, bone constantly regenerates itself. Bone cells called osteoclasts help remove old bone, while cells called osteoblasts rebuild the skeleton anew. That's fine so long as the osteoblasts prevail, but after the age of 35, the osteoclasts remove bone faster than osteoblasts can replace it. Eventually, bone can become so weak that it crumbles at the mildest of jars or jolts.

Calcium-rich foods and dietary supplements simply don't address the real causes of osteoporosis. You can chug a half-gallon of milk or chomp on chunks of cheese every day of your life and still get osteoporosis. In fact, these and other animal foods may be one reason for the epidemic proportions the disease has reached in the Western countries. High-protein diets—especially diets based on animal-protein foods—accelerate the loss of calcium from the body.

Trusting Americans have loved their dairy products blindly since the end of World War II, when the U.S. government decided to get rid of the dairy product surpluses by selling them to school lunch programs. Since then, dairy products have done little to stop the epidemic of osteoporosis and, ironically, may have added to it.

The Calcium Robbers in Your Diet

During midlife, you need to take additional steps to preserve your bone health. This is especially important for women during menopause, when a decline of estrogen production speeds bone loss. You can take steps now to prevent broken bones later.

While the conventional wisdom for keeping bones strong tells us to consume plenty of calcium, other nutrients can knock the mineral off-balance and undo its benefits by accelerating calcium loss from the body. The chief calcium robbers are excess dietary protein and sodium. Lifestyle risk factors for osteoporosis include lack of weight-bearing exercise, alcohol consumption, and tobacco use.

PROTEIN

When you eat protein in large amounts—especially from animal sources—the body must neutralize the toxic by-products of protein metabolism. As the kidney attempts to rid the body of these compounds, calcium is mobilized from the blood and bones to counter them. A recently published 12-year study of 86,000 nurses found that those who ate the most protein—more than 95 grams a day—had a 22% higher risk of suffering an arm fracture than those who ate the least—less than 68 grams a day. Women who ate five or more servings of red meat per week had a similar increase in risk of fractures, compared to those who ate red meat less than once a week.

SODIUM

When consumed in excess, sodium in table salt and food additives increases calcium losses through urine, which in turn decreases bone density. In a 2-year Australian study of 124 postmenopausal women, researchers found that at sodium intakes above 2,100 milligrams a day (slightly less than the amount in one teaspoon of salt), the more sodium a woman excreted (an indication of how much she consumed), the greater the loss of bone in her hips. The researchers conjecture that if you limit sodium to 2,400 milligrams a day, then 1,200 milligrams of calcium a day would be enough to protect against bone loss. If your diet is higher in sodium—as most American diets are—even that much extra calcium won't stop the daily depletion of calcium from your bones.

Got Milk?

Most people have never stopped to think about the health risks of cow's milk. And why should they? After all, most of us grew up with milk in our school lunch programs. Parents warned us to drink our milk to grow up to be big and strong. Role models on TV and in print advertising tout the benefits of milk. We are a nation of milk drinkers.

To some nutritionists and health faddists, attacking milk is akin to committing nutritional heresy. It's almost un-American. After all, Mom, milk, and apple pie are the sacred cows of American life. How can I tell you to abstain from consuming calcium-rich milk and milk products, such as cheese and ice cream, especially when osteoporosis is knocking at the door of so many American homes?

Pardon me for bursting your milk bubble, but the truth is that cow's milk was never part of the human diet until very recently in human existence. In fact, most people don't realize that it wasn't until just after World War II that milk was introduced into school lunch programs. Our government had to figure out what to do with a huge excess of dairy products that remained when our men came back from overseas. Someone got the bright idea to dump the surplus of dairy products down school kids' throats. It made perfect economic sense.

And it made nutritional sense to trusting parents, who were told that milk was the next best thing to sliced white bread (which is not so healthy either).

If milk products are effective at preventing osteoporosis, then why has this disease reached epidemic proportions? After all, Americans have been guzzling milk and eating chunks of cheese for a half-century—far more than other cultures in which osteoporosis is rare. Clearly, milk and other dairy products have done nothing to prevent the disease from running rampant. Don't get me wrong. Skim and very low-fat dairy products can be used, albeit sparingly, without jeopardizing health. But they must be used in relatively small amounts, as supplementary foods and as ingredients in recipes.

The good news is that consumption of milk has been steadily declining in recent years. The bad news is that sales of high-fat milk products, such as cheese and ice cream, increased during the same period (interesting aside: Americans drank as much beer as milk in 1992).

The vast majority of people in the world cannot digest milk because they don't have enough of the enzyme lactase to digest lactose, the sugar found in milk. Did Mother Nature err in making most of the adults in the world cow's milk–intolerant if it's so healthy and essential for strong bones? I think not. Even though a number of nutritionists believe that "cow's milk is for calves and human milk is for infants," I have no objection to using small amounts of skim milk and skim or very low-fat dairy products occasionally and in recipes. I do object, however, to the recommendations made by national health organizations to consume several servings of dairy foods each day. You can get all the calcium you need from vegetables, especially legumes, soy foods, and soy beverages—as well as from calcium supplements, if your doctor advises you to take them.

Calcium-Rich Foods for the Twenty-first Century

Cow's milk takes a backseat to soy milk and soy cocktails on the *Permanent Remissions* plan for two important reasons:

1. When you replace cow's milk with soy milk, cholesterol levels decline, especially in those people with the highest blood levels.

2. Soy milk contains phytonutrients that prevent and fight cancer, heart disease, and diabetes.

New recommendations for calcium intake, issued by the Institute of Medicine, a branch of the National Academy of Sciences, call for a daily dose of 1,000 mg, rather than 800 mg for most adults (including pregnant and lactating women). For those over 50, the new recommendation if 1,200 milligrams. For adolescents, the guidelines call for 1,300 milligrams.

Milk and milk products are rich sources of calcium. Consumption of skim milk and very low-fat dairy products, in small quantities, may actually help reduce risk of cancer. Skim milk is enriched in compounds called *sphingolipids,* which can protect against colon cancer. In contrast, whole-milk consumption has been linked to increased risk of developing lung cancer and heart disease. Several studies indicate that fermented-milk products, such as yogurt and buttermilk, may help reduce the risk of cancer by fostering the growth of healthy bacteria in the colon.

The *Permanent Remissions* Plan contains calcium-rich foods that lower the risk of developing cancer and heart disease, such as soymilk, legumes, and leafy vegetables. Skim milk and milk products may be used in small quantities and as called for in recipes. Used correctly, skim dairy products can be a part of your new way of eating. But soymilk beverages, soy cocktails, legumes, and calcium-rich vegetables provide most of the calcium (Table 9.1) on the *Permanent Remissions* Plan.

Are You at Risk for Developing Osteoporosis?

Answer the following questions yes or no:

1. Do you have a small, thin frame or are you white or Asian?
2. Are you fair-skinned, with blue eyes and blond hair?
3. Do you have a family history of osteoporosis?
4. Are you a postmenopausal woman?
5. Did you have an early or surgically induced menopause?
6. Have you taken steroids for asthma, arthritis, or cancer?
7. Is your diet deficient in such calcium-rich foods as beans, peas,

TABLE 9.1

Calcium Content of Selected Foods

Calcium (Milligrams)	Weight	Food
358	3.5 ounces	Smelt, Atlantic, canned
336	1 ounce	Parmesan cheese, hard
302	1 cup	Milk, skim
290	1 cup	Milk, whole, 3.7% fat
287	1 ounce	Gruyère cheese
285	1 cup	Buttermilk, 1% fat, cultured
297	4 ounces	Soy meal, defatted
269	5 ounces	Figs, dried
258	3 ounces	Tofu, raw, firm
244	½ cup	Winged beans, boiled
179	½ cup	Collards, frozen, boiled
175	½ cup	Soybeans, boiled
168	3.5 ounces	Seaweed, kelp (kombu/tangle), raw
161	½ cup	White beans, boiled
150	3.5 ounces	Seaweed, wakame, raw
148	½ cup	Collards, boiled
139	½ cup	Spinach, frozen, boiled
125	½ cup	Turnip greens, frozen, boiled
122	½ cup	Spinach, fresh, boiled

lentils, soy foods and beverages; such green leafy vegetables as kale, spinach, and broccoli; salmon; sardines; and dairy products?

8. Are you physically inactive?
9. Do you smoke cigarettes?
10. Do you drink more than one alcoholic beverage per day?

If you answered yes to just one of the above questions, you may be at risk of developing osteoporosis. Don't worry. Now that you're on the *Permanent Remissions* Plan, your chances of preventing further bone loss are greatly increased. The plan will help you prevent and reverse osteoporosis in two ways: by reducing calcium loss from the body and by restocking your bones with calcium and other vital minerals. You will be able to retain more calcium each day when you replace animal protein with soy protein and you will actually replace lost calcium and other minerals by eating the recommended calcium-rich foods. This is the only way, short of using drugs with harsh side effects, that you can actually send osteoporosis into remission.

Today, there are advanced methods of diagnosing and monitoring the progression of osteoporosis. Your doctor can use a bone densitometry or bone-density scan, which measures the amount of bone mineral content in specific areas of the body. With the information obtained from these tests, your doctor can predict whether you are at risk of suffering a bone fracture and then recommend appropriate treatments. If you receive or have received a diagnosis of osteoporosis, I strongly recommend that you give your doctor a copy of this book so that you can work with him or her to map out an effective treatment strategy.

The Calcium Supplement Myth

Less than half of the women in the United States who take calcium supplements will ultimately prevent the usual 2% loss in bone per year that occurs with aging. Why? Because calcium supplements alone don't provide the spectrum of nutrients the body needs to beat osteoporosis. Calcium supplements cannot override the primary diet and lifestyle risk factors that predispose you to osteoporosis:

- Alcohol intake
- Lack of exercise
- Cigarette smoking
- High protein intake
- High sugar intake
- High salt intake

Your ability to absorb calcium from foods and supplements declines with age. This is often due to a decrease in estrogen with menopause and the body's declining ability to convert vitamin D to the hormonal form that controls calcium absorption from foods and dietary supplements. The elderly may also experience an increase in the production of parathyroid hormone, which can accelerate the loss of calcium from the bones.

Calcium absorption from most foods, including most vegetables and grains, is similar to that of milk. You can absorb only between 10%

and 60% of the calcium in your diet. Only 20%–40% of the calcium in cow's milk is typically absorbed. The vitamin D added to milk and the natural sugar in milk (lactose) improve absorption.

While calcium supplementation is a good idea for some people, it is only a small part of the total strategy to prevent osteoporosis. Many people have a false sense of security because they believe that simply self-supplementing with calcium will protect them from the disease. There are at least a half-dozen nutrients that you'll need to know about in order to successfully defend yourself against osteoporosis or send it into a permanent remission.

Permanent Remissions Calcium Sources

Your goal is to retain the vital bone minerals that form the foundation of a healthy skeleton. To do this, you must follow the *Permanent Remissions* Plan, which includes supplemental minerals, including calcium, to prevent and reverse osteoporosis. By following the plan, you can reduce lifelong bone loss and keep your skeleton mineralized.

Calcium is readily available in tofu; leafy vegetables; legumes, such as beans, peas, and lentils; and vegetables, such as broccoli, kale, cabbage, mustard greens, rutabagas, cauliflower, and Brussels sprouts. Granted, most of these foods are hardly American diet mainstays, but on the *Permanent Remissions* Plan, you have three additional options to help you get enough calcium if you fail to eat calcium-rich foods:

1. Use MaxiLIFE Soy Cocktail (Twin Laboratories), which contains 50% of the daily recommended calcium requirement, to help you reach your goal of osteoporosis-fighting nutrients if you don't consume enough calcium-rich vegetables on any given day.
2. Use a soy milk beverage, such as White Wave's Silk, which contains 30% of the daily recommended calcium requirement per cup.
3. Use a calcium–magnesium supplement that contains a 2:1 ratio of calcium to magnesium (e.g., a supplement that supplies 500 milligrams of calcium and 250 milligrams of magnesium).

Permanent Remissions Nutrients That Fight Osteoporosis

Here is a list of nutrients—in addition to calcium—found in legumes, fruits, and vegetables that the body uses to build healthy bones:

BORON

Boron may play a role in keeping your bones healthy, but its role is most likely associated with its interactions with such other nutrients as calcium, magnesium, and vitamin D_3. In two human studies, a boron-deficient diet caused changes in calcium metabolism in a manner that was detrimental to bone formation and maintenance; these changes were exacerbated by low dietary magnesium. Changes caused by boron deprivation included increased urinary excretion of calcium. Because boron deprivation causes changes similar to those seen in women with postmenopausal osteoporosis, the mineral is apparently required for optimal calcium metabolism and is thus needed to prevent the excessive bone loss that often occurs in postmenopausal women. In one study, giving postmenopausal women 3 milligrams of boron each day raised sex hormone levels, which could help prevent osteoporosis. More research is required to elucidate boron's role in bone health.

CHROMIUM

Chromium helps normalize glucose and insulin levels in people suffering from type 2 diabetes, which accounts for 90%–95% of all cases of the disease in the United States. Diabetics usually have low chromium levels. Researchers gave 180 diabetics living in China a very high dose of chromium—1,000 micrograms—that successfully restored normal glucose and insulin levels. Other studies using 200 micro-grams—a level generally regarded as safe—have achieved clinically significant results. Chromium even helped people with impaired glucose tolerance, a prediabetic condition that affects an estimated 21 million Americans. Impaired glucose tolerance predisposes those with the condition to developing full-blown diabetes. The impact of chromium (alone or in conjunction with calcium and other micronutrients) on bone density and osteoporosis merits further evaluation in controlled studies. Chromium reduces urinary excretion of calcium in postmeno-pausal women, presumably indicative of a reduced rate of mineral loss from bone. Chromium can also increase blood levels of the hormone DHEA-S (dehydroepiandrosterone-sulfate), a metabolite of the hormone DHEA. Researchers suspect that DHEA may help preserve bone density in postmenopausal women. Foods rich in chromium include whole grains and cereals and legumes. But you'll need to take a chromium supplement in order to consume enough chromium to reach clinically effective levels.

MAGNESIUM

Magnesium influences bone health by indirectly affecting mineral metabolism through hormonal factors and by directly effecting the processes of bone formation and mineralization. Magnesium regulates the transportation of calcium into bone and other tissues. A 2-year study of menopausal women recently found that magnesium supplementation appeared to have prevented fractures and resulted in a significant increase in bone density. Magnesium is necessary for the synthesis of sex hormones. Magnesium-rich foods include seafood, avocados, apples, apricots, figs, peaches, beets, and whole grains.

Whether magnesium deficiency is a causal factor in osteoporosis is controversial, and there are conflicting reports as to the magnesium content of osteoporotic bone. One study has noted improved bone mineral density with use of a multinutrient supplement that contained 250 milligrams of magnesium. More research is needed on the role of magnesium in osteoporosis before any conclusions about this mineral and osteoporosis can be drawn.

Other Foods and Nutrients for Strong Bones

SOY PROTEIN

A growing body of evidence suggests that all protein is not created equal, and that soy protein has certain advantages for preventing and reversing osteoporosis. For example, a 1988 University of Texas Health Sciences Center study showed that volunteers excreted 50% less calcium in their urine when they replaced the animal-protein foods in their diet with soy foods. And a 1990 study at the United Medical and Dental School of Guy's and St Thomas's Hospitals in London found soy protein much easier on the kidneys than meat, which may be important for people with kidney disease.

VITAMIN C

Vitamin C helps build collagen, the substance bones use as an underlying structure. Recent research indicates that foods rich in vitamin C and vitamin C supplements may help postmenopausal women maintain healthy bone densities. More research is needed to confirm the role of vitamin C in preventing osteoporosis. Vitamin C–rich foods includes oranges, orange juice, papaya, grapefruit and grapefruit juice, strawberries, green bell pepper, broccoli, Brussels sprouts, cantaloupe, cabbage, and mustard greens.

VITAMIN D

Sunlight stimulates a hormone in skin that triggers the liver and kidney to make the active form of vitamin D_3. Two equally effective sources of vitamin D in humans are derived from plant ergosterol, which is converted to ergocalciferol (vitamin D_2) and cholecalciferol (vitamin D_3) by the action of sunlight on the skin. The body uses vitamin D_3 for normal immune system function, to control cellular growth, and to absorb calcium from the digestive tract. Vitamin D_3 can inhibit the growth of malignant melanoma, breast cancer, leukemia, and mammary tumors in laboratory animals. Vitamin D_3 can also inhibit angiogenesis, the growth of new blood vessels that permit the spread of cancer cells through the body. In warm weather, about 10–15 minutes of direct sun (in morning or late afternoon, to avoid skin damage) two to three times a week can produce sufficient vitamin D. As we age, however, our skin becomes less efficient at making vitamin D. People who live in cloudy climates with long winters may not get enough vitamin D. Many health experts believe that adults may benefit from 400 to 800 international units of vitamin D. But don't exceed this amount without your doctor's advice, since too much vitamin D can be toxic. Vitamin D can cause calcification in the kidneys, heart, and other tissues. Symptoms of vitamin D toxicity include anorexia, disorientation, dehydration, fatigue, weight loss, weakness, and vomiting.

New analogues of vitamin D_3 allow cancer victims to take high doses of the vitamin without fear of elevating calcium in the blood to dangerous levels. These new forms of vitamin D have very high potency in controlling cell proliferation and differentiation. One of these, calcipotriol, can be used topically to treat psoriasis and inhibit the growth of metastatic breast cancer in patients with whose tumors have vitamin D receptors. Foods rich in vitamin D include egg yolks, fatty fish, and liver.

Hormone Replacement Therapy:
Is It Right for You?

Since the 1940s, most health experts have believed that declining estrogen levels in the body were the primary cause of osteoporosis. Even today, medical students are taught that the proper treatment of osteoporosis is estrogen-replacement therapy. Estrogen does, in fact, inhibit the osteoclast cells that function to remove calcium and other minerals from bone. But estrogen alone cannot rebuild bone. The body also requires the hormone progesterone, and perhaps others as well, to replace bone by stimulating the osteoblast cells that remineralize and restore bone mass.

The use of estrogen without the balance of progesterone is fraught with side effects such as high blood pressure, increased tendency for blood clotting, promotion of fat synthesis, hypothyroidism, vaginal bleeding, painful breasts, fibrocystic breast disease, increased risk of development of gallbladder disease and gallstones, liver dysfunction, and increased risk of development of endometrial cancer of the uterus, pituitary tumors, and breast cancer.

Progesterone helps protect breast tissue from the cancer-promoting effects of estrogen-like hormones. Breast cancer may occur if normal or high amounts of estrogens are present without appropriate amounts of progesterone. Unfortunately, artificially synthesized progestins or progestenogens prescribed by many doctors cause harmful side effects and are not as effective as the natural progesterone made by the body.

To replace or not replace—that is the question. And therein lies the rub. This is a very personal decision that requires your physician's guidance. Only future research will be able to adequately answer this question, which depends, in part, on a number of factors, including family history of cancer, heart disease, osteoporosis, hypertension, and other health problems that could be affected by estrogen.

At present, there is no hormone-replacement therapy that can match the intricate way the body manufactures and releases hormones in the precise amounts under normal circumstances. That's why taking any hormone, such as insulin, DHEA*, melatonin, estrogen, progester-

---

*The hormone DHEA, available as an over-the-counter supplement, may play a role in preventing osteopo-

one, growth hormone, or testosterone, is fraught with side effects and serious health problems.

It remains to be proven that these hormone-replacement therapies are safe and effective. There is evidence, both pro and con, to persuade or dissuade women from embracing hormone-replacement therapy. Within the limits of present knowledge, it is simply too early to make sweeping generalizations.

Experimental Osteoporosis Diet and Protocol

DIET

The experimental protocol shown in Table 9.2 contains the phyto-nutrient-rich foods and nutrients that hold promise for being effective against osteoporosis. Phytonutrient-rich foods form the foundation of this protocol and should be eaten every day in the amounts listed. Supplementary nutrients should be used only with the permission and under the supervision of a physician.

Table 9.3 is a 3-day plan to use as a guide for constructing meals based on the experimental osteoporosis protocol. *Permanent Remissions* recipes are indicated in bold print.

FOODS TO AVOID

You don't have to completely eliminate any food from your new way of eating, but you should drastically reduce your intake of the following foods in order to achive optimal bone health and a permanent remission from osteoporosis if you have it.

METHIONINE-RICH FOODS

Most animal foods—such as red meats, eggs, milk, cheese, and fowl—contain high amounts the amino acid methionine. Methionine and other sulfur-containing amino acids can accelerate the loss of calcium from bones. In general, vegetables (with the exception of legumes) and fruits contain less methionine than animal foods.

---

rosis. When researchers fed DHEA to rats that had their ovaries removed, the hormone significantly increased bone density. Scientists suspect that DHEA may be converted to estrogen in bone cells, which could aid in the maintenance of bone mineral density. DHEA aids vitamin D_3 in maintaining bone mineral density, especially after menopause. At this time, I do not recommend that you use DHEA unless advised to do so by a physician. The long-term effects of hormone replacement with DHEA remain unknown.

TABLE 9.2

Experimental Osteoporosis Protocol*

Eat These Phytofoods Each Day	In These Amounts
Soy meat replacers: soy burgers, hot dogs, bacon, sausage, turkey, chicken, ground beef, tofu†	2 servings (as indicated on package) each day or 2½ ounces of tofu in place of all meat, chicken, most fish
Soy milk (nonfat or low-fat)	1 8-ounce serving each day
Broccoli, cabbage, kale, cauliflower, turnips, Brussels sprouts	½ cup, 2 servings each day
Skim-milk products	Up to 3 times each week
Legumes: beans, peas, lentils	Up to 1 cup each day
Olive oil, as a replacement for other vegetable oils, butter, and margarine	1–2 teaspoons
Salmon or tuna	1 4-ounce serving of salmon each week or 3 4-ounce servings of tuna
Citrus fruits: oranges, grapefruits	1 medium orange or ½ grapefruit

Take These Vitamins and Minerals

- Vitamin A complex (5,000 international units vitamin A; 1 milligram alpha-carotene; 5 milligrams lycopene; 6 milligrams lutein; 0.3 milligram zeaxanthin)
- Vitamin B complex (high-potency formula)[§]
- Vitamin C (1,000 milligrams)
- Vitamin D$_3$ (400 international units)
- Vitamin E complex (natural isomers: 400 international units)
- Calcium citrate (1,500 milligrams)
- Magnesium citrate (500 milligrams)
- Selenomax (200 micrograms)[‖]
- Boron (3 milligrams)
- Chromium picolinate (200 micrograms)

Take These Nutrients

- Soy cocktail (30 milligrams total isoflavones per serving)[‡]
- Bioflavonoid complex (500 milligrams citrus bioflavonoids; 30 milligrams grape-skin polyphenols; 200 milligrams quercetin; 50 milligrams rutin; 300 milligrams green-tea extract; anthocyanins; 5 milligrams Pycnogenol)
- Coenzyme Q$_{10}$ (90 milligrams)
- L-carnitine (500 milligrams)
- L-glutathione (250 milligrams)
- N-acetylcysteine (500 milligrams)

*A number of products, such as soy cocktails, phytonutrient cocktails, and choline cocktails, contain most or all of the vitamins, minerals, and other nutrients listed in this table.
[†]See brand-name soy-food meat replacers listed in Table 4.7, page 86.
[‡]See brand-name soy cocktails listed in Table 4.4, page 82.
[§]Use any brand of high-potency B-complex vitamin such as those made by Twinlab, Solgar Nature's Plus, or GNC.
[‖]Selenomax is the trade name for the organic form of selenium manufactured and licensed by Nutrition 21.

TABLE 9.3

Three-Day Sample Osteoporosis Diet

MEAL	DAY 1	DAY 2	DAY 3
Breakfast	• 2 Morningstar Farms Breakfast Strips • ¾ cup oatmeal with ½ banana • 6 ounces fresh orange juice	• **Pigs in the Blanket** • 1 cup soy milk (such as White Wave Silk Soy Beverage)	• **Buttermilk Pancakes with Banana** • 1 cup soy milk • 6 ounces fresh orange juice
Midmorning snacks	• ½ grapefruit	• Apple	• ½ grapefruit
Lunch	• **Hearty Lasagna** • 1 large wedge of watermelon	• **"Bacon" Cheese"burger"** on whole-grain bun, with lettuce and tomato • **Pasta e Fagiole** • Apple	• Green Giant Harvest Burger on whole-grain bun, with lettuce, tomato, and ketchup • ½ cup **Cajun Coleslaw** • 1 cup **Red Lentil Soup**
Midafternoon snacks	• **Super Soy Shake**	• **Super Soy Shake**	• **Super Soy Shake**
Dinners	• **Horseradish-Encrusted Salmon** • ½ cup steamed broccoli with lemon juice • Mixed-green salad with olive-oil-and-vinegar dressing • ½ grapefruit	• **"Beefy" Bean Burrito** • ½ cup brown rice	• **Lobster Malabar** • 1 slice **Chocolate Bundt Cake with Fruit Ribbon**
Evening snacks	• 1 cup **Fruit Yogurt Crunch**	• 1 cup **Strawberries and "Cream"**	• 1 cup **Pink Citrus Ice**

See pages 227–338 for *Permanent Remissions* recipes listed in this table (boldfaced items).

ALCOHOL

Alcohol consumption accelerates the loss of calcium and other minerals important to good bone health. Limit alcohol intake to no more than 3 drinks each week.

HIGH SODIUM FOODS

Foods that contain large amounts of sodium—such as salty snack foods (e.g., potato chips), canned soups and sauces, soy sauce, and pickles packed in brine— may accelerate the loss of calcium and other minerals from the body.

EXERCISE

Regular exercise can also play an important role in reducing the risk of recurrence of osteoporosis. Your goal should be to burn 1,500 calories a week through regular aerobic exercise such as walking. Recent research has shown that strength training, such as weight lifting, helps retain calcium and other minerals in the skeleton. If you do not currently exercise, obtain your doctor's permission and begin slowly, working up to a 45-minute walk at least 5 days each week.

SECTION II

Phytofood Recipes

Permanent Remissions

RECIPE HINTS

Here are a few suggestions, explanations, and general comments to help you make the most of this recipe section.

- Brand names are suggested for a reason. After repeated experimentation, I have found that just because an item is perfect for one recipe doesn't mean it can be plugged into every recipe with equal success. You will see many recurring favorites, but when another brand works better, that's what's suggested. For example, two different brands of nonfat cheddar cheese are called for at different times. The best one for each job is what's recommended. Of course, you may make substitutions. If you can't find something or it's out of stock, you're still way ahead of the game by preparing one of these recipes as closely as possible. The idea is to stay within the *Permanent Remissions* domain as often as you can.
- In order to assist you in finding as many recommended ingredients as possible, I have included a comprehensive list of all manufacturers and or distributors in the back of the book (pages 365–68). Whenever available, a toll-free number is listed. When that is not offered, an address and local phone number is listed. Many of these companies expect your call, so don't be shy.
- You've probably heard it before, but the best way to prepare a recipe is to lay out all the ingredients ahead of time. The French call it *mise en place*. This helps things move more quickly, avoids omissions, and lets you know if you have everything in the house before you begin, not after. Cover your work space or countertop with wax paper for

easy clean up. It's also a help to measure out teaspoons and table-spoons of dry ingredients (like spices and baking powder) and wet ingredients (like soy milk and olive oil) and put them in separate small dishes or ramekins so that you're not fumbling with the measuring spoons or separating egg whites at inopportune times. If you do your dicing, slicing, and measuring ahead of time, you'll be surprised at what a pleasure it can be to cook. You've seen cooking shows where they put together masterpieces in front of you and it looks easy, right? Well, the reason is that the prep work is all out of the way by the time they start. Be your own *sous*-chef and then switch hats. Both jobs can actually be enjoyable.

- Don't waste your efforts. You have a lot of things to do with your time. It's a valuable commodity, so treat it that way. People will spend an afternoon baking or cooking and then leave the results out on the counter or poorly wrapped in the refrigerator, only to have to throw away a good portion of what they made when it gets stale and hard a few days later. Freezer bags have really improved. They even have zippers on them now. Put all the baked goods you won't be using right away into one of these bags while they're still warm. (Do the same with many *Permanent Remissions* entrées.) Squeeze the air out of the bag or use a commercial sealer if you have one. You then have a few months of afternoons or evenings when the muffins or bread or lasagna you took the time to make are waiting with freshness and ingredients more healthful than any premade items currently offered.
- Many natural and organic foods are packaged without preservatives. Remember to keep your oils, flours, rice, and other grains in a cool, dark place so they retain their freshness longer. Some brands will even suggest refrigeration. Check the labels.
- You will notice that the baked-goods recipes often call for 1 or 2 teaspoons of wheat gluten. This is necessary because soy, oat, and whole-wheat flours don't rise or bake up with the same texture as all-purpose flour. The gluten allows the healthful substitutions to work out properly.
- Always use an olive oil–based cooking spray to coat your cookware; just don't use a garlic-flavored one for your sweet baked goods!
- Sometimes you will find another recipe called for within a recipe. The Taco Salad, for instance, calls for the *Permanent Remissions—PR—* Avocado Dressing Dip. The Pigs in the Blanket recipe calls for *PR* Buttermilk Pancakes. All recipes appear separately for your convenience.

- One of the most important and widely used "recipes within a recipe" in the book is the Soy Milk Blend (page 294). Memorize this one right away. (It has only two ingredients.)
- Here are a few specialty kitchen items that will help in the making of these recipes. They are not essential, but they will make things easier:

  - A food processor or blender
  - An electric mixer
  - A microwave oven
  - A mandoline or comparable vegetable slicer
  - A handheld immersion blender
  - A dumpling press
  - A garlic press
  - A 9½-inch springform pan
  - A bundt cake pan
  - Muffin tins

It is possible to get around all of this except for something that can purée foods and perhaps the muffin tins.

Don't be surprised when you start to feel better in general after eating the *Permanent Remissions* way for a while. When you get used to having meals that taste good and are filled with things that benefit you, you may look at restaurant menus and think that the rest of the world has some catching up to do. They do. You'll probably become accustomed to thinking of meal time as a healing time as well as a time for pleasure, and that may fly in the face of the standard guilt feelings that tend to go along with gastronomic enjoyment.

Until now, there's been that double-edged sword of "This is making me happy, but this is not making me healthy." And more often than not, ill health does become reality after years of indulgence. However, the advent of certain knowledge and the use of phytonutrients in general and soy products in particular has put the human diet on the edge of a revolution.

The tired adage "You are what you eat" takes on new meaning. So does the statement "One not willing to put bad fuel in a new car shouldn't then do so in the body." Until recently, this has been a hollow caveat, owing to its unlikely success. (Who could actually stomach the brewer's yeast and wheat grass of "health-food stores" in the seventies in the face of the sugary empty fat-free calories of grocery aisles in the nineties?) Even those with the best of intentions often lost steam

1 or 2 weeks into a New Year's resolution because there was no viable alternative.

Suddenly, though as if out of a science-fiction movie, it may become the new status symbol to eat like a king while consuming a meal of the best human fuel. And just as royalty of old were the first to get spices and fine delicacies, so too are the monarchs of today beginning to get functional foods—foods that separate them from the ignorance of the masses. Foods that heal and sustain them according to the owner's manual suggestion, much in the way automakers specify certain gasolines for vehicles. Foods that taste so good there isn't any desire to revert to the old way of eating.

The kings and queens in this case are ordained not by lineage or financial status but by knowledge. And those who are enlightened can stroll through the aisles of supermarkets and greengrocers with renewed purpose and make their selections with confidence and enthusiasm. Because research, development, and information are now making possible a new adage: You don't have to suffer at the table in order to thrive away from it. No, it doesn't have to be that way.

Permanent Remissions

RECIPE LIST

BREAKFAST

- APPLE CINNAMON OATMEAL / *231*
- BISCUITS 'N' "SAUSAGE" / *232*
- BUTTERMILK PANCAKES WITH BANANA / *234*
- CHEESE GRITS / *235*
- FRUIT YOGURT CRUNCH / *236*
- PIGS IN THE BLANKET / *237*
- ROBERT'S FAVORITE OMELET / *238*

APPETIZERS

- "CHICKEN" NUGGETS / *239*
- HUMMUS / *240*
- POTSTICKERS ("PORK" DUMPLINGS) / *241*
- SHRIMP WRAPPED IN "BACON" / *243*
- SPECIAL RESTAURANT SALSA / *244*
- SPINACH PITA PUFFS / *245*
- THAI NOODLES / *246*

SNACKS AND SANDWICHES

- "BACON" CHEESE "BURGER" / *249*
- "BEEFY" BEAN BURRITO / *251*
- EGG "FU" SALAD SANDWICHES / *252*
- "MEATBALL" OVEN GRINDER SUBS / *253*
- PO' BOY ("CHICKEN" STYLE) / *255*
- TRIPLE-DECKER CLUB / *256*

BREADS

- Aunt Jean's Zucchini Bread / *259*
- Buttermilk Biscuits / *261*
- Cheddar Jalapeño Corn Muffins / *262*
- Mandarin Orange Muffins / *263*
- Menopause Muffins / *264*
- Oat Bread (Baguettes and Rolls) / *266*
- Tuscan Garlic Bread / *269*
- Whole-Wheat Croutons / *270*

SOUPS

- Pasta e Fagiole / *271*
- Red Lentil Soup (Right Away) / *273*
- Rio Grande Pinto Bean Soup / *274*
- Southwestern Corn Chowder / *276*
- Sweet-and-Sour Cabbage Soup with "Beef" / *277*
- Tomato Rice Soup / *278*

SALADS

- Black-Eyed Salsa / *279*
- Cajun Coleslaw (and Dressing) / *280*
- Pita Salad Sandwich / *282*
- Spinach Salad with Warm "Bacon" Dressing / *283*
- Taco Salad / *284*
- Tuna Dijon Salad / *286*

DRESSINGS, SAUCES, AND DIPS

- Annato Vinaigrette / *287*
- Avocado Dressing Dip / *288*
- Creamy Garlic Dip / *289*
- "Creamy" Pink Tomato Sauce / *290*
- Honey Mustard Dip / *291*
- Nothing Lost Tartar Sauce / *292*

- Snappy Cocktail Sauce / 293
- Soy Milk Blend / 294

ENTRÉES

- Broccoli and Tofu Lo Mein with "Chicken" / 295
- Chili Con "Carne" / 297
- Hearty Lasagne / 298
- Horseradish-Encrusted Salmon / 300
- Lobster Malabar / 302
- Mrs. B's Chilies Rellenos / 303
- Ravioli di Liguria / 304
- Rigatoni with Garlic, Tomatoes, and Basil / 306
- "Sausage" Ratatouille à la Ann / 307
- Shrimp and "Scallops" Creole / 309
- Tricolor Pasta with Salmon (Skillet Dinner) / 311

SIDE DISHES

- Deluxe Refried Beans / 313
- Festive Kasmati Rice / 314
- Mexican "Beef" / 315
- Red Beans and Rice / 316
- Scalloped Potatoes / 318
- Spicy Couscous with Tomatoes / 319
- Sweet Carrot Side / 320
- Tangy Collard Greens / 321
- Tex-Mex Brown Rice / 322

DESSERTS

- Ambrosia / 323
- Chewy Oatmeal Chocolate Chip Cookies / 324
- Chocolate Bundt Cake with Fruit Ribbon and
  Mocha Frosting / 325
- Marzipan Cheese Tart / 327
- Pink Citrus Ice / 329
- Strawberries and "Cream" / 330

BLENDER DRINKS

- Berry Tofu Smoothie / *331*
- Café Espressoy Shake / *332*
- Double-Chocolate Malt / *333*
- Dreemsicle Shake / *334*
- Pure Fruit Smoothie / *335*
- Strawberry Banana Shake / *336*
- Super Soy Power Shake / *337*
- Tropical Fruit Shake / *338*

BREAKFASTS

Apple Cinnamon Oatmeal

YIELD: 1 SERVING

¾ cup pure apple juice
¼ cup *PR* Soy Milk Blend (page 294)
½ cup Quaker Old Fashioned Oats (cooks in 5 minutes)
⅛ teaspoon ground cinnamon
2 tablespoons golden raisins or dried apple pieces
1 tablespoon chopped walnuts (optional)

If you thought you could never eat oatmeal without brown sugar and cream, it's time to "feel your oats" in a new way.

In a saucepan combine the juice, milk, and cinnamon and bring mixture to a boil. Add the oats and bring mixture back to a boil. Heat it for 2 minutes on high, then 2 minutes on medium, and then 1 minute on low, stirring constantly. Remove oatmeal from heat and stir in raisins or apple (and walnuts, if using them). Drizzle oatmeal with pure maple syrup if desired.

For 2 servings: 1¼ cups juice, ½ cup Soy Milk Blend, 1 cup oats, ¼ teaspoon cinnamon, ¼ cup raisins or apple, 2 tablespoons walnuts

For 3 servings: 1¾ cups juice, ¾ cup soy milk, 1½ cups oats, ½ teaspoon cinnamon, ⅓ cup raisins or apple, 3 tablespoons walnuts

Calorie Breakdown per Serving	Nutrition Totals per Serving	
Protein: 7.5%	CALORIES:	261
Carbohydrate: 84.3%	PROTEIN:	4.9 grams
Fat: 8.2%	CARBOHYDRATE:	55.4 grams
	FAT:	2.4 grams
	SODIUM:	45 milligrams
	CHOLESTEROL:	0 milligrams

Biscuits 'n' "Sausage"

YIELD: 10 SERVINGS

PR Buttermilk Biscuits ingredients:
1½ cups unbleached all-purpose flour
¼ cup whole wheat flour
¼ cup Arrowhead Mills Organic Whole Grain Soy Flour
1 tablespoon baking powder
¼ teaspoons baking soda
2 teaspoons sugar
½ teaspoon cream of tartar
1 teaspoon Arrowhead Mills Wheat Gluten
¼ teaspoon sea salt
2 tablespoons Land O'Lakes Light Butter
2 tablespoons Sun Sweet Lighter Bake Butter and Oil
    Replacement
⅔ cup 1% buttermilk

Preheat oven to 425°F. In a bowl, stir together flours, baking powder, baking soda, sugar, cream of tartar, wheat gluten, and salt. Cut in butter and Lighter Bake until the mixture resembles coarse crumbs. Make a well in the center; pour in buttermilk all at once. Stir just until dough sticks together.

On a lightly floured surface, knead dough for about 12 strokes. Roll or pat out to ½-inch thickness. Cut with a 2½-inch biscuit cutter or use a clean, empty can (open on both ends) approximately 2½ inches in diameter.

Transfer biscuits to baking sheet. Bake for 10–12 minutes. These go well with *PR* Robert's Favorite Omelet (page 238) or *PR* "Chicken" Nuggets (page 239) drizzled with honey, but if you'd like to create a whole breakfast in a single package, keep reading.

SAUSAGE:
Cook as many Morningstar Farms Breakfast Patties as you will be using right away (up to 10) according to package instructions. When the biscuits have cooled slightly, slice them in half and place a warm sausage patty in the center.

These biscuits may be wrapped in plastic, placed in a freezer bag, and frozen. Preassemble your Biscuits 'n' Sausage by placing an uncooked patty in the center of those you plan to freeze. This allows you to reheat them in a single step. Simply microwave each sandwich on high for about 1 minute, turning it once midway through heating. Transfer it to a paper towel or napkin, and you're out the door with a breakfast that's compact, tasty, and very good for you.

Suggested Topping: Spread with *PR* Honey Mustard Dip (page 291).

Calorie Breakdown per Serving
Protein: 27.6%
Carbohydrate: 45.7%
Fat: 26.7%

Nutrition Totals per Serving

CALORIES:	179
PROTEIN:	11.8 grams
CARBOHYDRATE:	19.5 grams
FAT:	5.1 grams
SODIUM:	587 milligrams
CHOLESTEROL:	5 milligrams

◆

Buttermilk Pancakes with Banana

YIELD: 10 PANCAKES; SERVING SIZE: 2 PANCAKES

½ cup unbleached all-purpose flour
¼ cup Arrowhead Mills Whole Grain Organic Soy Flour
¼ cup whole-wheat flour
1 tablespoon sugar
1 teaspoon baking powder
½ teaspoon baking soda
1 teaspoon Arrowhead Mills Vital Wheat Gluten
¼ teaspoon sea salt
2 beaten egg whites
1¼ cups 1% buttermilk
1 tablespoon Sun Sweet Lighter Bake Butter and Oil
    Replacement
1 tablespoon Hain Organic Canola Oil
2 ripe bananas (thinly sliced)

In a large bowl, mix together flours, sugar, baking powder, baking soda, wheat gluten, and salt. In another bowl, combine egg whites, buttermilk, Lighter Bake, and oil. Add this to the flour mixture and stir till mixture is blended. Mix bananas into batter. Coat a skillet with olive-oil cooking spray (a nonstick skillet is preferable) and set it over medium heat. Pour ¼ cup of batter for each pancake onto the hot griddle. Cook pancakes until they are golden brown and bubbles form on their surface. Flip them to cook the other side. For best results, wipe and respray pan before each batch.

Drizzle pancakes with pure maple syrup, or dust with powdered sugar, if desired.

These make a surprisingly good match with the *PR* "Sausage" Ratatouille (page 307). Prepare the pancakes without the bananas and ladle the ratatouille on top.

Calorie Breakdown per Serving		Nutrition Totals per Serving	
Protein:	14.9%	CALORIES:	197
Carbohydrate:	63.9%	PROTEIN:	7.6 grams
Fat:	21.2%	CARBOHYDRATE:	32.6 grams
		FAT:	4.8 grams
		SODIUM:	201 milligrams
		CHOLESTEROL:	2 milligrams

Cheese Grits

YIELD: 4 SERVINGS

1 cup filtered water
1 cup Westsoy Non Fat Soy Beverage
½ cup Quaker Quick Grits
3 slices Kraft 2% Milk Singles (diced)
⅛ teaspoon garlic powder
Dash paprika

In a saucepan, combine the water and soy milk and bring the mixture to a boil. Slowly stir in the grits. Reduce heat and cover saucepan. Cook grits until they're thickened (5 to 7 minutes), stirring occasionally. Add cheese and garlic powder; continue stirring till grits are smooth and uniform in color. Top them with paprika.

Calorie Breakdown per Serving
Protein: 25.2%
Carbohydrate: 48.3%
Fat: 26.5%

Nutrition Totals per Serving

CALORIES:	76
PROTEIN:	5.0 grams
CARBOHYDRATE:	9.5 grams
FAT:	2.3 grams
SODIUM:	265 milligrams
CHOLESTEROL:	8 milligrams

Fruit Yogurt Crunch

YIELD: 1 SERVING

½ cup plain low-fat yogurt, 1½% milk fat
1 tablespoon clover honey
½ cup sliced or cubed fruit (Granny Smith apples work
    especially well)
¼ cup Grape Nuts–type cereal

This tastes fresher than store-bought versions. It's a better way to start your day.

In a small mixing bowl, blend yogurt with honey. Add fruit and stir all gently to combine. Transfer yogurt mix to a bowl or dish and top with cereal "crunchies."

Calorie Breakdown per Serving
Protein: 11.6%
Carbohydrate: 80.5%
Fat: 7.9%

Nutrition Totals per Serving

CALORIES:	272
PROTEIN:	8.4 grams
CARBOHYDRATE:	58.5 grams
FAT:	2.6 grams
SODIUM:	181 milligrams
CHOLESTEROL:	10 milligrams

Pigs in the Blanket

YIELD: 10 PIECES (5 SERVINGS)

PR Buttermilk Pancakes
10 Morningstar Farms Breakfast Links

Prepare the *PR* Buttermilk Pancakes (page 234) without the banana.

Cook 10 Morningstar Farms Breakfast Links according to package instructions. Wrap a pancake around each link and close it with a toothpick.

Serve with pure maple syrup if desired.

You can keep these warm in a 200°F oven while cooking the rest of the batch. Just be sure to use a plain wooden toothpick. Cellophane and plastic decorations may melt if put in the oven.

Calorie Breakdown per Serving
Protein: 27.5%
Carbohydrate: 43.5%
Fat: 29.1%

Nutrition Totals per Serving
CALORIES: 215
PROTEIN: 15.1 grams
CARBOHYDRATE: 23.9 grams
FAT: 7.1 grams
SODIUM: 540 milligrams
CHOLESTEROL: 2 milligrams

Robert's Favorite Omelet

YIELD: 1 SERVING

1 teaspoon olive oil

4 egg whites

¼ cup diced sweet onion (soaked in cold water several minutes, then drained)

⅓ cup ripe tomato, diced and seeded (if using canned, drain thoroughly)

2 tablespoons Heinz tomato ketchup

Sea salt

Freshly ground black pepper

Place the egg whites in a bowl and beat them with a fork or a whisk. Set them aside. In a skillet (preferably nonstick), sauté the onion and tomato in the oil over medium heat till tender. Add a dash of salt and pepper, if desired. Whisk the eggs again, briefly, and pour them into the pan. As they start to turn white, keep pushing the cooked portion to the side of the pan, allowing the clear portion to cook as well. When the omelet is done, transfer it to a plate. Add a dash more salt and pepper, if desired, and top with ketchup.

Egg whites tend to weep slightly while being cooked. If you keep them in the pan a few extra seconds, they will usually reabsorb the liquid.

Try serving this omelet with a *PR* bread selection such as a *PR* Buttermilk Biscuit (page 261), a *PR* Menopause Muffin (page 264), or a *PR* Oat Bread roll (page 266).

Calorie Breakdown per Serving	Nutrition Totals per Serving	
Protein: 33.8%	CALORIES:	183
Carbohydrate: 43.0%	PROTEIN:	16.0 grams
Fat: 23.2%	CARBOHYDRATE:	20.4 grams
	FAT:	4.9 grams
	SODIUM:	529 milligrams
	CHOLESTEROL:	0 milligrams

APPETIZERS

"Chicken" Nuggets

YIELD: 4 SERVINGS

1 package Morningstar Farms Chik Nuggets
Your choice of dipping sauces: *PR* Honey Mustard Dip (page
    291), *PR* Creamy Garlic Dip (page 289), Heinz tomato
    ketchup, *PR* Snappy Cocktail Sauce (page 293), or the
    dressing for the *PR* Cajun Coleslaw (page 280).

Prepare nuggets according to package instructions. Set the sauces
out in individual dipping cups.

When served with the suggested dips, these nuggets are irresistible.
Guests will love them, kids will love them, you will love them.

For a "better than take-out" meal, serve the "Chicken" Nuggets
along with the *PR* Red Beans and Rice and the *PR* Buttermilk Biscuits
(page 261).

Calorie Breakdown per Serving
Protein: 33.3%
Carbohydrate: 43.6%
Fat: 23.1%

Nutrition Totals per Serving

CALORIES:	160
PROTEIN:	13.0 grams
CARBOHYDRATE:	17.0 grams
FAT:	4.0 grams
SODIUM:	670 milligrams
CHOLESTEROL:	0 milligrams

Hummus

YIELD: 8 $^1/_4$-CUP SERVINGS

15-ounce can garbanzo beans (chickpeas), drained and rinsed
2 tablespoons fresh lemon juice
1 teaspoon lemon zest*
2 teaspoons Bertolli Extra Light Olive Oil
2 teaspoons Kame Dark Sesame Oil
$^1/_3$ cup Nasoya Extra Firm Tofu
2 cloves garlic, quartered
$^1/_4$ teaspoon paprika
$^1/_4$ teaspoon sea salt
1 tablespoon flaxseeds (preferably ground in spice grinder)

This is a very delicious—if slightly sneaky—way to give your family and friends the benefits of both soy and flaxseeds.

Combine all ingredients in a blender or food processor. (The seeds will remain whole if not preground.) Transfer the hummus to a bowl and cover. Chill it at least 2 hours to attain full flavor. Serve on whole-wheat pita bread or as a dip for fresh vegetables.

Calorie Breakdown per Serving
Protein: 15.3%
Carbohydrate: 50.8%
Fat: 33.9%

Nutrition Totals per Serving

CALORIES:	105
PROTEIN:	4.1 grams
CARBOHYDRATE:	13.6 grams
FAT:	4.0 grams
SODIUM:	242 milligrams
CHOLESTEROL:	0 milligrams

*If you're not frequently in the kitchen, you need to know that zest is finely grated lemon peel, used as flavoring.

Potstickers ("Pork" Dumplings)

YIELD: 16; SERVING SIZE: 4

3 Morningstar Farms Breakfast Patties
3 Morningstar Farms Breakfast Links
1–square inch cube of fresh ginger root, peeled
2 garlic cloves, minced
1 medium chopped scallion (white and green parts)
16 Nasoya Egg Roll Wrappers cut into 3½-inch–diameter
    circles
2 teaspoons Bertolli Extra Light Olive Oil

For best results, you will need a dumpling maker for this recipe. You can purchase one in most kitchen stores for under five dollars. If you don't want to buy one, you can still make the dumplings by hand; just be sure to pinch the seams together tightly.

Heat "sausage" patties and links enough to warm through. Cut each piece into quarters. Add them to the bowl of a food processor or blender along with the rest of the ingredients, except egg roll wrappers and the oil. Process the mixture until it resembles finely ground meat. Transfer into a medium-size bowl or dish.

Place a wrapper on the dumpling maker, then put 1 firmly packed teaspoon of the "sausage" mixture in the center of the circle. Moisten the edges with water and press them closed to seal. (If filling seeps into the crimped part after it's folded, use a little less filling.) Place dumplings on wax paper or foil as you finish them. You should have enough filling for 16 dumplings.

Put 1 teaspoon of the oil in an 8- or 9-inch skillet and bring it to medium high heat. Add ½ cup filtered water and half the dumplings to the pan. Cover loosely. Cook just until water evaporates (about 4–6 minutes). Gently loosen the dumplings with a spatula, being careful not to tear the skins. Wipe out the skillet and repeat the process with the remaining dumplings, starting with another teaspoon of oil.

Won ton wrappers may also be used for this recipe, but you may need to use less filling, as they are smaller than those called for here.

These taste delicious by themselves, but if you want a dipping sauce, try the *PR* Honey Mustard Dip (page 291), Kame Light Soy Sauce, or the sauce used for the *PR* Thai Noodles (page 246).

Calorie Breakdown per Serving
Protein: 28.9%
Carbohydrate: 40.4%
Fat: 30.7%

Nutrition Totals per Serving
CALORIES: 172
PROTEIN: 11.6 grams
CARBOHYDRATE: 16.3 grams
FAT: 5.5 grams
SODIUM: 515 milligrams
CHOLESTEROL: 4 milligrams

Shrimp Wrapped in "Bacon"

YIELD: 1 DOZEN; SERVING SIZE: 4

12 large shrimp, peeled and deveined
12 slices Morningstar Farms Breakfast Strips

Cook the shrimp in boiling water with a seafood seasoning till pink. Drain them, then rinse them with cold filtered water. (If you don't have a seafood seasoning, use a bay leaf in the boiling water along with a pinch of salt.)

Heat "bacon" according to package instructions (don't overcook; the strips need to remain pliable). When they are cool enough to handle, wrap 1 strip several times around the middle of each shrimp and close it with a toothpick.

Serve with *PR* Snappy Cocktail Sauce (page 293) or the *PR* Nothing Lost Tartar Sauce (page 292), or prepare the dressing for the *PR* Cajun Coleslaw (page 280) and use it as a dipping sauce.

For variety, you may want to add a slice of water chestnut or pineapple to the center of each appetizer.

This recipe can be prepared with precooked shrimp to save a step.

Calorie Breakdown per Serving	Nutrition Totals per Serving	
Protein: 25.8%	CALORIES:	71
Carbohydrate: 12.0%	PROTEIN:	4.3 grams
Fat: 62.3%	CARBOHYDRATE:	2.0 grams
	FAT:	4.6 grams
	SODIUM:	245 milligrams
	CHOLESTEROL:	21 milligrams

♦

Special Restaurant Salsa

YIELD: 5 SERVINGS; SERVING SIZE: ¼ CUP

6 plum tomatoes, peeled, seeded, and quartered
1 tablespoon finely minced jalapeno pepper, seeds and ridges
    removed
1 tablespoon fresh cilantro leaves, chopped
2 tablespoons scallion (white and green part), chopped
2 tablespoons fresh lime juice
½ teaspoon salt

Put all the ingredients in a food processor or blender. Run the blender on "pulse" just until blended; don't overprocess. Cover the salsa and chill it. Let the salsa warm slightly before serving.

To make your tomatoes easier to peel, score (make an X) at the stem end of each tomato with a knife: stab each one with a large fork on the scored end. Submerge it in boiling water for 30 seconds, then plunge it into a bowl of ice water for another 30 seconds. The skin will pull away easily.

Unlike Pico de Gallo, this is not a thick and chunky salsa. This is the kind of salsa you get at good Mexican restaurants but can never seem to duplicate at home. Make it a day ahead of time, if possible. The flavor keeps getting better.

Serve the salsa with flour tortillas or fat-free corn chips.

Calorie Breakdown per Serving	Nutrition Totals per Serving	
Protein: 15.1%	CALORIES:	25
Carbohydrate: 76.5%	PROTEIN:	1.1 grams
Fat: 8.4%	CARBOHYDRATE:	5.7 grams
	FAT:	0.3 grams
	SODIUM:	239 milligrams
	CHOLESTEROL:	0 milligrams

Spinach Pita Puffs
YIELD: 6 SERVINGS

3 cups fresh spinach leaves, washed and stems removed
1/3 cup chopped onion
2 teaspoons Bertolli Extra Light Olive Oil
1/4 cup Healthy Choice Non Fat Grated Mozzarella Cheese
1/2 cup Polly-O Non Fat Ricotta cheese
1 egg white
1/8 teaspoon salt
1/8 teaspoon freshly grated nutmeg *or* 1/4 teaspoon ground
    nutmeg
6 small pita pocket bread rounds (approximately 4 inches in
    diameter)

Preheat oven to 375°F. Sauté onion in oil over medium heat till it is tender. Add spinach and cook it till slightly wilted. Remove from heat and add to food processor or blender along with the rest of ingredients, except the pita. Blend mixture till the colors mingle but are still distinct. Set aside.

Dip each pita in filtered water briefly. Wrap it in a paper towel and microwave it on high for 15 seconds. This will plump up and separate the bread and make it easier to fill. Carefully remove it from the paper towel, waiting a few seconds to handle it if necessary (it will be hot). Cut a 2- to 3-inch slit in the seam of the pocket and spoon in about 3 heaping teaspoons of the spinach mixture; don't overstuff. As you complete each puff, wrap it in foil and place it on a cookie sheet. Bake puffs for 20 minutes.

Serve with *PR* Creamy Garlic Dip (page 289), if desired.

Calorie Breakdown per Serving	Nutrition Totals per Serving	
Protein: 58.8%	CALORIES:	120
Carbohydrate: 17.6%	PROTEIN:	9.3 grams
Fat: 23.6%	CARBOHYDRATE:	2.8 grams
	FAT:	1.7 grams
	SODIUM:	231 milligrams
	CHOLESTEROL:	2 milligrams

Thai Noodles

12-ounce package Nasoya Chinese Style Noodles (or 12
    ounces linguine pasta, preferably whole-wheat)

Thai Noodle Sauce:
2 chopped scallions, white part only
2-inch × 1-inch piece of peeled fresh ginger root, cut into
    quarters
2 garlic cloves, minced or cut into quarters
2 tablespoons smooth organic peanut butter (choose a peanut
    butter that is aflatoxin-free, such as the one made by
    Whole Foods Market)
8 ounces Nasoya Firm Tofu (half a block, cut into quarters)
1 teaspoon Kame Dark Sesame Oil
1/4 cup clover honey
1/4 cup Kame Light Soy Sauce
1/4 cup rice wine vinegar
1/4 teaspoon ground red pepper (optional)

Combine all the ingredients, except the noodles, together in a
food processor or blender till smooth. Pour into a bowl and chill.

Prepare the noodles according to the package's instructions. Drain
and rinse them in a colander with cold water. Empty colander into a
large bowl. Pour the Thai sauce over the noodles, tossing the noodles
until they are coated.

You may chill this dish briefly, but once the sauce is poured over
the noodles, it is best served within about 15 minutes. The pasta will
lose its texture if left coated with liquid for any length of time. You can
make the sauce in advance if you prefer and pour it over as many
servings of noodles as needed at a time.

To make entrée-size portions out of this appetizer, simply add pea
pods, broccoli florets, carrots, or other vegetables to the mix to increase
the volume and complete the meal.

The noodle sauce is also delicious used as a dip for the *PR* Potstickers ("Pork" Dumplings) (page 241).

Calorie Breakdown per Serving
Protein: 20.2%
Carbohydrate: 56.1%
Fat: 23.8%

Nutrition Totals per Serving

CALORIES:	273
PROTEIN:	14.0 grams
CARBOHYDRATE:	38.8 grams
FAT:	7.3 grams
SODIUM:	736 milligrams
CHOLESTEROL:	9 milligrams

SNACKS AND SANDWICHES

"Bacon" Cheese "Burger"

YIELD: 1 SANDWICH

1 whole-wheat or multigrain hamburger roll
1 Green Giant Harvest Burger (Original Flavor)
1 tablespoon Hellman's Low Fat Mayonnaise (1 gram per
    serving)
2 teaspoons prepared yellow mustard
1 tablespoon Heinz tomato ketchup
Pinch of dried dill weed
1 Morningstar Farms Breakfast Strip (cooked according to
    package's instructions)
1 slice Kraft 2% Milk Single
1 slice large ripe tomato
1 slice raw onion (optional)

Cook the Harvest Burger according to the package's instructions. Open the hamburger roll so that the 2 insides are face-up. Spread half the mayo on each side, spread half the ketchup on each side, and add 1 teaspoon of mustard to each side. Cut the bacon strip in 3 pieces and place them on 1 of the bun sides (the 1 that will be the bottom), along with a pinch of dill. Lay the cooked "burger" on the bacon. Unwrap the cheese and lay it on top of the burger, followed by the tomato slice and onion (if using). Carefully place the remaining bun half on top of the sandwich. Wrap the "burger" in a paper towel or wax paper and microwave on high for 20 seconds.

When making multiple sandwiches, lay all the buns out at once and add the condiments in the same way.

◆

These are fun to serve in wax paper. Rewrap them in a fresh sheet
after the final heating for an authentic drive-in diner experience.

Calorie Breakdown per Serving
Protein: 31.6%
Carbohydrate: 39.8%
Fat: 28.6%

Nutrition Totals per Serving

CALORIES:	357
PROTEIN:	29.3 grams
CARBOHYDRATE:	37.0 grams
FAT:	11.8 grams
SODIUM:	1,373 milligrams
CHOLESTEROL:	10 milligrams

"Beefy" Bean Burrito

YIELD: 1 BURRITO

1 burrito-sized flour tortilla (whole wheat or white)
¼ cup *PR* Deluxe Refried Beans (page 313)
¼ cup *PR* Mexican "Beef" (page 315)
2 tablespoons Alpine Lace Grated Skim Milk Cheddar Cheese
2 tablespoons Old El Paso Taco Sauce (hot or mild)
¼ cup diced tomato (if desired)
¼ cup diced onion (if desired)

Dip the tortilla in filtered water and lay it flat on a paper towel. Cover it with another paper towel and microwave it on high for 10–15 seconds. When the tortilla is cool enough to handle transfer it to a plate. Spread beans in the center. Top them with the "beef," cheese, taco sauce, and extra vegetables of your choice. Fold 2 sides in like a business letter, turn the plate a quarter turn, and repeat the folding process. Flip the burrito over so that the seams are on the bottom. Microwave it, covered with plastic, on medium for 30–60 seconds, then on high for 10–20 seconds, depending on how cold the fillings are. (The burrito can also be heated in a skillet coated with cooking spray or in the oven, wrapped in foil.)

This makes an appealing presentation when served with a side setup of shredded lettuce, diced tomato, *PR* Avocado Dressing Dip (page 288), *PR* Special Restaurant Salsa (page 244) in a ramekin, or *PR* Tex-Mex Brown Rice (page 322). Any or all of these will dress up the plate nicely and add to the flavor as well.

Calorie Breakdown per Serving
Protein: 23.0%
Carbohydrate: 59.8%
Fat: 17.2%

Nutrition Totals per Serving

CALORIES:	304
PROTEIN:	16.5 grams
CARBOHYDRATE:	42.9 grams
FAT:	5.5 grams
SODIUM:	1,140 milligrams
CHOLESTEROL:	2 milligrams

◆

Egg "Fu" Salad Sandwiches

YIELD: 4 SANDWICHES

6 hard-cooked egg whites
8 ounces Nasoya Firm Tofu
¼ teaspoon turmeric
¼ teaspoon mustard powder
¼ teaspoon sea salt
¼ cup Nasoya Nayonaise
1 tablespoon fresh lemon juice
¼ teaspoon Heinz Worcestershire Sauce
¼ teaspoon McIlhenny Tabasco Sauce
8 slices Pepperidge Farm Light Wheat Bread

Hold the cholesterol, bring on the soy. You've just found a healthier way to make this classic sandwich—and it's every bit as good to eat as the original.

To hard-boil the egg whites, place 6 eggs in the bottom of a saucepan, cover with cold water, and bring to a boil. Leave cover on and simmer the eggs for 15 minutes. Drain the water and allow the eggs to cool in ice water or the refrigerator. Discard the yolks and dice the whites into small pieces, then set them aside.

To make the egg "Fu" yolks, crumble 8 ounces of Nasoya Firm Tofu into a bowl. Add the turmeric, mustard powder, and salt. Stir to blend mixture. Set it aside.

To make the dressing, in a large mixing bowl combine Nayonaise, lemon juice, Worcestershire, and Tabasco. When all is thoroughly blended, add the egg whites and the "yolks" and toss them to coat them. Salt and pepper the dressing to taste.

Spread approximately ½ cup of the Egg "Fu" Salad on bread or toast, add tomato and lettuce if desired, and cover the salad with a second slice of bread. Slice the sandwich diagonally.

Calorie Breakdown per Serving	**Nutrition Totals per Serving**	
Protein: 30.5%	CALORIES;	205
Carbohydrate: 39.0%	PROTEIN:	15.5 grams
Fat: 30.5%	CARBOHYDRATE:	19.8 grams
	FAT:	6.9 grams
	SODIUM:	522 milligrams
	CHOLESTEROL:	0 milligrams

"Meatball" Oven Grinder Subs

YIELD: 4 SERVINGS

2 cups Green Giant Harvest Burgers For Recipes (at room temperature)

1/4 cup Progresso Plain Bread Crumbs

1 teaspoon sweet white onion flakes or dried minced onion

1/4 teaspoon herb seasoning such as Mrs. Dash

1/8 teaspoon garlic powder

1/8 teaspoon salt

1/8 teaspoon freshly ground black pepper

1 egg white

1/2 teaspoon Heinz Worcestershire Sauce

1 tablespoon *PR* Soy Milk Blend (page 294)

1 cup Classico Tomato and Basil Pasta Sauce

3/4 cup Healthy Choice Shredded Non Fat Mozzarella Cheese

2 tablespoons Lite & Less Grated Parmesan Cheese Substitute

4 *PR* Oat Bread sandwich rolls (page 266) or 4 6-inch whole-wheat sub rolls, unsliced

Preheat the oven to 450°F. Line an 8- or 9-inch baking dish with foil and coat it with cooking spray. In a medium bowl, combine ground "meat," bread crumbs, onion, herb seasoning, garlic powder, salt, pepper, egg white, Worcestershire sauce, 1/4 cup pasta sauce and soy milk. Shape mixture into 12 balls and place them into the foil-lined pan. Bake the balls for 8–10 minutes, then remove them. Turn the oven down to 350°F.

Warm the remaining spaghetti sauce over medium heat. Arrange the bread on a foil-lined baking sheet. Slice out a 2-inch–wide and 1-inch–deep trough in the center of each roll, stopping 1 inch from the ends. Spoon a little sauce and some shredded mozzarella on each roll. Place three "meatballs" per sandwich into the premade holes. Cover the "meatballs" with a little more sauce, then top them with more mozzarella cheese and a sprinkling of the Parmesan cheese substitute. Bake the subs in a 350°F oven for 5–10 minutes. If you wish, finish cooking them under the broiler till cheese starts to brown slightly.

Make spaghetti and "meatballs" with these, too! Heat them up with some extra pasta sauce and ladle over al dente Contadina Protein

Enriched Pasta. Serve with *PR* Oat Bread garlic rolls (page 266) and a salad with *PR* Creamy Garlic Dip dressing (page 289), or *PR* Annato Vinaigrette (page 287) and you have an Italian feast that follows the rules.

Calorie Breakdown per Serving

Protein: 30.9%
Carbohydrate: 63.4%
Fat: 5.8%

Nutrition Totals per Serving

CALORIES:	380
PROTEIN:	29.2 grams
CARBOHYDRATE:	60.0 grams
FAT:	2.4 grams
SODIUM:	1,671 milligrams
CHOLESTEROL:	3 milligrams

Po' Boy Sandwich ("Chicken" Style)

YIELD: 4 SANDWICHES

4 whole-wheat sub rolls or *PR* Oat Bread sandwich rolls (page
    266)
16 (One Package) Morningstar Farms Chik Nuggets
½ teaspoon Creole seasoning (1 whole teaspoon for extra
    spicy)
1 recipe *PR* Nothing Lost Tartar Sauce (page 292)
½ cup shredded lettuce
1 medium ripe tomato, thinly sliced

One of the major fast-food restaurants served a sandwich similar to this one a few years back. It still tastes delicious, but in this form, it's good for you.

Prepare the tartar sauce. Cover it and chill it.

Cook the "chicken" pieces according to package instructions (preferably in the microwave). While they're still warm, place them into a large heat-proof plastic bag along with the Creole seasoning, then close the bag securely and shake it. Open the bag so it can breathe and set it aside.

Slice open the sub or sandwich rolls and scoop out a portion of the bottom halves to make room for the sandwich fillings.

Spread tartar sauce on both halves of each roll and lay 4 "chicken" pieces widthwise in each premade trough. Top the pieces with tomato and shredded lettuce. Close each sandwich with 2 toothpicks and slice it in half on an angle.

Calorie Breakdown per Serving	Nutrition Totals per Serving	
Protein: 22.5%	CALORIES:	395
Carbohydrate: 54.3%	PROTEIN:	22.9 grams
Fat: 23.2%	CARBOHYDRATE:	55.4 grams
	FAT:	10.5 grams
	SODIUM:	1,178 milligrams
	CHOLESTEROL:	0 milligrams

◆

Triple-Decker Club

YIELD: 1 SANDWICH (2 SERVINGS)

3 slices Pepperidge Farm Light Wheat Bread (lightly toasted)
2 teaspoons Heinz tomato ketchup
4 leaves lettuce
1 Morningstar Farms Breakfast Strip, cooked according to
    package instructions and cut in half
1 Slice White Wave Meatless Chicken Style Sandwich Slices
2 slices large ripe tomato
2 slices Soya Kaas Monterey Jack Style Cheese Substitute, ⅛-
    inch thick each
2 tablespoons *PR* Avocado Dressing Dip (page 288)
4 teaspoons Hellman's Reduced Fat Mayonnaise (1 gram of fat
    per serving)
1 slice Kraft 2% Milk Singles
2 slices Lightlife Meatless Smart Deli Country Ham
4 toothpicks

Arrange all the ingredients, including the toasted bread, in front
of you. Build the sandwich in the following order:

- 1 slice bread
- Ketchup
- 2 leaves lettuce
- Breakfast Strip (2 halves side by side)
- "Chicken"
- 1 slice tomato
- "Monterey Jack Cheese" (2 slices side by side)
- Avocado Dressing Dip
- 1 slice bread
- 2 teaspoons mayo
- 2 leaves lettuce
- "American cheese"
- 2 slices "ham"
- 1 slice tomato
- 2 teaspoons mayo
- 1 slice bread

Stick the toothpicks all the way through the sandwich layers in the center of what will become the 4 triangles. Cut the sandwich diagonally with a sharp knife, crossing in the middle. Arrange 2 wedges per plate with the crust side down and the corners sticking up. Serve sandwiches with fat-free chips and *PR* Black-Eyed Salsa (page 279) if desired.

Calorie Breakdown per Serving	Nutrition Totals per Serving	
Protein: 28.0%	CALORIES:	235
Carbohydrate: 41.8%	PROTEIN:	17.2 grams
Fat: 30.2%	CARBOHYDRATE:	25.7 grams
	FAT:	8.3 grams
	SODIUM:	839 milligrams
	CHOLESTEROL:	6 milligrams

BREADS

Aunt Jean's Zucchini Bread

YIELD: 16 SLICES

1 cup zucchini squash, shredded, with skin on
3 egg whites
1 cup sugar
½ cup plus 2 tablespoons Sunsweet Lighter Bake Butter and
    Oil Replacement
3 tablespoons smooth organic peanut butter (choose a peanut
    butter that is aflatoxin-free, such as the one made by
    Whole Foods Market)
1 tablespoon Hain Expeller Pressed Canola Oil
1 teaspoon pure vanilla extract
1 cup unbleached all-purpose flour
½ cup Arrowhead Mills Organic Whole Grain Soy Flour
1 teaspoon Arrowhead Mills Vital Wheat Gluten
½ teaspoon baking powder
½ teaspoon baking soda
1½ teaspoons ground cinnamon
¼ cup chopped walnuts (optional)

Preheat oven to 325°F. In a bowl, beat together zucchini, eggs, sugar, Lighter Bake, peanut butter, oil, and vanilla, till blended thoroughly. In another bowl, combine flours, wheat gluten, baking powder, baking soda, cinnamon, and nuts (if using). Gradually add dry ingredients to the zucchini mixture. Blend them thoroughly. Coat a 12-inch × 3-inch loaf pan with cooking spray. Pour in batter and smooth top. Bake bread for 1 hour to 1 hour 10 minutes. Bread is done when a toothpick inserted in the center comes out with a few crumbs.

A crack may form on the top of the loaf. Although this will not affect the bread, it can be lessened by loosely covering the pan with foil for the last 20 minutes of baking.

This bread is delicious sliced thinly and toasted. Spread with a little nonfat cream cheese or a thin layer of Land O'Lakes Light Butter, if desired. Tastes equally good for breakfast, snack time, or dessert.

Calorie Breakdown per Serving		Nutrition Totals per Serving	
Protein:	9.2%	CALORIES:	143
Carbohydrate:	68.1%	PROTEIN:	3.4 grams
Fat:	22.7%	CARBOHYDRATE:	25.4 grams
		FAT:	3.8 grams
		SODIUM:	52 milligrams
		CHOLESTEROL:	0 milligrams

Buttermilk Biscuits

YIELD: 10 SERVINGS

These go well with PR Robert's Favorite Omelet and PR "Chicken" Nuggets (drizzled with honey). They are also called for in the PR Biscuits 'n' "Sausage" recipe.

1 ½ cups unbleached all-purpose flour
¼ cup whole wheat flour
¼ Arrowhead Mills Organic Whole Grain Soy Flour
1 tablespoon baking powder
¼ teaspoon baking soda
2 teaspoons sugar
½ teaspoon cream of tartar
1 teaspoon Arrowhead Mills Wheat Gluten
¼ teaspoon sea salt
2 tablespoons Land O'Lakes Light Butter
2 tablespoons Sun Sweet Lighter Bake Butter and Oil
    Replacement
⅔ cup 1% Buttermilk

Preheat oven to 425°F. In a bowl stir together flours, baking powder, baking soda, sugar, cream of tartar, wheat gluten, and salt. Cut in butter and Lighter Bake until mixture resembles coarse crumbs. Make a well in the center; pour in buttermilk all at once. Stir just until dough sticks together.

On a lighly floured surface knead dough for about 12 strokes. Roll or pat out to ½-inch thickness. Cut with a 2½-inch biscuit cutter, or use a clean empty can (open on both ends) approximately 2½ inches in diameter.

Transfer biscuits to a baking sheet. Bake for 10 to 12 minutes.

Calorie Breakdown per Serving	Nutrition Totals per Serving	
Protein: 13.5%	CALORIES:	109
Carbohydrate: 69.8%	PROTEIN:	3.8 grams
Fat: 16.7%	CARBOHYDRATE:	19.5 grams
	FAT:	2.1 grams
	SODIUM:	317 milligrams
	CHOLESTEROL:	5 milligrams

Cheddar Jalapeño Corn Muffins

YIELD: 12 SERVINGS

1 cup unbleached all-purpose flour
½ cup Quaker Yellow Corn Meal
¼ cup Bob's Red Mill Golden Corn Masa Flour
⅓ cup sugar
2 teaspoons baking powder
1 teaspoon Arrowhead Mills Vital Wheat Gluten
¼ teaspoon sea salt
2 beaten egg whites
¾ cup *PR* Soy Milk Blend (page 294)
2 tablespoons Sunsweet Lighter Bake Butter and Oil
    Replacement
1 tablespoon Hain Canola Oil
½ cup Green Giant Extra Sweet Niblets Corn (thawed if frozen)
⅓ cup Alpine Lace Grated Skim Milk Cheddar Cheese
1 heaping tablespoon finely minced jalapeño pepper, seeded
    and rinsed

Preheat oven to 400°F. Combine flour, corn meal, corn flour, sugar, baking powder, wheat gluten, and salt. Make a well in the center. In another bowl, combine eggs, soy milk, Lighter Bake, and oil, then add all at once to flour mixture. Stir mixture just till moistened, making sure to incorporate all the corn meal and flour. Add corn, cheese, and peppers, distributing them evenly, but don't overmix. Coat 12 muffin cups with olive-oil cooking spray. Fill with batter to just below the rim. Bake 20 minutes or till golden. Serve warm.

Freeze the muffins that you're not going to use right away in a good freezer bag while they're slightly warm. Reheat them in the microwave, wrapped in plastic or in a 350°F oven, wrapped in foil, for fresh-baked muffins anytime.

Calorie Breakdown per Serving	Nutrition Totals per Serving	
Protein: 12.7%	CALORIES:	116
Carbohydrate: 74.7%	PROTEIN:	3.8 grams
Fat: 12.7%	CARBOHYDRATE:	22.3 grams
	FAT:	1.7 grams
	SODIUM:	166 milligrams
	CHOLESTEROL:	0 milligrams

Mandarin Orange Muffins

YIELD: 12 SERVINGS

1 cup unbleached all-purpose flour

½ cup whole-wheat flour

⅓ cup sugar

2 teaspoons baking powder

2 egg whites

⅓ cup *PR* Soy Milk Blend (page 294)

⅓ cup Tropicana Pure Premium Orange Juice

1 tablespoon orange oil *or* 1 tablespoon canola oil and 1
     teaspoon orange extract

2 tablespoons Sunsweet Lighter Bake Butter and Oil
     Replacement

1 teaspoon dried orange peel *or* 1 teaspoon orange zest*

11-ounce can mandarin orange slices in light syrup, drained

Preheat oven to 350°F. In a mixing bowl, combine flours, sugar, and baking powder. Make a well in the center. In another bowl, combine egg whites, soy milk, orange juice, orange oil, Lighter Bake, and peel or zest. Add wet mixture all at once to dry mixture. Stir it just until moistened. Set aside 12 of the orange slices and add the rest to the batter. Stir the batter to blend. Don't worry if the orange sections break apart. Coat 12 muffin cups with olive-oil cooking spray. Fill each cup evenly with batter. Top with 1 reserved orange slice per cup. Bake 20 minutes or till muffins are done. Drizzle the tops with honey if you wish.

Freeze the muffins you're not going to use immediately in a good freezer bag while they're slightly warm. Reheat them in the microwave, wrapped in plastic, or in a 350°F oven, wrapped in foil, for fresh-baked muffins anytime.

Calorie Breakdown per Serving	Nutrition Totals per Serving	
Protein: 9.5%	CALORIES:	111
Carbohydrate: 78.6%	PROTEIN:	2.7 grams
Fat: 11.9%	CARBOHYDRATE:	22.4 grams
	FAT:	1.5 grams
	SODIUM:	85 milligrams
	CHOLESTEROL:	0 milligrams

*If you're not frequently in the kitchen, you need to know that zest is finely ground orange peel, used as flavoring.

Menopause Muffins

YIELD: 12 SERVINGS

2½ cups whole-wheat flour
1 package active dry yeast
¾ cup 1% cottage cheese
3 tablespoons packed brown sugar
2 tablespoons Land O'Lakes Light Butter
⅓ cup *PR* Soy Milk Blend (page 294)
2 egg whites
½ teaspoon sea salt
2 Morningstar Farms Breakfast Strips, cut into small pieces
    (optional)
2 tablespoons flaxseeds

Combine 1½ cups flour and the yeast. Heat and stir cottage cheese, soy milk, brown sugar, butter, and salt till warm and butter almost melts, then add these ingredients to the flour mixture along with eggs and Breakfast Strips "bacon," if using. Beat the mixture with an electric mixer on low speed for 30 seconds, scraping bowl constantly. Then beat it on high speed for 2 minutes. Using a spoon, stir in as much of the remaining flour as you can.

Turn the batter out onto a lightly floured surface. Knead in enough remaining flour to make a moderately stiff dough that is smooth and elastic (8–10 minutes total). Shape the dough into a ball. Place it in a bowl coated with cooking spray. Cover the bowl with plastic wrap; let the dough rise in a warm place till it doubles in size (30–45 minutes).

Preheat oven to 375°F. Punch the dough down. Turn it out onto a lightly floured surface. Cover it and let it rest 10 minutes. Shape it into 12 smooth balls. Place the flaxseeds in a small shallow dish. Dip the top of each ball into warm soy milk, then into the seeds (you may add some coarse sea salt to the seed mixture if you wish). Place the dough in muffin tins that have been coated with cooking spray. Cover the dough and let it rise 20 more minutes. Bake the muffins for 10–12 minutes.

These are a little more work than most muffins, but they're good—and good for you! The kneading of the dough doubles as your weight-resistance exercise of the day.

Menopause Muffins make the perfect afternoon snack. They can also serve as dinner rolls for many of the *Permanent Remissions* entrées. Men will love them, too! Try making mini "ham" or "chicken" sandwiches with Lightlife meatless deli slices. Don't forget to freeze what muffins you won't be using right away so that you can have them ready for reheating anytime.

Calorie Breakdown per Serving	Nutrition Totals per Serving	
Protein: 20.5%	CALORIES:	142
Carbohydrate: 61.7%	PROTEIN:	7.2 grams
Fat: 17.8%	CARBOHYDRATE:	21.6 grams
	FAT:	2.8 grams
	SODIUM:	195 milligrams
	CHOLESTEROL:	4 milligrams

Oat Bread (Baguettes and Rolls)

YIELD: 2 BAGUETTES, 4 SANDWICH ROLLS, 12 DINNER ROLLS, OR
18 GARLIC ROLLS—RECIPE PROVIDES 8 SERVINGS

1½–2 cups unbleached all-purpose flour
1 package active dry yeast
1 teaspoon Arrowhead Mills Vital Wheat Gluten
1½ teaspoons sea salt
½ cup Arrowhead Mills Organic Oat Flour
1 cup warm filtered water (120°–130°F)
1 egg white
2 tablespoons *PR* Soy Milk Blend (page 294)
2 tablespoons Quaker Yellow Corn Meal

In a large mixng bowl, combine 1 cup of the all-purpose flour, yeast, wheat gluten, and salt. Add the cup of warm water and beat the mixture with an electric mixer on low for 30 seconds, scraping down the bowl constantly. Beat the mixture on high speed for 2 minutes. Stir in the oat flour with a spoon. When it is thoroughly combined, stir in ¼–½ cup more of the all-purpose flour or as much as the dough will take on.

Turn out the dough onto a lightly floured surface. Knead in enough all-purpose flour to make a stiff, elastic dough. The dough should remain somewhat sticky (don't add too much flour or the bread will be dry). Continue kneading it for about 5 minutes, dusting your hands with flour as needed to prevent sticking. Shape the dough into a ball. Place it into a bowl coated with olive-oil cooking spray. Turn it once to coat dough with oil. Cover it and let it rise in a warm place till doubled (about 1 hour).

Punch the dough down and turn it out onto a lightly floured surface. Divide it into the appropriate number of pieces (see below). Cover it and let it rest 10 minutes.

- For baguettes: 10-inch tapered loaves (2 each)
- For sandwich rolls: 5-inch tapered loaves (4 each)
- For dinner rolls: round balls (12 each)
- For garlic rolls: small round balls (18 each)

Shape the dough according to which size you have chosen. Coat a baking sheet or sided pan (for rolls) with olive-oil cooking spray and dust with cornmeal. Combine egg white and soy milk and brush the mixture over loaves. Cover the dough and let it rise till nearly doubled (35–45 minutes). With a very sharp knife, make several diagonal cuts about ¼ inch deep into the baguettes, or 1 cut down the middle (lengthwise) of the sandwich rolls, or X's on the dinner rolls. The garlic rolls should remain uncut until the end of baking.

Bake the bread in a 375°F oven for 12 minutes for dinner rolls and garlic rolls, 15 minutes for sandwich rolls, or 20 minutes for baguette loaves. Brush the bread again with egg and soy mixture. Continue baking it for 10–15 more minutes or till bread tests done. (It is helpful to have a spray bottle filled with filtered water, to "steam" the bread every few minutes during the second half of the baking. Open the oven door and spray the bread 4 or 5 times with the nozzle set on the mist setting).

You will really enjoy sandwiches made on these oat rolls. Be sure to use the Whitewave and Lightlife meatless sandwich slices of your choice and Kraft Fat Free Singles or Soya Kaas Soy Cheeses for a healthy deli experience.

The smaller homemade oat rolls go beautifully with any of the *Permanent Remissions* soup selections. Or you can slice yourself a piece off the baguette, if that's what you decide to make.

Remember, except for the garlic rolls, this bread is made without any fats or oils. It should be eaten the day of baking or frozen for later use.

Calorie Breakdown per Serving
Protein: 14.2%
Carbohydrate: 80.1%
Fat: 5.8%

Nutrition Totals per Serving
CALORIES: 108
PROTEIN: 3.8 grams
CARBOHYDRATE: 21.6 grams
FAT: 0.7 grams
SODIUM: 439 milligrams
CHOLESTEROL: 0 milligrams

TO MAKE THE GARLIC ROLLS:

Combine 3 tablespoons Bertolli Extra Light Olive Oil with 3 cloves of minced garlic. Heat it in the microwave 20–30 seconds on high. Remove the rolls from the oven a few minutes early; prick all 18 rolls several times each with a fork and pour oil-and-garlic mixture over them for the last few minutes of baking. Try to distribute the garlic as evenly as possible.

Calorie Breakdown per Serving		Nutrition Totals per Serving	
Protein:	10.0%	CALORIES:	69
Carbohydrate:	56.6%	PROTEIN:	1.7 grams
Fat:	33.5%	CARBOHYDRATE:	9.8 grams
		FAT:	2.6 grams
		SODIUM:	196 milligrams
		CHOLESTEROL:	0 milligrams

Tuscan Garlic Bread

YIELD: 10 PIECES

1 loaf *PR* Oat Bread (page 266), baguette size, cut into 10
  slices, *or* 1 small loaf French bread (multigrain if possible),
  cut into 10 slices, *or* 1 regular-size piece whole-wheat pita
  pocket bread, split open and cut into 10 or 12 triangles
2 tablespoons Bertolli Extra Light Olive Oil
2 garlic cloves, minced
¼ teaspoon garlic powder
¼ teaspoon sea salt
1 teaspoon dried oregano, crushed
Freshly ground black pepper
1 tablespoon Soyco Lite & Less Grated Parmesan Cheese
  Substitute
1 teaspoon sesame seeds

Slice the bread into 1-inch-thick rounds. Don't use the ends of the loaf. Combine oil, garlic, garlic powder, and salt in a small dish. With a basting brush, swipe the top of each bread round (or pita triangle) with the mixture, making sure to scoop up the minced garlic. Arrange the slices closely together on a baking sheet covered with foil. Sprinkle them with oregano, pepper, soy cheese, sesame seeds, and a pinch more salt. Broil the bread till it is golden and bubbling.

Calorie Breakdown per Serving
Protein: 9.3%
Carbohydrate: 48.5%
Fat: 42.2%

Nutrition Totals per Serving
CALORIES: 64
PROTEIN: 1.5 grams
CARBOHYDRATE: 7.9 grams
FAT: 3.0 grams
SODIUM: 216 milligrams
CHOLESTEROL: 0 milligrams

Whole-Wheat Croutons

YIELD: 8 SERVINGS; SERVING SIZE: 1 TABLESPOON

3 Slices Pepperidge Farm Very Thin Wheat Bread
1 tablespoon Land O'Lakes Light Butter, at room temperature
¼ teaspoon garlic powder
1 teaspoon sesame seeds (optional)

Preheat oven to 300°F. Spread a thin layer of softened butter on both sides of the bread slices. Sprinkle the bread slices with garlic powder on both sides and place them on a baking pan or sided baking sheet covered with foil. Distribute the seeds over the bread, if using them, and press them with the back of a spoon or spatula so that they stick to the bread. Bake bread for 10 minutes. Remove it from the oven and cut it with kitchen scissors into ½-inch to 1-inch squares. Place bread squares back onto the foil. Return the pan to the oven and bake for 15 more minutes. Shake the pan every 5 minutes or so to redistribute the croutons to toast them evenly. (It may be necessary to use an egg-white wash in order to hold all the sesame seeds in place.)

For plumper croutons, substitute Pepperidge Farm Light Style Wheat Bread.

These croutons are used on the *PR* Spinach Salad with Warm "Bacon" Dressing (page 283). Try them on a variety of salads.

Calorie Breakdown per Serving	Nutrition Totals per Serving	
Protein: 11.7%	CALORIES:	22
Carbohydrate: 45.6%	PROTEIN:	0.7 grams
Fat: 42.7%	CARBOHYDRATE:	2.8 grams
	FAT:	1.2 grams
	SODIUM:	38 milligrams
	CHOLESTEROL:	3 milligrams

SOUPS

Pasta e Fagiole

YIELD: 7 CUPS

1 tablespoon Bertolli Extra Light Olive Oil
1 cup dried cannellini or Great Northern beans, picked
    through, rinsed, and soaked overnight
¾ cup chopped carrots
¾ cup chopped celery
¾ cup chopped onion
2 cloves garlic, minced
¼ teaspoon sea salt
¼ teaspoon freshly ground black pepper
14½-ounce can Del Monte Fresh Cut Diced Tomatoes,
    undrained
3 ounces or about 6 slices Lightlife Meatless Smart Deli
    Country Ham
4 cups vegetable stock made with 2 cubes of bouillon, such as
    Morga Vegetable Bouillon with Sea Salt
3 sprigs fresh thyme
1 bay leaf
Rind of hard Italian Parmesan cheese wedge (slice the rind off
    the block of cheese)
1 cup dry small tube-shaped pasta noodles (tubettini or
    ditalini)

Heat oil in a Dutch oven or a large pot. Add carrots, celery, onion, and garlic. Sauté vegetables till they are tender. Add salt, pepper, drained beans, tomatoes, "ham," vegetable stock, thyme, bay leaf, and rind. Simmer the soup in covered pot for 1 hour, stirring occasionally.

Cook the pasta according to the package's instructions. After draining the pasta, lower the colander into warm water to keep pasta ready to use. Remove the thyme sprigs, bay leaf, and cheese rind from the pot. Bring a hand-held immersion blender to the pot and blend most of the solid into a smooth purée, or remove 1 cup of the bean mixture and set it aside while you purée the rest of the soup in a food processor or blender. Return the blended liquid to the pot along with the cup of bean mixture and bring it back to the desired temperature. Ladle soup into bowls and top with $1/4-1/2$ cup drained pasta and chopped fresh basil. Mix the soup before eating it.

Note: The beans should be tender before they are added to the soup. If they are still too firm after soaking overnight, heat them in fresh water on the stove (covered) while you prepare the other ingredients. They should be soft enough by the time you're ready for them.

When storing the soup, keep the pasta separated from the rest of the soup. The pasta will lose its texture if it is left with the liquid. Rinse the pasta with warm water and serve it over reheated soup or make a small fresh batch.

Thanks to David Rosengarten of the TV Food Network for his inspiration in this recipe.

Calorie Breakdown per Serving
Protein: 24.3%
Carbohydrate: 59.8%
Fat: 15.9%

Nutrition Totals per Serving

CALORIES:	206
PROTEIN:	12.0 grams
CARBOHYDRATE:	29.6 grams
FAT:	3.5 grams
SODIUM:	584 milligrams
CHOLESTEROL:	1 milligrams

Red Lentil Soup (Right Away)

YIELD: 10 CUPS

14½-ounce can Del Monte Fresh Cut Diced Tomatoes
2 cups red lentils
¼ cup Old El Paso Chopped Green Chilies
1 package (tube) Manischewitz Split Pea Soup Mix with Barley
8 cups filtered water

In a Dutch oven or large pot, begin heating the water on a medium-high setting. Rinse the lentils and add them to the pot along with the tomatoes. Bring the mixture to a boil. Reduce heat. Cover the pot and simmer the mixture for 10 minutes, stirring once midway through.

Open the package of pea soup at the end where the flavor packet is. Carefully remove the packet and set it aside. Separate the red and green peas from the white barley. You can do this by pinching the tube before the barley and letting the peas drop out into a cup, then pinching the tube after the barley and letting it fall out into another cup. A few stray peas in the barley won't matter. Save the separated peas for another use.

When the soup has simmered 10 minutes or so, open the flavor packet and add the contents to the pot along with the barley and chilies. Let the mixture simmer another 10–30 minutes. The longer, the better, but if you're in a hurry, it will be soup in 10 more minutes, guaranteed.

How about serving this with one of the *Permanent Remissions* breads or muffins you made on a day when you *did* have the time? They can defrost in the microwave or conventional oven while you make the soup.

Green lentils are not interchangeable with red lentils in this recipe because they are larger and take longer to cook.

Calorie Breakdown per Serving	Nutrition Totals per Serving	
Protein: 27.3%	CALORIES:	134
Carbohydrate: 71.5%	PROTEIN:	8.8 grams
Fat: 1.3%	CARBOHYDRATE:	23.1 grams
	FAT:	0.2 grams
	SODIUM:	474 milligrams
	CHOLESTEROL:	0 milligrams

Rio Grande Pinto Bean Soup

YIELD: 8 SERVINGS; SERVING SIZE: 1 CUP

1 tablespoon Bertolli Extra Light Olive Oil
¼ cup onion, diced
1 cup celery, diced
2 cloves garlic, minced
1 teaspoon freshly ground black pepper
14½-ounce can Hunt's Choice Cut Tomatoes with Roasted
     Garlic
1 medium baking potato, peeled and sliced into 1-inch rounds
2 15-ounce cans Progresso pinto beans (drained)
5 cups filtered water
6 slices Morningstar Farms Breakfast Strips, cut into 1-inch
     pieces
1½ teaspoons McIlhenny Tabasco Sauce
1 teaspoon ground cumin
6 ounces nonalcoholic beer
8 3-inch sprigs fresh cilantro

You can get soup similar to this one in a legendary New York restaurant, but you can bet they put real bacon in it. Enjoy the similarity in taste of this version while you benefit from the substituted ingredients.

Heat oil in a large pot or Dutch oven over medium heat. Add the onion, celery, garlic, and black pepper, and sauté till the mixture is tender. Add potato slices, undrained tomatoes, beans, and water, then stir. Add the Breakfast Strips "bacon," Tabasco, cumin, beer, and 4 sprigs of cilantro. Stir the mixture to combine and cover the pot. Simmer the soup over low heat for 45 minutes, stirring occasionally.

With a slotted spoon, ladle as many of the potato pieces as possible and some of the bean, tomato, and "bacon" mixture into the bowl of a blender or food processor. Blend the mixture till it is smooth but not overblended. Return the mixture to the pot along with 4 more sprigs of cilantro. Stir the soup, cover the pot, and simmer the soup for 20 more minutes.

Calorie Breakdown per Serving
Protein: 17.4%
Carbohydrate: 60.8%
Fat: 21.9%

Nutrition Totals per Serving

CALORIES:	162
PROTEIN:	6.9 grams
CARBOHYDRATE:	24.3 grams
FAT:	3.9 grams
SODIUM:	780 milligrams
CHOLESTEROL:	0 milligrams

♦

Southwestern Corn Chowder

YIELD: 6 SERVINGS; SERVING SIZE: 1 CUP

2 teaspoons Bertolli Extra Light Olive Oil

¾ cup celery, diced

⅓ cup chopped scallion (white and green parts)

¼ cup Old El Paso Chopped Green Chilies

⅛ teaspoon white pepper

1 teaspoon sea salt

⅛ teaspoon freshly ground black pepper

¼ teaspoon turmeric

Dash red pepper

Dash paprika

1 tablespoon chopped fresh cilantro leaves

4 cups *PR* Soy Milk Blend (page 294)

4 slices Morningstar Farms Breakfast Strips, thawed and diced

2 tablespoons Argo Corn Starch dissolved in ¼ cup cold water

2 tablespoons Bob's Red Mill Golden Corn Masa Flour
   dissolved in ¼ cup warm water

2½ cups Green Giant Frozen Extra Sweet Niblets Corn rinsed
   with warm water in colander

Heat the oil in a Dutch oven or large pot. Add the celery and scallions and sauté them until they're tender. Add the chilies, white pepper, salt, black pepper, red pepper, paprika, tumeric, and cilantro. Pour in the milk and add the Breakfast Strips. Cook the mixture over medium heat till it's simmering. Add the cornstarch mixture, then gradually add the masa. Add the corn and bring the chowder to a rolling boil. Turn the heat to low. Cover and simmer 15 minutes, stirring occasionally.

This rich and flavorful chowder is even better with a teaspoon or two of sweet vermouth mixed into each cup.

Calorie Breakdown per Serving	Nutrition Totals per Serving	
Protein: 16.0%	CALORIES:	183
Carbohydrate: 62.3%	PROTEIN:	7.6 grams
Fat: 21.7%	CARBOHYDRATE:	29.6 grams
	FAT:	4.6 grams
	SODIUM:	577 milligrams
	CHOLESTEROL:	0 milligrams

Sweet-and-Sour Cabbage Soup with "Beef"

YIELD: 8 SERVINGS; SIZE: 1 CUP

1 tablespoon Bertolli Extra Light Olive Oil

1 cup onion, diced

6 cups sliced red cabbage, core removed

2 garlic cloves, minced

2 tablespoons brown sugar

1/4 cup balsamic vinegar

1 cup diced tomatoes, seeds removed

6 cups vegetable broth made with 3 cubes of Morga Vegetable
    Bouillon with Sea Salt (or equivalent)

1 1/2 cups Green Giant Harvest Burgers for Recipes

In a Dutch oven or large pot, heat the oil and add the onion and garlic. Sauté onion and garlic till they're tender. Add the cabbage and tomatoes and stir the mixture. Add the broth, brown sugar, and vinegar; heat everything to a near boil. Reduce the heat and cover the pot. Simmer the soup for 20–30 minutes, stirring occasionally. Add the Harvest Burger "beef" and simmer the soup for another 20–30 minutes, stirring it occasionally.

If you like less cabbage in your soup, you may remove some of the strips before adding the "beef." The cabbage will already have filled the broth with its share of phytonutrients.

Calorie Breakdown per Serving		Nutrition Totals per Serving	
Protein:	25.7%	CALORIES:	86
Carbohydrate:	49.0%	PROTEIN:	5.7 grams
Fat:	25.3%	CARBOHYDRATE:	10.9 grams
		FAT:	2.5 grams
		SODIUM:	489 milligrams
		CHOLESTEROL:	0 milligrams

Tomato Rice Soup

YIELD: 6 SERVINGS

28-ounce can Progresso Crushed Tomatoes With Added Puree
¼ cup unbleached all-purpose flour
½ cup Karo Light Corn Syrup
1 tablespoon Bertolli Extra Light Olive Oil
¼ teaspoon sea salt
2 cups *PR* Soy Milk Blend (page 294)
1 tablespoon dry onion flakes
1 cup cooked Rice Select Teximati Brown Rice or Basmati Rice

You've experienced this taste before. Can you place it? Here's a hint: you probably weren't very tall. There is a difference, though. If you had been served this version regularly back then, you'd be better off for it today.

Combine the tomatoes, flour, corn syrup, oil, and salt in a food processor or blender till smooth. Empty the contents into a saucepan and add soy milk. Bring the mixture to a boil, then reduce heat. Add the onion flakes. Let the mixture simmer approximately 10 minutes, stirring it occasionally. Add the rice and cook 5 more minutes.

Calorie Breakdown per Serving	Nutrition Totals per Serving	
Protein: 10.8%	CALORIES:	208
Carbohydrate: 75.3%	PROTEIN:	5.8 grams
Fat: 13.9%	CARBOHYDRATE:	40.8 grams
	FAT:	3.3 grams
	SODIUM:	260 milligrams
	CHOLESTEROL:	0 milligrams

SALADS

Black-Eyed Salsa

2 cups frozen black-eyed peas, cooked till tender (or canned)
1 cup red onion, diced
1 cup tomato, diced and seeded (drained if canned)
2 tablespoons fresh cilantro leaves
1 heaping tablespoon jalapeño pepper, diced, seeds and
    ridges removed
1 teaspoon ground cumin
1 teaspoon sea salt
¼ cup fresh lemon juice
3 tablespoons balsamic vinegar

Blend all the ingredients except the peas in a blender or food processor (don't liquefy them). Pour the mixture over the peas in a mixing bowl and stir to coat the peas. For best flavor, chill the salsa, covered, overnight and then let it warm slightly before serving.

Calorie Breakdown per Serving
Protein: 21.3%
Carbohydrate: 73.2%
Fat: 5.6%

Nutrition Totals per Serving

CALORIES:	76
PROTEIN:	4.2 grams
CARBOHYDRATE:	14.6 grams
FAT:	0.5 grams
SODIUM:	294 milligrams
CHOLESTEROL:	0 milligrams

♦

Cajun Coleslaw (and Dressing)

YIELD: 6 SERVINGS

Slaw:
2 cups white cabbage, shredded
½ cup red cabbage, shredded
½ cup carrots, shredded

Cajun dressing:
1 tablespoon Bertolli Extra Light Olive Oil
⅓ cup Heinz tomato ketchup
1 tablespoon sugar
1 tablespoon white wine vinegar
2 tablespoons *PR* Soy Milk Blend (page 294)
2 tablespoons Sunsweet Lighter Bake Butter and Oil
    Replacement
1 tablespoon fresh lemon juice
1 teaspoon Worcestershire sauce
½ teaspoon celery seeds (optional)
½ teaspoon paprika
¼ teaspoon sea salt
⅛ teaspoon freshly ground black pepper
⅛–¼ teaspoon red pepper

Place the white and red cabbage, along with the carrots, into a large mixing bowl. Set it aside.

Add the rest of the ingredients to another bowl and stir them to combine. Pour the mixture over the cabbage and carrots and toss to coat the cabbage. Cover and chill the slaw.

For convenience, you may also use preshredded slaw available in the produce section of most grocery stores. Use 3 cups per batch of coleslaw.

Try the spicy dressing as a dipping sauce for the *PR* Shrimp Wrapped in "Bacon" (page 243) and the *PR* "Chicken" Nuggets (page 239), or instead of ketchup on the *PR* "Bacon" Cheese"burger" (page 249). It also makes a nice dressing poured over a wedge of head lettuce topped with *PR* Whole-Wheat Croutons (page 270).

Calorie Breakdown per Serving
Protein: 5.4%
Carbohydrate: 66.1%
Fat: 28.5%

Nutrition Totals per Serving
CALORIES: 76
PROTEIN: 1.1 grams
CARBOHYDRATE: 13.4 grams
FAT: 2.6 grams
SODIUM: 263 milligrams
CHOLESTEROL: 0 milligrams

Pita Salad Sandwich

YIELD: 4 SANDWICHES

4 pieces regular-size whole-wheat pita pocket bread
3 cups chopped head lettuce (or salad greens of your choice)
3 medium carrots, shredded
1 tablespoon plus 1 teaspoon raw sunflower seeds, without
    shells
¾ cup Healthy Choice Non Fat Grated Cheddar Cheese
½ cup green pepper, cut julienne style (optional)
¾ cup *PR* Creamy Garlic Dip (page 289)

In a medium bowl, combine lettuce, carrots, seeds, cheese, and green pepper (if using). Add the dressing dip and toss the salad to coat it. Set it aside.

Wet the pitas with filtered water, wrap them in a paper towel and heat each of them separately in the microwave on high for 10–15 seconds. When they are cool enough to handle, cut a 4-inch opening in the side seam of each. Spoon ¼ of the salad mixture into the opening of each pocket and press the seam closed.

Customize this sandwich with the fresh vegetables of your choice. For a Middle Eastern flavor, try this Pita Salad Sandwich with lettuce, onion, tomato, and 3 Morningstar Farms "Chik" Nuggets heated according to package instructions. To season, combine 1 tablespoon Fantastic Foods Falafel mix with warm "Chik" Nuggets in a plastic bag and shake the bag till the nuggets are coated.

Although the Pita Salad Sandwiches will keep a short while in the refrigerator if they are wrapped in foil or plastic, they are best eaten right away to avoid wilted lettuce.

Calorie Breakdown per Serving
Protein: 34.9%
Carbohydrate: 45.2%
Fat: 19.9%

Nutrition Totals per Serving
CALORIES: 279
PROTEIN: 16.2 grams
CARBOHYDRATE: 21.0 grams
FAT: 4.1 grams
SODIUM: 864 milligrams
CHOLESTEROL: 5 milligrams

Spinach Salad with Warm "Bacon" Dressing

YIELD: 4 SIDE SERVINGS OR 2 MAIN-COURSE SALADS

6 cups torn fresh spinach leaves, rinsed thoroughly and patted
    dry
¼ cup sliced scallion (white and green parts)
⅛ teaspoon freshly ground black pepper
4 Morningstar Farms Breakfast Strips
3 tablespoons white wine vinegar
2 teaspoons sugar
¼ teaspoon sea salt
2 hard-cooked egg whites, chopped
¼ cup *PR* Whole-Wheat Croutons (optional) (page 270)

Combine spinach, scallion, and ground pepper in a large salad
bowl. Set the bowl aside. Cook Breakfast Strip "bacon" according to
the package's instructions. When they are cool enough to handle, cut
them into small pieces and put them in microwave-safe bowl along
with the vinegar, sugar, and salt. Microwave the mixture on high for
30 seconds or till it is warmed through. (This may also be done in a
saucepan on the stovetop.) Once the dressing is heated, pour it over
the spinach mixture and toss to coat the mixture. Top with chopped
egg and *PR* Whole-Wheat Croutons, if using.

Try serving this salad with warm *PR* Menopause Muffins (page
264) or *PR* Oat Bread rolls (page 266).

As in the *PR* Egg "Fu" Salad Sandwich (page 252), you may also
include some tofu "egg yolk" in this salad. Simply crumble 2 ounces of
Nasoya Firm Tofu into a small dish and add a dash of turmeric and
mustard powder. When mixed together, it will resemble hard-boiled yolk.
Use this along with the hard-boiled egg white (if desired) on all the dishes
you would ordinarily garnish with crumbled egg. You will eliminate the
cholesterol and add valuable isoflavones by making this substitution.

Calorie Breakdown per Serving	Nutrition Totals per Serving	
Protein: 28.7%	CALORIES:	67
Carbohydrate: 39.8%	PROTEIN:	5.3 grams
Fat: 31.5%	CARBOHYDRATE:	7.3 grams
	FAT:	2.6 grams
	SODIUM:	345 milligrams
	CHOLESTEROL:	0 milligrams

Taco Salad

YIELD: 4 SALADS

4 burrito-size flour tortillas
1 cup *PR* Deluxe Refried Beans (page 313)
2 cups *PR* Mexican "Beef" (page 315)
½ cup plus 1 tablespoon chopped scallion (white and green
    parts)
2 cups lettuce, shredded or chopped
1 cup Alpine Lace Skim Milk Cheddar Cheese
1 cup tomato, diced
1 cup *PR* Avocado Dressing Dip (page 288)
¼ cup black olives, sliced (optional)

This looks like a professionally catered meal. Dig deep to experience all the flavors at once.

SHELLS:
Preheat the oven to 350°F. Spray a tortilla with olive-oil cooking spray on both sides. Push into a Pyrex or oven-safe bowl (9-inch diameter works best) and arrange the sides into scalloped edges as symmetrically as possible. Bake for 15 minutes. Repeat with the other 3 tortillas. When the last shell is cool enough to handle, put each salad "bowl" on a plate and fill in the order listed below.

FILLING:
- ¼ cup of refried beans spread on the bottom
- ½ cup of "beef"
- 2 tablespoons scallion
- ½ cup lettuce
- ¼ cup cheese
- ¼ cup tomato
- ¼ cup avocado dressing (in the center)
- Scallion pieces or sliced black olive, or both as garnish

If you make all your fillings and bake your tortilla "bowls" ahead of time, these salads can be assembled in a matter of minutes.

Calorie Breakdown per Serving

Protein: 27.0%

Carbohydrate: 53.1%

Fat: 19.9%

Nutrition Totals per Serving

CALORIES:	450
PROTEIN:	28.6 grams
CARBOHYDRATE:	56.2 grams
FAT:	9.4 grams
SODIUM:	1,739 milligrams
CHOLESTEROL:	6 milligrams

Tuna Dijon Salad

YIELD: 2 SALADS OR 4 SANDWICHES

6-ounce can solid white tuna, packed in spring water
1/4 cup low-fat yogurt (1 1/2% milk fat)
2 tablespoons Nasoya Nayonaise
1 tablespoon Dijon mustard
1/4 cup finely chopped celery
1/4 cup finely chopped red onion
1/8 teaspoon dried dill weed
1/8 teaspoon celery seed
Pepper to taste

Drain water from the tuna and place the tuna in a bowl. Mash it with hands or a fork until the fibers are separate and feathery. Add the rest of the ingredients and mix well. Chill the salad. Serve it on a bed of lettuce with brown-rice crackers or use for sandwiches on whole-wheat toast or *PR* Oat Bread rolls (page 266).

Calorie Breakdown per Serving
Protein: 58.1%
Carbohydrate: 10.5%
Fat: 31.4%

Nutrition Totals per Serving

CALORIES:	92
PROTEIN:	12.5 grams
CARBOHYDRATE:	2.3 grams
FAT:	3.0 grams
SODIUM:	282 milligrams
CHOLESTEROL:	19 milligrams

DRESSINGS, SAUCES, AND DIPS

Annato Vinaigrette

YIELD: 20 SERVINGS; SERVING SIZE: 2 TABLESPOONS

2 tablespoons Bertolli Extra Light Olive Oil
1 tablespoon annato seeds
¾ cup balsamic vinegar
¼ cup apple cider vinegar
¼ cup red wine vinegar
1½ teaspoons celery seeds
½ teaspoon dried sweet basil, crushed

Heat the oil with the annato seeds. This can be done on the stovetop or in a microwave oven on high for 30 seconds. Stir the seeds around to infuse the oil and let them cool.

In a shaker bottle or jar with a tight-fitting lid, combine the vinegars, celery seeds, and basil. Strain the oil through a sieve or small colander and discard the annato seeds. Add the infused oil to the shaker bottle, cover, and shake to combine.

Makes approximately 20 2-tablespoon servings.

This dressing goes well on a salad of mixed organic baby greens. Top with *PR* Whole-Wheat Croutons (page 270) and Lite & Less Grated Parmesan Cheese Substitute for a first course that starts the meal out with gourmet flair.

Calorie Breakdown per Serving	Nutrition Totals per Serving	
Protein: 0.7%	CALORIES:	19
Carbohydrate: 33.6%	PROTEIN:	0.0 grams
Fat: 65.7%	CARBOHYDRATE:	1.6 grams
	FAT:	1.4 grams
	SODIUM:	0 milligrams
	CHOLESTEROL:	0 milligrams

♦

Avocado Dressing Dip

YIELD: 8 SERVINGS; SERVING SIZE: 2 TABLESPOONS

1 ripe Haas avocado
½ cup Breakstone Fat Free Sour Cream
¼ teaspoon garlic powder
¼ teaspoon sea salt
1 teaspoon fresh lime juice

Scoop out the pulp of the avocado and discard the skin. Add the avocado to a food processor or blender with remaining ingredients and combine them thoroughly.

This is used in the *PR* Taco Salad (page 284) and the *PR* Triple-Decker Club (page 256). It also makes an excellent topping for any low-fat, high-soy Mexican dishes you may prepare using the *PR* Mexican "Beef" (page 315), the *PR* Deluxe Refried Beans (page 313), and the *PR* Special Restaurant Salsa (page 244).

This should be stored in a tall, narrow container covered with plastic. After several hours, the surface of the dip may discolor slightly owing to its exposure to oxygen. Simply skim off a thin layer with a spoon and the bright green color will be revealed just below the surface.

Calorie Breakdown per Serving
Protein: 10.2%
Carbohydrate: 32.1%
Fat: 57.8%

Nutrition Totals per Serving
CALORIES:	56
PROTEIN:	1.5 grams
CARBOHYDRATE:	4.7 grams
FAT:	3.8 grams
SODIUM:	303 milligrams
CHOLESTEROL:	2 milligrams

Creamy Garlic Dip

YIELD: 8 SERVINGS; SERVING SIZE: 2 TBSP

3/4 cup Hellman's Low Fat Mayonnaise (1 gram per serving)
1/4 cup Breakstone Non Fat Sour Cream
2 teaspoons white wine vinegar
2 tablespoons *PR* Soy Milk Blend (page 294)
1/4 teaspoon dried basil, crushed
1/4 teaspoon dry mustard
1/8 teaspoon sea salt
2 garlic cloves, finely minced

In a food processor, blender, or mixing bowl blend together mayonnaise, sour cream, vinegar, soy milk, basil, mustard, salt, and garlic. Chill the dip.

This recipe is called for in the *PR* Pita Salad Sandwich (page 282) and the *PR* "Chicken" Nuggets (page 239). It also works well as a dip for crudités. Serve it in a small bowl surrounded by fresh-cut vegetables on a chilled platter.

To make a creamy dressing, stir in some additional *PR* Soy Milk Blend (starting with 2 tablespoons) till the dressing is of desired consistency.

Calorie Breakdown per Serving
Protein: 5.5%
Carbohydrate: 65.9%
Fat: 28.6%

Nutrition Totals per Serving
CALORIES: 50
PROTEIN: 0.7 grams
CARBOHYDRATE: 8.1 grams
FAT: 1.6 grams
SODIUM: 253 milligrams
CHOLESTEROL: 1 milligrams

♦

"Creamy" Pink Tomato Sauce

YIELD: 4 SERVINGS; SERVING SIZE: ½ CUP

2 cups Classico Tomato and Basil Pasta Sauce
½ cup Edensoy Original Organic Soy Beverage

Combine the sauce and the soy milk in a saucepan. Warm the mixture over medium heat.

This sauce is used on the *PR* Ravioli di Liguria (page 304). It is also a good basic sauce served over any shape Contadina protein-enriched pasta. Try bow ties, linguini, or rigatoni.

Calorie Breakdown per Serving
Protein: 18.8%
Carbohydrate: 61.6%
Fat: 19.6%

Nutrition Totals per Serving

CALORIES:	66
PROTEIN:	3.3 grams
CARBOHYDRATE:	10.6 grams
FAT:	1.5 grams
SODIUM:	403 milligrams
CHOLESTEROL:	0 milligrams

Honey Mustard Dip

YIELD: 12 SERVINGS; SERVING SIZE: 1 TABLESPOON

½ cup Hellman's Dijonnaise
3 tablespoons clover honey
2 teaspoons prepared horseradish

In a mixing bowl, stir together all ingredients.

This is the perfect dip for *PR* "Chicken" Nuggets (page 239). It's also delicious spread in the center of the *PR* Biscuits 'n' Sausage sandwich (page 232).

Calorie Breakdown per Serving
Protein: 0.3%
Carbohydrate: 82.1%
Fat: 17.6%

Nutrition Totals per Serving
CALORIES: 33
PROTEIN: 0.0 grams
CARBOHYDRATE: 7.0 grams
FAT: 0.7 grams
SODIUM: 97 milligrams
CHOLESTEROL: 0 milligrams

Nothing Lost Tartar Sauce

YIELD: 10 SERVINGS; SERVING SIZE: 1 TABLESPOON

⅓ cup Nasoya Nayonaise
¼ cup celery, extra finely chopped
½ teaspoon sugar
¼ teaspoon dried dill weed
1 finely chopped scallion (white and some of the green parts)

Combine all the ingredients in a small mixing bowl. Stir them until they are thoroughly blended.

This is the sauce used on the *PR* Po' Boy Sandwich ("Chicken" Style) (page 255). It can also be used as a dip for the *PR* Shrimp Wrapped in "Bacon" (page 243).

Calorie Breakdown per Serving
Protein: 1.4%
Carbohydrate: 9.7%
Fat: 88.8%

Nutrition Totals per Serving

CALORIES:	20
PROTEIN:	0.1 grams
CARBOHYDRATE:	0.4 grams
FAT:	1.6 grams
SODIUM:	56 milligrams
CHOLESTEROL:	0 milligrams

Snappy Cocktail Sauce

YIELD: 9 SERVINGS; SERVING SIZE: 2 TABLESPOONS

1 cup Heinz tomato ketchup
2 tablespoons prepared horseradish
3/4 teaspoon Heinz Worcestershire sauce

Mix all ingredients together in a bowl. Chill sauce, then serve.
Try this with the *PR* Shrimp Wrapped in "Bacon" (page 243) and
the *PR* "Chicken" Nuggets (page 239).

Calorie Breakdown per Serving
Protein: 7.0%
Carbohydrate: 87.9%
Fat: 5.1%

Nutrition Totals per Serving
CALORIES:	29
PROTEIN:	0.5 grams
CARBOHYDRATE:	6.8 grams
FAT:	0.2 grams
SODIUM:	288 milligrams
CHOLESTEROL:	0 milligrams

◆

Soy Milk Blend

YIELD: 8 SERVINGS; SERVING SIZE 1 CUP

32-ounce carton Westsoy Non Fat Soy Beverage
33.8-ounce carton Edensoy Original Organic Soy Beverage

Combine these soy beverages into a single container and keep in your refrigerator for use in many of the *Permanent Remissions* recipes and any time you would use milk (for example, on cereal or in coffee). Make it anew once a week; don't add leftovers to the new batch. (You should also keep separate cartons of each beverage on hand when possible, as they are called for undiluted in certain recipes.)

If you are ever in a pinch and are unable to make this recipe or use this much soy milk in a week, you may substitute Westsoy 1% Lite Soy Beverage (2 grams of fat per cup) for Soy Milk Blend.

Calorie Breakdown per Serving
Protein: 25.7%
Carbohydrate: 56.3%
Fat: 18.0%

Nutrition Totals per Serving
CALORIES: 109
PROTEIN: 6.8 grams
CARBOHYDRATE: 14.9 grams
FAT: 2.1 grams
SODIUM: 105 milligrams
CHOLESTEROL: 0 milligrams

ENTRÉES

Broccoli and Tofu Lo Mein with "Chicken"

YIELD: 4 SERVINGS

8-ounce package of Contadina Protein Enriched Linguine
8 ounces Nasoya Extra Firm Tofu (half a block)
2 cups frozen broccoli florets
⅓ cup Karo Light Corn Syrup
2 teaspoons Kame Dark Sesame Oil
3 tablespoons Kame Oyster Sauce
3 tablespoons Kame Light Soy Sauce
2 tablespoons Argo Corn Starch
¼ cup cold filtered water
2 cloves garlic, minced
⅓ cup scallion, chopped
2 teaspoons Bertolli Extra Light Olive Oil
8 ounces Chicken Style Wheat Meat (half a package) *or* 8
    Morningstar Farms Chik Nuggets, cut into strips

You may make this recipe with or without the "chicken." But definitely enjoy this Asia-inspired phytonutrient feast without guilt—it's got all the right stuff.

If using Wheat Meat, dice it and brown it briefly in the skillet, then remove it and set it aside. If using Chik Nuggets, place them in a 375°F oven and let them cook while you prepare the rest of the dish. They should be turned once during baking and removed after 18 minutes. (If microwaving the nuggets, wait until the end of the recipe to do so.)

Cook the linguine according to the package's instructions. Drain it and set it aside in warm water. Slice the tofu into bite-size pieces. Place the tofu on a microwave-safe plate and microwave the tofu on high for 5 minutes, turning it once halfway through cooking. (This step is to make the tofu firmer and is optional.) Rinse the broccoli with warm water and drain it. Set it aside.

In a small mixing bowl, combine corn syrup, sesame oil, oyster sauce, and soy sauce. Dissolve the cornstarch in the filtered water, add it to the bowl, and stir it.

Heat the olive oil in a large skillet or wok and add the scallion and garlic. Sauté the onion and garlic for 1–2 minutes. Add the tofu to the pan, then the broccoli. As the vegetables start to sizzle, pour in the corn-syrup mixture. Add the drained linguine and Wheat Meat, if using, and toss the mixture (like a salad) to coat it. When the ingredients are hot and blended and the sauce begins to thicken, remove the pan from the heat. Place the lo mein on a serving platter. If using Chik Nuggets place them on top of the dish at this time.

Calorie Breakdown per Serving
Protein: 29.5%
Carbohydrate: 54.4%
Fat: 16.1%

Nutrition Totals per Serving

CALORIES:	539
PROTEIN:	39.9 grams
CARBOHYDRATE:	73.6 grams
FAT:	9.7 grams
SODIUM:	988 milligrams
CHOLESTEROL:	0 milligrams

◆

Chili Con "Carne"

YIELD: 4 SERVINGS

2 teaspoons Bertolli Extra Light Olive Oil
1/3 cup diced onion
14 1/2-ounce can Del Monte Fresh Cut Diced Tomatoes (No Salt
   Added)
2 2/3 cups Green Giant Harvest Burgers for Recipes
15 1/2-ounce can Bush's Chili Magic (flavor of your choice)
2 tablespoons Bob's Red Mill Golden Corn Masa Flour
4 ounces (1/2 cup) nonalcoholic beer

In a saucepan sauté the onion in the oil till it's tender. Add un-drained tomatoes, "beef" Harvest Burgers, and Chili Magic. Stir ingredients together and cook them over medium heat. When they are hot, gradually stir in corn flour a little at a time. Add beer, reduce heat, cover the pot, and simmer the chili, stirring occasionally. Cook it at least 10 minutes, but the longer, the better—up to 1 hour. If the chili is too thick, add more beer; if it's too thin, add more masa and leave the lid off for a while.

Serve with your choice of diced onion, nonfat grated cheddar cheese, fat-free sour cream, soy-enriched elbow macaroni, or low-fat crackers, such as soda, oyster, or rice crackers. Or how about *all* of these?

Spoon the leftover chili over a Morningstar Farms Deli Frank or Lightlife Smart Dog and serve on a whole-wheat bun with the toppings suggested above for a healthy chili dog that tastes like the real thing.

Calorie Breakdown per Serving	Nutrition Totals per Serving	
Protein: 49.5%	CALORIES:	258
Carbohydrate: 29.9%	PROTEIN:	20.8 grams
Fat: 20.6%	CARBOHYDRATE:	12.6 grams
	FAT:	3.9 grams
	SODIUM:	1,384 milligrams
	CHOLESTEROL:	0 milligrams

♦

Hearty Lasagne

YIELD: 8 SERVINGS

26-ounce jar Classico Four Cheese Pasta Sauce
3 cups Green Giant Harvest Burgers For Recipes *or* 2½ cups
    Green Giant Harvest Burgers For Recipes and 2
    Morningstar Farms Breakfast Patties, finely chopped
2 cups Polly-O Fat Free Ricotta Cheese
2 cups Healthy Choice Fat Free Grated Mozzarella cheese
2 tablespoons Soyco Lite & Less Grated Parmesan Cheese
    Substitute
3 egg whites
2 tablespoons fresh parsley, finely chopped
⅛ teaspoon freshly ground black pepper
9 curly-edged lasagne noodles

Preheat the oven to 350°F. Cook the lasagna noodles according to the package's instructions. Noodles should be drained and laid out in a single layer on wax paper or tin foil, till needed. Place the frozen meat substitute—with or without chopped "sausage"—in a saucepan and cover it with approximately half the spaghetti sauce. Warm the meat and sauce over medium heat, stirring occasionally, until the crumbles thaw (about 5 minutes). Remove it from heat. In a mixing bowl, combine ricotta, mozzarella (reserve 2 tablespoons for topping), soy Parmesan, egg whites, parsley, and pepper.

Spread ⅓ cup of the remaining spaghetti sauce in the bottom of a 2-quart oven-proof baking dish. Arrange 3 lasagne noodles in the dish lengthwise. Add half the "meat" mixture, then half the cheese mixture. Spread it out evenly. Add another layer of noodles, "meat," and cheese. Finish with a third layer of noodles, topped with the remaining sauce and two tablespoons of mozzarella. Cover the pan (use foil if you don't have a lid) and bake the lasagne for 25 minutes. Uncover the pan and bake the lasagna for 10 more minutes.

You may use precooked lasagne noodles if you are in a hurry, but if you have the time, it pays to do it the old-fashioned way.

Freeze any unused lasagne in individual-portion sizes for home-made microwavable meals (with only 3 grams of fat per serving) that can be used for quick dinners or taken to work or school and heated at lunchtime.

Calorie Breakdown per Serving

Protein: 46.3%
Carbohydrate: 43.1%
Fat: 10.6%

Nutrition Totals per Serving

CALORIES:	309
PROTEIN:	34.0 grams
CARBOHYDRATE:	30.3 grams
FAT:	3.5 grams
SODIUM:	894 milligrams
CHOLESTEROL:	11 milligrams

Horseradish-Encrusted Salmon

YIELD: 4 SERVINGS

3 teaspoons Bertolli Extra Light Olive Oil
1 pound fresh Norwegian salmon filet
½ cup prepared horseradish
2 garlic cloves, minced
Salt
Freshly ground black pepper

Rub the entire top surface of the filet with 1 teaspoon of the oil and remove any bones. Salt and pepper the fish, cover it loosely with plastic wrap, and refrigerate it for 15–20 minutes.

Adjust oven racks to the middle and broil positions. Preheat the oven to 400°F.

In a small bowl, mix the horseradish, garlic, the remaining 2 teaspoons of oil, and a dash of salt and pepper till blended. Remove the fish from the refrigerator and take the plastic off. Spoon dollops of the horseradish mixture over the filet, creating a ¼-inch–thick coating. Pat it firmly with the back of a spoon and make sure that no pink shows through except along the vertical sides. Cover the roasting pan or deep-dish pie pan with foil and gently place the salmon into the center. Cover it loosely with more foil (balance on the edge of the pan) and bake it for 15 minutes. Remove the foil cover and bake the salmon for another 10–15 minutes or until it is cooked through; the time will depend on thickness of the filet. (You may insert a knife through the horseradish coating and into the salmon to determine if the fish has turned from dark transparent pink to light opaque pink in the center.) Remove the pan from the oven and increase the heat to broil.

Carefully fold the edges of the foil away from the sides of the pan toward the fish so that the pan juices are completely covered and all you see is the coated salmon. (This is necessary to keep the juices from burning while the horseradish browns.) Broil the fish for 2–3 minutes on low or until you see the first signs of browning. (The coating is still damp, so most of it won't actually char.) Remove the fish and let it sit for 5–10 minutes. Remove the bottom skin before serving.

This dish can be made ahead of time and served cold. Make sure you choose a horseradish to your liking, whether it be hot and spicy or mild.

Calorie Breakdown per Serving
Protein: 47.8%
Carbohydrate: 2.1%
Fat: 50.1%

Nutrition Totals per Serving

CALORIES:	195
PROTEIN:	22.7 grams
CARBOHYDRATE:	1.0 grams
FAT:	10.6 grams
SODIUM:	170 milligrams
CHOLESTEROL:	63 milligrams

♦

Lobster Malabar

YIELD: 4 SERVINGS

2 lobster tails, approximately 8 ounces each
2 teaspoons Bertolli Extra Light Olive Oil
Dash freshly ground black pepper
Dash sea salt
4 fresh thyme sprigs
Dash Indian asafoetida (optional)
1 cup Thai Kitchen LIte Coconut Milk
1 cup Edensoy Original Organic Soy Beverage
2 teaspoons Thai Kitchen Green Curry Paste
1 tablespoon plus 1 teaspoon curry powder
2 tablespoons cornstarch dissoved in ½ cup cold filtered water

Place the oven racks in the middle and broil positions and preheat the oven to 350°F.

Take the lobster tails out of the shells. Cut a ½-inch–deep slit down the middle of the back of each tail. Rub each piece with 1 teaspoon of oil. Break up the thyme sprigs and distribute them evenly over each tail. Add a dash of salt, pepper, and asafoetida (if using). Place the lobster tails in a baking pan or sided sheet lined with foil and bake for 10–12 minutes or until the lobster is cooked through (flesh will no longer be transparent—it will be solid white). Turn on the broiler and broil the tails until they are lightly browned. Remove any large twigs of the thyme. Cut the lobster into bite-size pieces and set them aside.

In a large skillet over medium heat, combine coconut milk, soy milk, curry paste, and curry powder. Stir until the ingredients are hot and blended. Add the dissolved cornstarch and stir it briskly to avoid lumping. Add the lobster pieces to the skillet and cook for approximately 5 more minutes. Serve alongside or over *PR* Festive Kasmati Rice (page 314).

Calorie Breakdown per Serving	Nutrition Totals per Serving	
Protein: 45.4%	CALORIES:	240
Carbohydrate: 19.0%	PROTEIN:	26.5 grams
Fat: 35.7%	CARBOHYDRATE:	11.1 grams
	FAT:	9.3 grams
	SODIUM:	578 milligrams
	CHOLESTEROL:	81 milligrams

Mrs. B's Chilies Rellenos

YIELD: 8 SERVINGS

2 cups Healthy Choice Grated Non Fat Cheddar Cheese
1 cup Healthy Choice Grated Non Fat Mozzarella Cheese
4 ounces Soya Kaas Monterey Jack Cheese Substitute (grated)
2 4½-ounce cans Old El Paso Chopped Green Chilies
4 egg whites
¼ cup Edensoy Original Organic Soy Beverage
¼ cup unbleached all-purpose flour
8-ounce can Contadina Tomato Sauce

This dish is adapted from an exquisitely good but very high fat recipe. Without sacrificing too much in the taste department, it is now available to those who are making more careful culinary choices.

Preheat the oven to 350°F. Combine cheeses in a mixing bowl; set aside 2 tablespoons for the top. Drain chilies and set them aside. In another bowl, beat together egg whites, soy milk, and flour.

Coat a 2-quart casserole with olive-oil cooking spray. Cover the bottom with approximately ⅓ of the cheese mixture, followed by ⅓ of the chilies and ⅓ of the soy-milk mixture. Repeat twice more. Pour the entire can of tomato sauce over the top. Smooth it out with the back of a spoon and sprinkle with the reserved cheese. Bake the chilies, covered, for 50 minutes. Remove the lid and bake the chilies for another 10 minutes.

Calorie Breakdown per Serving
Protein: 54.3%
Carbohydrate: 28.5%
Fat: 17.2%

Nutrition Totals per Serving

CALORIES:	142
PROTEIN:	19.3 grams
CARBOHYDRATE:	10.1 grams
FAT:	2.7 grams
SODIUM:	762 milligrams
CHOLESTEROL:	6 milligrams

Ravioli di Liguria

YIELD: 4 SERVINGS; SERVING SIZE: 3 RAVIOLI

1 large baking potato
2 Morningstar Farms Breakfast Patties
2 Morningstar Farms Breakfast Links
1 tablespoon Lite & Less Grated Parmesan Cheese Substitute
½ teaspoon fennel seeds (optional)
⅛ teaspoon sea salt
⅛ teaspoon freshly ground black pepper
24 Nasoya Won Ton Wrappers
Half recipe *PR* "Creamy" Pink Tomato Sauce (page 290)

Bake, boil, or microwave the potato till tender. Remove the skin. Place the potato in a mixing bowl and mash by hand, then set aside.

Cook the patties and links according to the packages' instructions. Cut each piece into thirds. Place them in a food processor or blender and blend into a coarse purée. Combine the ground sausage into the mashed potato with a spoon. Add the grated cheese, fennel seeds, salt, and pepper. Mix well.

Preheat the oven to 350°F. Coat 2 baking sheets with cooking spray.

Fill a small container with filtered water and place it near you. On a clean working surface, lay out 2 wonton wrappers. Dip your index finger in the water and draw it along all 4 sides of 1 of the square wrappers. Keep wetting your finger as necessary. Take 1 heaping tablespoon of the potato-and-sausage mixture out of the bowl. Leave it on the spoon while you cup it with your palm and pack it firmly. Push the filling out onto the middle of the wonton wrapper. Cover it with the second wrapper and line up the sides. Pinch the edges together, trying not to leave any openings. Place the ravioli on a cookie sheet. Repeat the filling process with the remaining pouches. Bake them for 10 minutes.

Fill a skillet with water and bring to a simmer. Remove the ravioli from the baking sheet and lower into the water, letting them cook for approximately 3 minutes, carefully turning once or twice. Remove them with a slotted spoon and place them on a serving dish. Ladle approximately ⅓ cup *PR* "Creamy" Pink Tomato Sauce on top of 3 ravioli per serving. Serve with a side of Italian green beans if desired.

Make sure you press the sides of the wonton wrappers together firmly and completely when you stuff the ravioli. This will keep them from "blowing out" (water seeping in) when they are simmered.

Calorie Breakdown per Serving	Nutrition Totals per Serving	
Protein: 26.3%	CALORIES:	232
Carbohydrate: 59.1%	PROTEIN:	12.4 grams
Fat: 14.6%	CARBOHYDRATE:	27.8 grams
	FAT:	3.0 grams
	SODIUM:	792 milligrams
	CHOLESTEROL:	6 milligrams

Rigatoni with Garlic, Tomatoes, and Basil

YIELD: 6 SERVINGS

16-ounce package Rigatoni pasta (preferably imported from
    Italy)
3 tablespoons Bertolli Extra Light Olive Oil
4 cloves garlic (minced)
2 14½-ounce cans Hunt's Choice Cut Tomatoes with Roasted
    Garlic
¼ cup chopped fresh basil leaves

Cook the pasta to the al dente stage and rinse it with cold water. Set it aside.

In a large pot, heat 1 tablespoon of the oil, along with the tomatoes. When the tomatoes are heated through, add the pasta and toss it with the tomatoes and oil to distribute evenly.

Heat the remaining 2 tablespoons of oil with the garlic in the microwave on high for 30 seconds or on the stovetop. Pour it over the pasta mixture and stir it in well. When all the ingredients are sufficiently heated, add the basil and toss a final time to blend. Salt and pepper to taste.

For a special addition, sprinkle a few pine nuts on each serving to add flavor and texture or cut up a few cubes of fresh mozzarella and garnish each bowl with the cheese and a fresh basil leaf.

This may also be served cold. Try it alongside the *PR* Horseradish-Encrusted Salmon (page 300), which is also served hot or cold.

Calorie Breakdown per Serving
Protein: 11.7%
Carbohydrate: 68.9%
Fat: 19.4%

Nutrition Totals per Serving

CALORIES:	364
PROTEIN:	10.6 grams
CARBOHYDRATE:	62.0 grams
FAT:	7.7 grams
SODIUM:	596 milligrams
CHOLESTEROL:	0 milligrams

"Sausage" Ratatouille à la Ann

YIELD: 4 SERVINGS

1 tablespoon Bertolli Extra Light Olive Oil
⅓ cup onion, diced
2 cups zucchini squash,unpeeled, cut in half lengthwise and
    then into ½-inch–wide semicircles
1 cup eggplant, peeled and cubed
1 cup green pepper, seeded, rinsed, and cubed
1 cup red pepper, seeded, rinsed, and cubed
¼ teaspoon sugar
½ teaspoon salt
½ teaspoon freshly ground black pepper
3 sprigs of fresh thyme *or* ½ teaspoon dried thyme
3 fresh chopped basil leaves *or* ½ teaspoon dried basil
14½-ounce can Hunt's Choice Cut Diced Tomatoes With
    Roasted Garlic
2 tablespoons Contadina Tomato Paste
5 Morningstar Farms Breakfast Links

In a large skillet, sauté the onions in the oil till they are tender. Add the remaining ingredients, except tomatoes, tomato paste, sausages, and basil (if using fresh). Stir well. Reduce heat, cover the skillet, and simmer the ingredients approximately 15 minutes until the vegetables soften. Cook the sausages according to package instructions. When they are cool enough to handle, slice Breakfast Link "sausages" into 1-inch pieces on the bias (diagonally), leaving off the ends. Mash the ends into a pulp resembling ground sausage. Add sausage slices and pulp to the skillet along with tomatoes, tomato paste, and fresh basil, if using. Simmer the ratatouille uncovered about 7 minutes. Remove fresh thyme sprigs.

Try this ratatouille over brown rice or over the *PR* Buttermilk Pancakes (page 234) prepared without the banana.

This recipe also makes a perfect side dish or appetizer for 6–8 people. It is a superb starter for the *PR* Ravioli di Liguria (page 304) or side for the *PR* Horseradish-Encrusted Salmon entrée (page 300).

Calorie Breakdown per Serving
Protein: 23.4%
Carbohydrate: 39.4%
Fat: 37.3%

Nutrition Totals per Serving

CALORIES:	120
PROTEIN:	7.4 grams
CARBOHYDRATE:	12.5 grams
FAT:	5.3 grams
SODIUM:	942 milligrams
CHOLESTEROL:	0 milligrams

Shrimp and "Scallops" Creole

YIELD: 4 SERVINGS

8 ounces fresh peeled and deveined shrimp, uncooked

8 ounces Nasoya Extra Firm Tofu

½ cup chopped onion

½ cup chopped celery

½ cup chopped green pepper

½ cup sliced okra

2 cloves garlic, minced

1 tablespoon Bertolli Extra Light Olive Oil

14½-ounce can Hunt's Choice Cut Diced Tomatoes with
  Roasted Garlic

½ cup filtered water

2 tablespoons parsley, chopped

½ teaspoon sea salt

½ teaspoon paprika

¼ teaspoon ground red pepper

1 bay leaf

4 teaspoons cornstarch dissoved in 2 tablespoons cold filtered
  water

2 cups hot cooked Rice Select Basmati or Teximati brown rice

Slice the tofu block widthwise into ½-inch–deep sheets and cut out scallop-size circles 2–3 inches in diameter. (It will take approximately ⅔ of the block to yield 8 ounces of "scallops.") Use a small cookie cutter or a fluted champagne glass (carefully) or do it by hand. Save the scraps in filtered water for another recipe. Microwave the disks on a large oven-safe plate for 5 minutes on high, flipping the tofu halfway through cooking. (Careful—the tofu and plate will be hot.) Set the tofu aside. Heat the oil in a large skillet. Add onion, celery, green pepper, okra, and garlic. Sauté the mixture till the ingredients start to soften. Stir in undrained tomatoes, ½ cup water, parsley, salt, paprika, red pepper, and bay leaf. Bring the mixture to a boil, then reduce heat to low. Cover the skillet and simmer the mixture for 15 minutes.

Stir together the 2 tablespoons water and the cornstarch. Add the cornstarch mixture to the tomato mixture in the skillet, along with the shrimp and "scallops." Cook and stir the mixture for several more minutes until shrimp turn pink. Remove the bay leaf. Serve the dish over rice.

In order to avoid the slippery feel of the okra, it helps to boil it (after it's sliced) for 1–2 minutes before adding it to the skillet. When it's drained, it will lose a lot of its stickiness but none of its flavor or health benefits.

This dish can be made with precooked shrimp to save a step.

You may also leave out the shrimp and double the "scallop" amount for a completely vegetarian Creole with extra isoflavones.

Calorie Breakdown per Serving
Protein: 20.7%
Carbohydrate: 54.2%
Fat: 25.1%

Nutrition Totals per Serving

CALORIES:	278
PROTEIN:	14.3 grams
CARBOHYDRATE:	37.4 grams
FAT:	7.7 grams
SODIUM:	1,054 milligrams
CHOLESTEROL:	33 milligrams

Tricolor Pasta with Salmon (Skillet Dinner)

YIELD: 4 SERVINGS

2 cups vegetable broth made with 1 bouillon cube, such as
    Morga Vegetable Bouillon with Sea Salt
2½ cups tricolor rotini pasta (preferably imported from Italy)
¼ cup Kraft Whipped Cream Cheese with Chives
½ cup Edensoy Organic Soy Beverage
1 tablespoon Lite & Less Grated Parmesan Cheese Substitute
1 teaspoon prepared mustard
½ teaspoon dried basil, crushed
Dash freshly ground black pepper
14.75-ounce can red salmon (sockeye), drained, skin and
    bones removed, and cut into bite-size pieces

In a large skillet, bring the vegetable broth to a boil. Add the pasta. Cover the skillet and simmer the mixture for 10 minutes or till the pasta is just tender. Stir in the cream cheese till combined. Stir in the soy milk, Parmesan substitute, mustard, basil, and pepper. Gently stir in salmon and cook till heated.

For a complete "one-pan" dinner, thaw 1–2 cups of frozen vegetables in warm water, then drain. Add them to the skillet along with the salmon. Heat and serve.

Calorie Breakdown per Serving
Protein: 27.4%
Carbohydrate: 51.6%
Fat: 21.0%

Nutrition Totals per Serving

CALORIES:	431
PROTEIN:	28.9 grams
CARBOHYDRATE:	54.4 grams
FAT:	9.8 grams
SODIUM:	818 milligrams
CHOLESTEROL:	43 milligrams

SIDE DISHES

Deluxe Refried Beans

YIELD: 4 SERVINGS

2 teaspoons Bertolli Extra Light Olive Oil
15-ounce can Progresso Black Beans, drained of most but not
    all liquid
½ teaspoon onion powder
2 slices Morningstar Farms Breakfast Strips, thawed and diced

In a saucepan, sauté the beans, Breakfast Strip "bacon" pieces, and onion powder in the oil till heated through. Mash the mixture with a potato masher or fork until few if any whole beans remain. Continue cooking over medium heat till of desired consistency. (The bean mixture gets thicker the longer it's cooked.)

This is used in the *PR* Taco Salad (page 284) and the *PR* "Beefy" Bean Burrito (page 251). Try adding it to tostadas and nachos, too. Just be sure to use a nonfat cheese and don't forget the *PR* Mexican Beef (page 315) and *PR* Avocado Dressing Dip (page 288).

Calorie Breakdown per Serving	Nutrition Totals per Serving	
Protein: 19.8%	CALORIES:	133
Carbohydrate: 56.6%	PROTEIN:	6.3 grams
Fat: 23.7%	CARBOHYDRATE:	18.2 grams
	FAT:	3.4 grams
	SODIUM:	559 milligrams
	CHOLESTEROL:	0 milligrams

Festive Kasmati Rice

YIELD: 4 SERVINGS

1 cup dry rice (Rice Select Kasmati Rice)
2 tablespoons toasted slivered almonds
¼ cup golden raisins
⅓ cup small carrots, sliced into thin rounds

Cook the rice according to the package's instructions. Transfer the rice to a large bowl and stir in almonds, raisins, and carrots. Mix to blend, then serve.

Serve this rice with *PR* Lobster Malabar (page 302).

Calorie Breakdown per Serving
Protein: 8.1%
Carbohydrate: 77.9%
Fat: 14.0%

Nutrition Totals per Serving

CALORIES:	252
PROTEIN:	5.0 grams
CARBOHYDRATE:	48.1 grams
FAT:	3.8 grams
SODIUM:	584 milligrams
CHOLESTEROL:	0 milligrams

Mexican "Beef"

YIELD: 4 SERVINGS

2 cups Green Giant Harvest Burgers For Recipes
1 packet Old El Paso Taco Seasoning (reduced sodium if
    possible)
¾ cup filtered water

In a large skillet over medium heat, combine ground "meat" with taco flavor packet and ¾ cup water until hot and well blended.

This is used in the *PR* "Beefy" Bean Burrito (page 251) and the *PR* Taco Salad (page 284). It can also be used for nachos, enchiladas, tostados, and any other Mexican recipe that calls for spicy ground beef.

Calorie Breakdown per Serving	Nutrition Totals per Serving	
Protein: 53.7%	CALORIES:	106
Carbohydrate: 46.3%	PROTEIN:	11.4 grams
Fat: 0.0%	CARBOHYDRATE:	9.8 grams
	FAT:	0.0 grams
	SODIUM:	730 milligrams
	CHOLESTEROL:	0 milligrams

Red Beans and Rice

YIELD: 6 SERVINGS

1 cup (dry) Rice Select Teximati Brown Rice or Basmati Rice
2 teaspoons Bertolli Extra Light Olive Oil
1/3 cup onion, chopped
2 scallions (white and green parts), chopped
2 tablespoons whole-wheat flour
6 slices Lightlife Meatless Smart Deli Country Ham, diced
2 slices Morningstar Farms Breakfast Strips, thawed and diced
1 Morningstar Farms Meatless Deli Frank, thawed and diced
1 teaspoon spicy Creole seasoning
15-ounce can Progresso Pinto Beans, drained of most—but
　　　not all—of the liquid
1 cup filtered water

The item this recipe is meant to replace is a seductively delicious side dish served at a popular chicken restaurant. The only difference is, over time the fast-food version can be harmful to your health. This recipe is the healthful alternative.

Cook the rice according to the package's instructions, including the teaspoon of (sea) salt. Meanwhile, heat the oil in a medium skillet. Add the onions and scallions and sauté them till they're tender. Add the flour, the Creole spice, and 1/3 cup of the water and make a paste. Add the beans, "ham," Breakfast Strips "bacon," and "frank" and stir while adding the final 2/3 cup of water, 1/3 cup at a time. When all is well blended, reduce heat and cover the skillet, stirring the mixture occasionally. After 15 minutes, remove 1/2 cup of the bean mixture from the skillet and set it aside. Purée the remaining mixture either in a blender or food processor or preferably by bringing a hand blender to the skillet. When blending is completed, combine the 1/2 cup whole-bean mixture with the puréed bean mixture in the skillet and bring back up the heat. If the mixture is too thick, add 1–2 tablespoons water. Serve the beans over or alongside the steamed rice.

If you already have cooked rice in the refrigerator, simply reheat it when the beans are ready to serve (about 30 minutes altogether).

Calorie Breakdown per Serving
Protein: 19.1%
Carbohydrate: 65.1%
Fat: 15.8%

Nutrition Totals per Serving

CALORIES:	250
PROTEIN:	12.0 grams
CARBOHYDRATE:	40.8 grams
FAT:	4.4 grams
SODIUM:	546 milligrams
CHOLESTEROL:	0 milligrams

Scalloped Potatoes

YIELD: 6 SERVINGS

3 medium *or* 2 large baking potatoes, peeled and thinly sliced
1 tablespoon Bertolli Extra Light Olive Oil
¼ cup onion, chopped
2 tablespoons whole-wheat flour
1 bouillon cube, such as Morga Vegetable Bouillon with Sea
   Salt
1¼ cups *PR* Soy Milk Blend (page 294)
1 tablespoon Land O'Lakes Light Butter
¾ cup Healthy Choice Non Fat Grated Mozzarella Cheese
¼ teaspoon salt
⅛ teaspoon freshly ground pepper

Preheat oven to 350°F. In a saucepan, sauté the onion in oil till tender. Gradually stir in flour, bouillon, soy milk, butter, cheese, salt, and pepper. Continue stirring mixture till it's smooth and slightly thickened. Remove the saucepan from heat.

Coat a 1-quart casserole dish with olive-oil cooking spray. Place half the potatoes in the bottom and cover with half the sauce. Add the remaining potatoes and the rest of the sauce. Cook the potatoes covered in a 350°F oven for 35 minutes. Uncover the dish and bake the potatoes 30 minutes more or till they are tender.

Calorie Breakdown per Serving		Nutrition Totals per Serving	
Protein:	34.3%	CALORIES:	161
Carbohydrate:	26.9%	PROTEIN:	8.2 grams
Fat:	38.8%	CARBOHYDRATE:	6.4 grams
		FAT:	4.1 grams
		SODIUM:	400 milligrams
		CHOLESTEROL:	5 milligrams

Spicy Couscous with Tomatoes

YIELD: 6 SERVINGS

14½-ounce can Hunt's Choice Cut Diced Tomatoes with
   Roasted Garlic
¼ cup scallion (white and green parts), chopped
¼ teaspoon ground red pepper
½ teaspoon sea salt
1 cup filtered water
⅔ cup instant couscous

This comes together in less than 10 minutes, but it tastes like it simmered all afternoon.

In a saucepan, combine undrained tomatoes, scallion, red pepper, salt, and water. Bring the mixture to a boil. Stir in couscous. Cover the pan and remove it from heat. Let it stand 5 minutes.

Calorie Breakdown per Serving
Protein: 17.5%
Carbohydrate: 78.7%
Fat: 3.8%

Nutrition Totals per Serving

CALORIES:	86
PROTEIN:	3.7 grams
CARBOHYDRATE:	16.5 grams
FAT:	0.4 grams
SODIUM:	292 milligrams
CHOLESTEROL:	0 milligrams

Sweet Carrot Side

YIELD: 6 SERVINGS

2 teaspoons Bertolli Extra Light Olive Oil

3 cups carrots, peeled and sliced thinly on the bias (diagonally)

½ cup celery stalk, leaves removed, sliced thinly on the bias

¼ cup onion, diced

¼ cup firmly packed brown sugar

1 tablespoon cornstarch dissolved in ¼ cup filtered water

⅛ teaspoon sea salt

⅛ teaspoon freshly ground black pepper

¼ cup filtered water

⅛ teaspoon ground cinnamon

⅛ teaspoon nutmeg *or* ½ a nut freshly grated

In a skillet, heat the oil and sauté the onion briefly. Add the carrots and celery, and stir while heating them. Add the salt, pepper, and ¼ cup filtered water. Cover the skillet loosely. When the water evaporates and vegetables soften, distribute the sugar over the top, then the cornstarch mixture. As mixture thickens, add cinnamon and nutmeg. Stir to blend, then serve.

The vegetables in this recipe should be sliced thinly for best results. Use a mandoline or vegetable slicer if possible.

Calorie Breakdown per Serving		Nutrition Totals per Serving	
Protein:	3.6%	CALORIES:	73
Carbohydrate:	77.0%	PROTEIN:	0.7 grams
Fat:	19.4%	CARBOHYDRATE:	14.6 grams
		FAT:	1.6 grams
		SODIUM:	76 milligrams
		CHOLESTEROL:	0 milligrams

Tangy Collard Greens

YIELD: 6 SERVINGS

2 teaspoons Bertolli Extra Light Olive Oil
8 cups collard greens
1/8 teaspoon sea salt
1/8 teaspoon freshly ground black pepper
3/4 cup Tropicana Pure Premium Ruby Red Grapefruit Juice
1 tablespoon plus 1 teaspoon prepared yellow mustard
2 teaspoons prepared whole-grain mustard (organic if
    possible)
1/8 teaspoon McIlhenny Tabasco Sauce

Wash the collard greens and remove the stems and large ridges. Stack 3 or 4 leaves at a time and roll into a cylinder. Cut 1/2-inch slices off the roll, placing the greens in a pile as you cut them free. Continue stacking, rolling, and cutting until you accumulate 8 cups' worth of strips.

In a large skillet, heat the oil, then sauté the greens along with the salt and pepper. Continue to move the greens around so they heat evenly. When the greens begin to wilt and the volume starts to reduce, add the grapefruit juice. Let the juice come to a boil. Add both the mustards and the Tabasco. Stir to blend. Reduce heat and cover the skillet loosely. Simmer to desired tenderness (usually 1–2 minutes), stirring occasionally.

Calorie Breakdown per Serving	Nutrition Totals per Serving	
Protein: 13.9%	CALORIES:	48
Carbohydrate: 51.7%	PROTEIN:	1.8 grams
Fat: 34.4%	CARBOHYDRATE:	6.5 grams
	FAT:	1.9 grams
	SODIUM:	134 milligrams
	CHOLESTEROL:	0 milligrams

♦

Tex-Mex Brown Rice

YIELD: 6 SERVINGS

1 cup rice (Rice Select Teximati Brown Rice), uncooked
2 cups V-8 Picante (mild flavor)
⅓ cup Old El Paso Taco Sauce (mild or hot)
½ teaspoon sea salt (optional)

Put all the ingredients into a saucepan along with the sea salt, if you wish. Bring the mixture to a boil and stir it once. Reduce heat, cover the saucepan, and simmer the mixture for 45 minutes. Remove it from heat and let sit covered for 5–10 minutes.

This is a perfect side dish for the *PR* "Beefy" Bean Burrito (page 251).

Calorie Breakdown per Serving
Protein: 10.2%
Carbohydrate: 85.3%
Fat: 4.5%

Nutrition Totals per Serving

CALORIES:	139
PROTEIN:	3.1 grams
CARBOHYDRATE:	26.2 grams
FAT:	0.6 grams
SODIUM:	301 milligrams
CHOLESTEROL:	0 milligrams

DESSERTS

Ambrosia

YIELD: 6 SERVINGS

¼ cup unsweetened coconut chips, toasted
1½ cups plain low-fat yogurt (1½% milk fat)
3 tablespoons clover honey
1 cup orange, peeled and cubed
1 cup red seedless grapes
1 cup cubed Granny Smith apple (with skin on)
1 cup banana, peeled and sliced
1 cup fresh pineapple, cut into triangles approximately 1 inch
    across at the bottom

Unlike other versions, this fresh fruit dessert truly deserves the name "food of the gods."

For best results, chill the fruit before starting to make this dish.

Toast the coconut on a pie tin or cookie sheet in a 300°F oven for 5–10 minutes or until the coconut is golden. Set it aside.

In a mixing bowl, combine the yogurt and honey. In another large bowl, toss all the fruit together to integrate it. Pour the yogurt mixture over the fruit and continue tossing it until the fruit is thoroughly coated. Assemble 6 parfait glasses or large wineglasses. Distribute the fruit evenly between the glasses and top each serving with 2 teaspoons of coconut. Chill the ambrosia briefly if desired. Serve it within 1 hour.

Calorie Breakdown per Serving		Nutrition Totals per Serving	
Protein:	8.5%	CALORIES:	194
Carbohydrate:	70.7%	PROTEIN:	4.5 grams
Fat:	20.8%	CARBOHYDRATE:	37.3 grams
		FAT:	4.9 grams
		SODIUM:	47 milligrams
		CHOLESTEROL:	5 milligrams

♦

Chewy Oatmeal Chocolate Chip Cookies

YIELD: 18 COOKIES

½ cup firmly packed light brown sugar
¼ cup sugar
⅓ cup Sunsweet Lighter Bake Butter and Oil Replacement
2 egg whites
2 tablespoons Land O'Lakes Light Butter, cut into pieces
1 teaspoon pure vanilla extract
½ cup all-purpose flour
¼ cup whole-wheat flour
½ teaspoon baking soda
¼ teaspoon baking powder
¼ teaspoon sea salt
1½ cups Quaker Old Fashioned Oats (you may also use Quick
    but not instant)
⅓ cup Hershey Reduced Fat Baking Chips, chocolate

Preheat the oven to 375°F. Coat baking sheets with olive-oil cooking spray, then set them aside. In a mixing bowl, beat together sugars, Lighter Bake, eggs, butter, and vanilla. In another bowl, combine flours, baking soda, baking powder, and salt, then stir this mixture into the wet mixture. Stir in the oats and chocolate chips. Drop dough by rounded spoonfuls onto the baking sheets. Bake cookies approximately 12 minutes or till they're done.

For added flavor and texture, stir in 1–2 tablespoons of chopped walnuts into the batter.

Calorie Breakdown per Serving	Nutrition Totals per Serving	
Protein: 6.1%	CALORIES:	95
Carbohydrate: 79.0%	PROTEIN:	1.5 grams
Fat: 14.9%	CARBOHYDRATE:	19.2 grams
	FAT:	1.6 grams
	SODIUM:	78 milligrams
	CHOLESTEROL:	2 milligrams

Chocolate Bundt Cake with Fruit Ribbon and Mocha Frosting

YIELD: 16 SLICES

Cake:
¾ cup unsweetened cocoa powder
¾ cup *PR* Soy Milk Blend (page 294)
6 egg whites
1 teaspoon pure vanilla extract
2 cups sugar
¼ cup plus 2 tablespoons Sunsweet Lighter Bake Butter and
    Oil Replacement
1½ cups unbleached all-purpose flour
½ cup Arrowhead Mills Whole Grain Organic Soy Flour
1½ teaspoons Arrowhead Mills Vital Wheat Gluten
1 teaspoon baking powder
¼ teaspoons baking soda
½ teaspoon sea salt
⅓ cup Breakstone's Fat Free Sour Cream
⅓ cup Hershey Reduced Fat Baking Chips, chocolate
½ cup fruit preserves or jam (preferably no sugar added)—try
    raspberry, orange, or apricot

Frosting:
1 cup powdered sugar
3 tablespoons cocoa
½ shot espresso, regular or decaffeinated, *or* 1 teaspoon
    espresso crystals and 1–3 tablespoons hot water *or* 1
    tablespoon coffee flavoring

This dense, dark cake is low in fat and full of soy, but that's not what you'll be thinking about while you eat it. You'll probably be trying to talk yourself out of a second slice.

CAKE:
Preheat the oven to 350°F. In a microwave-safe bowl, combine cocoa and ½ cup soy milk. Heat the mixture on 50% power until the milk is warm. Stir it into a thick paste. Separate the whites of 6 large eggs and

set them aside. In a large bowl, combine sugar, Lighter Bake, and ¼ cup soy milk. Blend the ingredients with an electric mixer till they're smooth. Pour in the egg whites approximately 2 at a time, scraping down the bowl and mixing after each addition. Add the cocoa mixture and the vanilla.

In another large bowl, whisk together both flours, wheat gluten, baking soda, baking powder, and salt. Add half the dry mixture to the wet ingredients and blend them. Mix in the sour cream. Add the rest of the dry mixture and blend all. Add the chocolate chips and stir them in.

Coat a bundt pan with olive-oil cooking spray. Fill a pastry bag with fruit preserves or use a plastic storage bag and snip off the corner to use as a nozzle. Pour half the cake batter into the bundt pan. Squeeze out a ribbon of fruit preserves over the batter in a full circle, trying to stay in the center by avoiding the inside and outside edges of the pan. Go around again if you don't use up all the preserves the first time. Pour the remaining cake batter on top. Bake for approximately 45 minutes or until a toothpick comes out with a few crumbs. The cake should spring back when touched. Let it cool for 15 minutes. Invert it onto a serving plate, let it cool 5–10 more minutes, and frost it.

FROSTING:

Whisk together the powdered sugar and cocoa. Stir in 1 tablespoon brewed espresso (or flavoring diluted with water) at a time, till the mixture is of desired consistency. The frosting should be firm, not runny. Place dollops of it on the top ridge of the warm cake and let them slowly melt down the sides.

Calorie Breakdown per Serving	Nutrition Totals per Serving	
Protein: 5.9%	CALORIES:	172
Carbohydrate: 87.3%	PROTEIN:	2.7 grams
Fat: 6.8%	CARBOHYDRATE:	39.2 grams
	FAT:	1.4 grams
	SODIUM:	55 milligrams
	CHOLESTEROL:	0 milligrams

Marzipan Cheese Tart

YIELD: 12 SERVINGS

Crust:
1 cup reduced fat graham cracker crumbs (usually equal to 6
    whole double grahams)
3 large *or* 4 medium pitted dates (organic if possible)
1 tablespoon Land O'Lakes Light Butter
1 tablespoon *PR* Soy Milk Blend (page 294)
1 tablespoon wheat bran (organic if possible)
1 tablespoon slivered almonds, lightly toasted

Filling:
1 package Jell-O brand flan (Spanish-style custard)
1 packet Knox unflavored gelatine
3/4 cup *PR* Soy Milk Blend (page 294)
3/4 cup sugar
1 cup Polly-O fat-free ricotta cheese
6 ounces Nasoya Extra Firm Tofu (a little less than half the
    block)
2 teaspoons almond extract

This dessert has fooled many unsuspecting people who would
never dream of eating tofu or drinking soy milk.

Preheat the oven to 375°F. Place graham cracker crumbs, dates,
wheat bran, and almonds in a blender or food processor. Melt the butter together with the soy milk and gradually pour the mixture into the
dry ingredients while processing. When the mixture is blended, transfer
it to a flat-bottom springform pan or tart pan and press evenly out to
the sides, covering the seam if possible. (If you don't have a springform
pan, you may use an 8-inch or 9-inch cake pan). Bake the crust 8–10
minutes. Let it cool to room temperature. (Small cracks may form in
the crust, but they are not a problem.)

Open the box of Jell-O flan. Set aside the smaller caramel pouch
that comes with the flan. It will be used later for the topping.

In a saucepan, add contents of the flan packet, gelatine, and soy
milk. Let the mixture sit for 5 minutes. Place the saucepan on a burner
over medium high heat and stir to blend ingredients. Gradually add
the sugar. Bring the mixture to a boil, then remove the saucepan from

heat, stirring the mixture once or twice. When it is no longer steaming (pan can be placed in a large bowl filled with ice cubes and water to hasten cooling), process with ricotta, tofu, and almond flavoring till the mixture is smooth. Pour it into the prepared crust. Let the tart sit for about 5 minutes to firm up slightly. Snip a corner of the caramel packet and drizzle over the filling.

TO DECORATE:

Try making a spiral with the caramel that starts in the center and makes its way out to the sides. Next, take a toothpick and draw straight lines out away from the center and back in from the edges. (Shoot for 2-inch-wide intervals at the perimeter of the tart.) The lines should all meet in the center like the spokes of a wheel. This will turn the original spiral into a marble- or weblike design. Chill the tart overnight or for at least 6 hours.

Calorie Breakdown per Serving	Nutrition Totals per Serving	
Protein:　17.4%	CALORIES:	144
Carbohydrate:　69.0%	PROTEIN:	6.4 grams
Fat:　13.6%	CARBOHYDRATE:	25.3 grams
	FAT:	2.2 grams
	SODIUM:	75 milligrams
	CHOLESTEROL:	3 milligrams

Pink Citrus Ice

YIELD: 4 SERVINGS

1 cup filtered water
½ cup sugar
½ cup Ocean Spray Ruby Red & Tangerine Grapefruit Juice
    Cocktail
½ cup Tropicana Pure Premium Ruby Red Grapefruit Juice

For this dessert, use a durable pint container from a frozen dessert you may have purchased previously, but treat it carefully. Once you taste how good your own homemade fruit ice can be, you may never want to buy another one.

In a saucepan, heat the water and sugar to a boil. Stir the mixture constantly for 2 minutes, then remove the pan from the heat. When the mixture is no longer hot, add both juices. Pour the mixture into a pint container and freeze a minimum of 4 hours. (Don't overfill your container as the liquid will expand in volume when frozen. You may have 1–2 extra tablespoons of liquid.)

Let the ice thaw a few minutes before serving.

Calorie Breakdown per Serving
Protein: 0.4%
Carbohydrate: 99.6%
Fat: 0.0%

Nutrition Totals per Serving
CALORIES: 119
PROTEIN: 0.1 grams
CARBOHYDRATE: 30.9 grams
FAT: 0.0 grams
SODIUM: 4 milligrams
CHOLESTEROL: 0 milligrams

Strawberries and "Cream"

YIELD: 6 SERVINGS

2 pints fresh strawberries
2 cups Breakstone's Fat Free Sour Cream
½ cup firmly packed light brown sugar

Wash the strawberries thoroughly and cut out the stems on all but 6. (Choose the largest and best-shaped strawberries to leave the stems on because they will be used as the garnish.) Pat them dry, then chill them. You may slice the strawberries in half before layering your parfait if you prefer smaller pieces.

In a mixing bowl combine the sour cream with the sugar. Assemble 6 parfait glasses. Place a spoonful of cream in the bottom of each glass, then 3 or 4 strawberries (6–8 halves). Add several spoonfuls of cream, then 3 or 4 more strawberries. Finish with a dollop of the cream mixture topped with a reserved strawberry with its stem attached.

Serve immediately or chill for up to 2 hours.

For a different serving idea, place the "cream" in 6 individual ramekins. Set them on 6 plates surrounded by whole strawberries (with stems on) that may be used for dipping.

Calorie Breakdown per Serving	Nutrition Totals per Serving	
Protein: 13.5%	CALORIES:	177
Carbohydrate: 84.4%	PROTEIN:	5.9 grams
Fat: 2.1%	CARBOHYDRATE:	37.0 grams
	FAT:	0.4 grams
	SODIUM:	72 milligrams
	CHOLESTEROL:	11 milligrams

BLENDER DRINKS

Berry Tofu Smoothie

YIELD: 1 SERVING

1 cup frozen mixed berries
½ cup Mori-Nu Silken Soft Tofu
1 small banana (chilled or partially frozen if possible)
¼ cup plain low-fat yogurt
¼ cup pure apple juice
1 to 3 tablespoons clover honey (optional)

Place all the ingredients into a blender and combine till smooth.

Calorie Breakdown per Serving
Protein: 14.7%
Carbohydrate: 68.7%
Fat: 16.6%

Nutrition Totals per Serving
CALORIES: 258
PROTEIN: 10.2 grams
CARBOHYDRATE: 47.9 grams
FAT: 5.1 grams
SODIUM: 56 milligrams
CHOLESTEROL: 5 milligrams

Café Espressoy Shake

YIELD: 1 SERVING

8-ounce container Café Westbrae Coffee Drink (soy beverage)
½ cup fat-free coffee-flavored frozen yogurt
¼ cup plain low-fat yogurt
1 serving Twinlab's MaxiLIFE Soy Cocktail
1–3 ice cubes

Place all the ingredients except the ice cubes into a blender and combine them. Add the ice cubes if needed for texture, 1 at a time through the hole in the top of the lid. Mix till the shake is smooth.

Calorie Breakdown per Serving		Nutrition Totals per Serving	
Protein:	39%	CALORIES:	428
Carbohydrate:	50.9%	PROTEIN:	39.3 grams
Fat:	10.1%	CARBOHYDRATE:	51.3 grams
		FAT:	4.5 grams
		SODIUM:	203 milligrams
		CHOLESTEROL:	5 milligrams

Double Chocolate Malt

YIELD: 1 SERVING

¾ cup White Wave Chocolate Silk (soy beverage)
¾ cup fat-free light chocolate frozen yogurt
¼ cup plain low-fat yogurt
1 tablespoon malted milk powder
1 serving Twinlab's MaxiLIFE Soy Cocktail
1–3 ice cubes

Place all the ingredients except the ice cubes into a blender and combine them. Add the ice cubes, if needed for texture, 1 at a time through the hole in the top of the lid. Mix till the shake is smooth.

Calorie Breakdown per Serving
Protein: 37.4%
Carbohydrate: 52.7%
Fat: 9.9%

Nutrition Totals per Serving
CALORIES: 493
PROTEIN: 44 grams
CARBOHYDRATE: 62.0 grams
FAT: 5.2 grams
SODIUM: 278 milligrams
CHOLESTEROL: 8 milligrams

Dreemsicle Shake

YIELD: 1 SERVING

¾ cup Tropicana Pure Premium Orange Juice
¾ cup fat-free light vanilla frozen yogurt
½ cup Edensoy Organic Soy Beverage (vanilla flavored if
    possible)
1 serving Twinlab's MaxiLIFE Choline Cocktail
1–3 ice cubes

Place all the ingredients except the ice cubes into a blender and combine them. Add the ice cubes, if needed for texture, 1 at a time through the hole in the top of the lid. Mix till the shake is smooth.

Calorie Breakdown per Serving
Protein: 17.1%
Carbohydrate: 76.7%
Fat: 6.2%

Nutrition Totals per Serving

CALORIES:	408
PROTEIN:	12.5 grams
CARBOHYDRATE:	56.0 grams
FAT:	2.0 grams
SODIUM:	143 milligrams
CHOLESTEROL:	0 milligrams

Pure Fruit Smoothie

YIELD: 1 SERVING

½ cup watermelon, cubed and seeded
½ cup apple, cubed and peeled
½ cup strawberries, stems removed
1 small banana
1 serving Twinlab's MaxiLIFE Choline Cocktail
1–3 ice cubes

Because there is no added sugar in this recipe, it is the natural choice for diabetics.

Place all the ingredients except the ice cubes into a blender and combine them. Add the ice cubes, if needed for texture, 1 at a time through the hole in the top of the lid. Mix till the drink is smooth.

For best results, use refrigerated fruit in this recipe. If you have the time, slice the fruit and put it in the freezer for 10–15 minutes before blending.

Calorie Breakdown per Serving		Nutrition Totals per Serving	
Protein:	6.4%	CALORIES:	243
Carbohydrate:	86.8%	PROTEIN:	3.0 grams
Fat:	6.7%	CARBOHYDRATE:	40.6 grams
		FAT:	1.4 grams
		SODIUM:	14 milligrams
		CHOLESTEROL:	0 milligrams

Strawberry Banana Shake

YIELD: 1 SERVING

½ cup chilled fresh strawberries, stems removed
1 small ripe banana (chilled if possible)
½ cup fat-free frozen strawberry sorbet
¼ cup *PR* Soy Milk Blend (page 294)
¼ cup plain low-fat yogurt
1 serving Twinlab MaxiLIFE Choline Cocktail
1–3 ice cubes

Place all the ingredients except the ice cubes into a blender and combine them. Add the ice cubes, if needed for texture, 1 at a time through the hole in the top of the lid. Mix till the shake is smooth.

Calorie Breakdown per Serving
Protein: 8.2%
Carbohydrate: 85.1%
Fat: 6.7%

Nutrition Totals per Serving
CALORIES: 436
PROTEIN: 6.4 grams
CARBOHYDRATE: 66.2 grams
FAT: 2.3 grams
SODIUM: 71 milligrams
CHOLESTEROL: 5 milligrams

Super Soy Power Shake

YIELD: 1 SERVING

¾ cup ice cold Tropicana Pure Premium Orange Juice
½ medium banana (chilled if possible)
1 serving Twinlab MaxiLIFE Soy Cocktail
¼ cup crushed ice or 2 ice cubes

Place all the ingredients in a blender and combine. Serve immediately.

Calorie Breakdown per Serving	Nutrition Totals per Serving	
Protein: 47.3%	CALORIES:	286
Carbohydrate: 48.4%	PROTEIN:	32.1 grams
Fat: 4.3%	CARBOHYDRATE:	32.9 grams
	FAT:	1.3 grams
	SODIUM:	1 milligram

Tropical Fruit Shake

YIELD: 1 SERVING

½ cup fat-free frozen mango sorbet
½ cup pineapple (fresh or canned in juice), cubed and chilled
½ cup kiwi–strawberry juice cocktail (or tropical juice
     combination of choice)
1 teaspoon fresh lime juice
1 serving Twinlab's MaxiLIFE Choline Cocktail
2–4 ice cubes

Place all the ingredients except the ice cubes into a blender and combine them. Add the ice cubes, if needed for texture, 1 at a time through the hole in the top of the lid. Mix till the shake is smooth.

Calorie Breakdown per Serving
Protein: 5.0%
Carbohydrate: 91.8%
Fat: 3.2%

Nutrition Totals per Serving
CALORIES: 314
PROTEIN: 3.8 grams
CARBOHYDRATE: 69.9 grams
FAT: 1.1 grams
SODIUM: 50 milligrams
CHOLESTEROL: 5 milligrams

SECTION III

SECTION III

GLOSSARY

Adjuvant therapy: A treatment used to increase the effectiveness of the primary therapy, such as radiotherapy or chemotherapy. The drug tamoxifen is often used as adjuvant therapy following surgery for breast cancer.

Amino acid: A molecule that contains an ammonia-like compound (amine group) coupled to an organic acid (carboxyl group) that forms the building blocks of all proteins. The human body requires 22 specific amino acids. Twelve of them can be synthesized by the body (called nonessential amino acids), whereas 10 must be obtained from foods (essential amino acids).

Androgen: A hormone that produces male characteristics. See **testosterone.**

Angiogenesis: The process by which the body builds new blood vessels. Malignant tumors can trick the body into building blood vessels in order to bring in vital nutrients that allow cancer cells to grow and spread. See **Metastasis.**

Antiandrogen: A drug that blocks the activity of androgens at the cellular receptor sites.

Antibody: A protein produced by the immune system that counteracts the toxic effects of a foreign organism, substance, or disease.

Antioxidant: A natural or synthetic chemical or a nutrient that inactivates the damaging portion (active site) of free radicals. Antioxidants also help neutralize chemicals that cause free-radical formation. Such phytonutrients as lycopene, alpha- and beta-carotene; vitamins B_1, B_5, B_6, C, and E; the minerals selenium and zinc; coenzyme Q_{10}, uric acid; and three enzymes in your body—superoxide dismutase, catalase, and glutathione peroxidase—are all antioxidants. By neutralizing free radicals, antioxidants prevent damage to cell membranes and genetic material, such as DNA (deoxyribonucleic acid).

Apoptosis: The process of genetically programmed cell death, normally triggered after 50–60 cell divisions. Certain genes can trigger premature cell death if cells have become damaged, thereby preventing the cell from turning cancerous.

Ascorbic acid: See **Vitamin C (ascorbic acid).**

ATP (adenosine triphosphate): The universal energy molecule in nature. ATP is created in the mitochondria (energy center of each cell) using energy-derived foods consumed. When ATP is split by enzymes, energy is released for various cellular functions and muscular contractions.

Benign prostatic hyperplasia (BPH): Also benign prostatic hypertrophy. A non-cancerous enlargement of the prostate gland.

Benign: A noncancerous state used to describe a tumorous growth.

Beta-carotene (provitamin A): A yellowish pigment found in such plants as carrots, squash, and pumpkins. A liver enzyme splits one molecule of beta-carotene in half, forming two molecules of active vitamin A. Beta-carotene is just one of at least 10 or so carotenes found in human blood. Beta-carotene is also a powerful antioxidant that neutralizes a damaging type of activated oxygen called singlet oxygen.

Bioflavonoids: A group of compounds, including hesperidin and rutin, that work synergistically with vitamin C to maintain healthy blood vessels and a healthy immune system. Bioflavonoids are commonly found in many fruits, vegetables, wine, and tea.

Biopsy: A surgical procedure involving the removal of tissue for the purposes of microscopic examination by a pathologist in order to make a diagnosis.

Boron: A trace mineral required for bone and muscle growth. Boron may help in preventing osteoporosis by stimulating bone mineralization.

BPH: See **Benign prostatic hyperplasia.**

Brachytherapy: A type of radiotherapy in which radioactive seeds are implanted into the prostate to deliver radiation directly to a tumor.

Cancer: One or more cells that have lost their ability to stop dividing. Unlike benign tumors, cancerous tumors tend to invade surrounding tissues and spread to distant sites of the body. See **Metastasis.**

Carcinoma: A malignant tumor composed primarily of epithelial cells that form the lining of an organ or cavity.

Chemotherapy: The treatment of cancer using drugs designed to kill tumor cells or deter their growth.

Cholesterol: A sterol manufactured in the liver and other cells found only in animal protein and fats and oils (one exception: spirulina, a blue-green algae, contains cholesterol). The body uses cholesterol to synthesize hormones and cell membranes. High levels of plasma cholesterol (called LDL, or low-density lipoprotein) are associated with an increased risk of developing cardiovascular disease. Oxidized cholesterol is suspected as the primary culprit in artery damage.

Chromium: An element required for normal carbohydrate metabolism. Chromium helps the hormone insulin clear the blood of glucose and move it into cells.

Chromium picolinate: A special form of chromium developed by a scientist at the U.S. Department of Agriculture that is several times more effective than chromium. Chromium picolinate seems to aid muscle building in people who use it during periods of intense exercise and caloric control.

Cobalamin: See **Vitamin B$_{12}$ (cobalamin).**

Coenzyme Q$_{10}$: A substance synthesized by the body responsible for the synthesis of adenosine triphosphate (ATP), the universal energy molecule. Research suggests that coenzyme Q$_{10}$ acts as a fat-soluble free-radical neutralizer and helps regulate the electrical conduction system of the heart.

Complementary therapy: The use of conventional medical treatments, such as surgery, chemotherapy, and radiotherapy combined with diet or other nonmedical intervention, to create a more powerful treatment strategy than either medical or nonmedical could provide alone.

Cryosurgery: The freezing of tissue with liquid nitrogen. Cryosurgery is often used to treat prostate cancer.

Daidzein: An isoflavone found in soy foods and beverages that inhibits the growth of cancer cells.

D-alpha tocopherol: Natural vitamin E. This is the preferred form to use as a dietary supplement because it contains all of the natural isomers, or chemical forms, of vitamin E required by the body to fight such diseases as cancer and atherosclerosis.

DHT (dihydrotestosterone): A metabolite of testosterone that stimulates the growth of prostate gland cells and leads to benign prostatic hyperplasia (BPH) and may be a cause of prostate cancer.

Digital rectal examination (DRE): A procedure in which a physician inserts a gloved, lubricated finger into the rectum to examine the prostate gland for signs of enlargement or tumors.

DNA: Deoxyribonucleic acid, the genetic blueprint that resides in the nucleus of every cell of every living organism ever studied. Many researchers believe that free radical damage is responsible for the cellular damage that leads to cancer, heart disease, and many other degenerative diseases.

Double-blind: A method of designing a scientific experiment so that neither the experimental subjects nor the investigator knows what treatment, if any, a subject is getting until after the experiment is over. This method of experimental design attempts to eliminate bias on the part of both subjects and investigators.

DRE: See **Digital rectal exam.**

Enzymes: Complex proteins that are capable of inducing chemical changes in other substances without being changed themselves.

Estrogen: A steroid sex hormone made from cholesterol in the body, often used as a drug to replace estrogen during menopause and to inhibit the production of testosterone in patients diagnosed with prostate cancer. Overproduction of estrogen, synthetic estrogens given as drugs, or environmental estrogens (see **Xenoestrogens**) may stimulate the growth of cancer, especially in the reproductive organs.

Free radical: A highly chemically reactive atom, molecule, or molecular fragment with a free or unpaired electron. Free radicals are produced in many different ways, such as normal metabolic processes, ultraviolet radiation from the sun, nuclear radiation, and the breakdown in the body of spoiled fats. Free radicals have been implicated in aging, cancer, cardiovascular disease, and other kinds of damage to the body. See **Antioxidants.**

Free-radical reaction: The cascade of chemical reactions that occurs when a free radical reacts with another molecule in order to gain an electron. The molecule that loses an electron to the free radical then becomes a free radical, repeating the process until the energy of the free radical is spent or the reaction is stopped by an antioxidant.

Genistein: An isoflavone found only in soy foods and beverages that inhibits enzymes that promote tumor growth.

Gland: An aggregation of cells that secretes a chemical or hormone for use by the body.

Gleason score: A diagnostic method for classifying the cellular differentiation of cancerous tissue. The more cells differ in appearance from normal, the more malignant the cancer. Two grades of 1–5, identifying the two most common degrees of differentiation present in the examined tissue sample, are added together to produce the Gleason score.

Glutathione peroxidase: A sulfur-containing enzyme that possesses powerful antioxidant properties. Each molecule of glutathione peroxidase contains four molecules of selenium.

Hormone: A chemical messenger such as growth hormone, testosterone, or insulin.

Impotence: The loss of ability to achieve and maintain a penile erection.

Isoflavone: A phytonutrient found in legumes and vegetables that can prevent sex hormones from stimulating cellular growth that leads to cancer. Soybeans and garbanzo beans (chickpeas) are rich sources of isoflavones.

L-cysteine: A sulfur-containing amino acid with antioxidant properties.

L-methionine: A sulfur-containing amino acid with antioxidant properties.

L-taurine: A nonessential amino acid that possesses antioxidant properties and helps stabilize the conduction of electrical impulses in the heart, nervous system, and brain.

Lymph node: A small mass of tissue along the vessels of the lymphatic system that filter out microorganisms, toxins, and cancer cells.

Malignant: A classification for tumor cells that possess invasive and metastatic properties.

Manganese: A cofactor in many enzyme-mediated reactions. It is essential for the production of the antioxidant enzyme superoxidase dismutase (SOD).

Metastasis: The spread of cancer cells, through the bloodstream or lymphatic system, beyond the boundaries of the organ or tissue where the cancer originated.

Methylation: The combining of methyl groups (CH3-) derived from vitamin B_{12}, folic acid, and dietary compounds, such as the amino acids L-methionine and L-cysteine, and betaine, with DNA (deoxyribonucleic acid). This coupling turns certain genes on or off, thereby preventing run-away cellular growth that can lead to cancer. Inadequate methylation of DNA can lead to tumor cell formation.

Mitochondria: The "power plants" inside cells where oxygen and nutrients are metabolized to water, carbon dioxide, and energy.

Niacin: See **Vitamin B₃ (niacin).**

Oncology: The branch of medical science dealing with cancer. An oncologist specializes in diagnosing and treating cancerous tumors.

Oxidation: A type of chemical reaction in which an electron is removed from the compound being oxidized. Removing an electron creates a free radical (a compound lacking an electron or with an unpaired electron). Oxygen is the most common oxidizing compound.

Pantothenic acid: See **Vitamin B₅ (pantothenic acid).**

Phosphatidylcholine: A phospholipid (a fat) that the body can use as a precursor to make choline.

Phytic acid: An antioxidant found in vegetables that chelates, or ties up, such minerals as iron or cadmium that may promote tumor growth. Phytic acid can also reduce the size and number of tumors in laboratory animals fed carcinogens.

Placebo: An inert compound usually given to a portion of the test subjects in a scientific experiment in order to distinguish the psychological effects of the experiment from the physiological effects of the drug being tested.

Potassium: Potassium is responsible for transmitting electrical impulses. It is highly active in the tissues of the brain and nervous system.

Precursor: A chemical that can be converted by the body into another is a precursor of the latter chemical.

Prostate-specific antigen (PSA): A blood test that measures a compound manufactured solely by the prostate gland, used to detect an abnormal condition of the prostate gland, either benign or malignant.

Protease Inhibitors: Phytonutrients found in soybeans and other vegetables that block the actions of enzymes that promote tumor growth.

PSA: See **Prostate-specific antigen (PSA).**

Pyridoxine: See **Vitamin B₆ (pyridoxine).**

Radiotherapy: Use of high-energy rays to kill cancer cells. Radiotherapy may be used externally (external beam) or internally (see **Brachytherapy**).

Radical prostatectomy: A surgical procedure used to remove the entire prostate gland and seminal vesicles.

Radiosensitivity: The degree to which a type of cancer responds to radiotherapy.

Receptors: Sites on the outside of cells where particular messenger molecules, such as hormones, can attach. This attachment to the receptor site causes corresponding changes inside the cell.

Recurrence: The return of the cancer following treatment or remission. When the cancer is at a site distant from the original site, the recurrence indicates the appearance of one or more metastases of the disease.

Refractory: A term indicating that a disease, such as cancer, no longer responds to current therapy.

Retinol: See **Vitamin A (retinol).**

Riboflavin: See **Vitamin B₂ (riboflavin).**

Selenium: An important trace mineral with antioxidant properties. Selenium and antioxidant enzymes containing selenium have shown strong anticancer properties.

SOD: See **Superoxidase dismutase (SOD).**

Stroke: A rupture or blockage in a blood vessel in the brain, often with disastrous effects, depending on where the rupture or blockage occurs.

Superoxide dismutase (SOD): An antioxidant enzyme containing zinc and copper or manganese. Its main function is to scavenge and neutralize the superoxide free radical.

Synergy: The action of two or more compounds combined such that their effects are greater than the sum of their individual effects.

Testosterone: A steroid sex hormone made from cholesterol in the body, often used as a drug to replace testosterone during old age. Overproduction of testosterone may encourage the growth of cancer cells, especially in the prostate gland.

Thiamin: See **Vitamin B₁ (thiamin).**

Unsaturated fats: Fats that contain double bonds between some of their carbon atoms. These double bond positions are very vulnerable to attack by oxygen and free radicals.

Vitamin A (retinol): One of the fat-soluble vitamins and an important antioxidant. The form of vitamin A that is found in animals, it is essential to growth, healthy skin and epithelial tissue, and the prevention of night blindness.

Vitamin B₁ (thiamin): A member of the B complex of vitamins that is essential for the health of brain and nerve tissue.

Vitamin B₁₂ (cobalamin): A member of the B complex of vitamins that is particularly important in the brain and nerve tissues. It is a powerful water-soluble antioxidant that helps protect against cancer and atherosclerosis.

Vitamin B₂ (riboflavin): A member of the B complex of vitamins that functions as an antioxidant cofactor, taking part in metabolic reactions involving proteins, fats, and carbohydrates.

Vitamin B₃ (niacin): A member of the B complex of vitamins that is a particularly important coenzyme in the brain and nerve tissues. It is necessary for the synthesis of DNA (deoxyribonucleic acid), enhances the action of vitamin C and several amino acids, and is required for building the walls of brain cells.

Vitamin B₅ (pantothenic acid): A member of the B complex of vitamins that acts an antioxidant. It is also required for the conversion of choline to the neurotransmitter acetylcholine.

Vitamin B₆ (pyridoxine): A member of the B complex of vitamins that acts as an antioxidant. It is necessary for the synthesis of DNA (deoxyribonucleic acid) and enhances the action of vitamin C and amino acids in the body and their conversion into neurotransmitters in the brain.

Vitamin C (ascorbic acid): One of the most important antioxidant nutrients. It is essential in building strong, healthy connective tissue, especially in capillary walls.

Vitamin E: A fat-soluble antioxidant vitamin chemically known as D-alpha-tocopherol. It is a necessary factor in over 20 enzymatic reactions and is essential for the production of the antioxidant enzyme SOD (superoxidant dismutase).

Xenobiotic: A compound not ordinarily found in the body, such as a pesticide, drug, or environmental pollutant.

Xenoestrogen: A chemical in the environment that mimics the effect of the body's estrogen. Xenoestrogens can promote the unchecked cell growth that leads to cancer. Pesticides are examples of xenoestrogens.

Zinc: A mineral that is found in substantial concentrations in the prostate gland. It is a necessary factor in over 20 different enzymatic reactions and is essential for the production of the antioxidant enzyme SOD (superoxide dismutase).

APPENDIX I

Permanent Remissions
Computer Software

The *Permanent Remissions* computer program for Microsoft Windows (Windows 3.1, Windows 95, or higher) creates phytonutrient-rich meals based your favorite foods, beverages, recipes, spices, and fresh, canned, and frozen foods. The *Permanent Remissions* software program can help you find the vital nutrients you need to prevent or achieve remission from cancer, heart disease, diabetes, and osteoporosis.

The *Permanent Remissions* program contains the latest information on the carotene content including lycopene, alpha- and beta-carotene, lutein, and xeaxanthin, of foods and supermarket food products. The *Permanent Remissions* program will help build you a healthy diet based on the latest phytonutrient research on these disease-fighting compounds from vegetables and fruits.

The program will graph the amino-acid content of foods and recipes. It also produces easy-to-read graphs and pie charts revealing foods' and recipes' nutritional content, including vitamins, minerals, cholesterol, fat, protein, calories, and carbohydrates.

The program easily converts units of measure (such as grams, ounces, pounds, teaspoons, and tablespoons) and lets you make "what if" changes to food quantities and see the nutritional effects of such changes on recipes and menus.

All of the nutritional graphs and charts and the recipe analyses in this book were created using the program.

You may order a copy of the program by sending check or money order for $19.95 (includes shipping and handling) to:

Small Planet Systems Corporation
P.O. Box 80-0102
Aventura, FL 33280

For information on this program and other health software, call: (305) 443-6011.

APPENDIX II

Directory of Selected Cancer Associations and Support Groups

American Academy of Pain Medicine
5700 Old Orchard Road
Skokie, IL 60077
phone: (847) 966-9510

American Brain Tumor Association
2720 River Road, suite 146
Des Plaines, IL 60018
phone: (800) 886-2282;
fax: (847) 827-9918
e-mail address: ABTA@aol.com
website address: http://
pubweb.acns.nwu.edu/~lberko/
abta_html/abta l.htm

American Cancer Society, Inc.
National Headquarters
1599 Clifton Road, N.E.
Atlanta, GA 30329
phone: (800) ACS-2345
website address: http://
www.cancer.org

American Brain Tumor Association
3725 North Talman Avenue
Chicago, IL 60618
phone: (800) 886-2282 or
(312) 286-5571 (in Chicago)

American Foundation for Urologic Disease
300 West Pratt Street
Baltimore, MD 21201
phone: (410) 727-2908;
fax: (410) 528-0550
e-mail address: admin@atud.org
website address: http://
www.acess.digex.net.~afud

American Institute for Cancer Research
1759 R Street, NW
Washington, D.C. 20009
phone: (800) 843-8114 (nutrition hotline) or (202) 328-7744 (in Washington, D.C.);
fax: (202) 328-7226
website address: http://www.aicr.org

American Lung Association
1740 Broadway, 14th floor
New York, NY 10019-4374
phone: (800) LUNG-USA or (212) 315-8700 (in New York City);
fax: (212) 265-5642
America On Line (AOL) key word:
ALA

American Melanoma Foundation
c/o Malcolm Mitchell, M.D.
Center for Biological Therapy and
Melanoma Research
University of California San Diego
9500 Gilman Drive
La Jolla, CA 92093

American Pain Society
5700 Old Orchard Road
Skokie, IL 60077
phone: (847) 966-5595

**Biological Therapy Institute
Foundation**
P.O. Box 681700
Franklin, TN 37068
phone: (615) 790-7535;
fax: (615) 794-9110

**Blood and Marrow Transplant
Newsletter**
1985 Spruce Avenue
Highland Park, IL 60035
phone: (847) 831-1913;
fax: (847) 831-1943
e-mail address:
bmtnews@transit.nyser.net

**Bone Marrow Transplant Family
Support Network**
P.O. Box 845
Avon, CT 06001
phone: (800) 826-9376

Breast Cancer Advisory Center
11426 Rockville Pike, suite 406
Rockville, MD 20859
phone: (301) 984-1020

Cancer Care, Inc.
1180 Avenue of the Americas
New York, NY 10036
phone: (800) 813-HOPE or
(212) 302-2400 (in New York City);

fax: (212) 719-0263
e-mail address: info@cancercareinc.org
website address: http://
www.cancercareinc.org

Cancer Guidance Institute
5604 Solway Street
Pittsburgh, PA 15217
phone: (412) 521-2291 or
(412) 782-4023

Cancer Information Service
National Cancer Institute
Bethesda, MD
phone: (800) 4-CANCER

Cancer Research Institute
681 Fifth Avenue
New York, NY 10022
phone: (800) 99-CANCER or
(212) 688-7515 (in New York City);
fax: (212) 832-9376
website address: http://
www.cancerresearch.org

Cancer Support Network
802 East Jefferson
Bloomington, IL 61701
phone: (309) 829-2273

**Candlelighters Childhood Cancer
Foundation**
7910 Woodmont Avenue, suite 460
Bethesda, MD 20814
phone: (800) 366-2223 or (301) 657-
8401 (in Bethesda); fax: (301) 718-2686

CHEMOcare
231 North Avenue West
Westfield, NJ 07090-1428
phone: (800) 55-CHEMO or
(908) 233-1103 (inside New Jersey);
fax: (908) 233-0228

Children's Hospice International
1101 King Street, suite 131
Alexandria, VA 22314
phone: (800) 242-4453 or
(703) 684-0330 (in Alexandria)

Choice in Dying
200 Varick Street, 10th floor, room
1001
New York, NY 10014-4810
phone: (800) 989-WILL or
(212) 366-5540 (in New York City);
fax: (212) 366-5337
e-mail addresses: cid@choices.org
website address: http://www.choices.org

Coping Magazine
P.O. Box 682268
Franklin, TN 37068-2268
phone: (615) 790-2400;
fax: (615) 794-0179
e-mail address: Copingmag@aol.com

Colon Cancer Support Group
c/o Andrew Kneier
UCSF/Mt. Zion Cancer Center
2356 Sutter Street
San Francisco, CA 94120
phone: (415) 885-7546

Corporate Angel Network (CAN)
Westchester County Airport Building I
White Plains, NY 10604
phone: (914) 328-1313;
fax: (914) 328-3938
e-mail address:
corpangl@ix.netcom.com
website address:
www.mach2media.cam/can

Cure for Lymphoma Foundation
215 Lexington Avenue
New York, NY 10016
phone: (212) 213-9595;
fax: (212) 213-1987

ENCORE
YWCA of the U.S.A.
726 Broadway, 5th floor
New York, NY 10003
phone: (212) 614-2700

International Cancer Alliance (ICA)
4853 Cordell Avenue, suite 11
Bethesda, MD 20814
phone: (800) 1 CARE-61;
fax: (301) 654-8684
website address: http://www.icare.org/
icare

**The Helping Hand Melanoma
Newsletter**
12 Arlington Avenue
Portland, ME 04101

Hospicelink
Hospice Education Institute
5 Essex Square, suite 3-B
P.O. Box 713
Essex, CT 06426-0713
phone: (800) 331-1620 or
(203) 767-1620 (in Essex)

**International Association for
Enterostomal Therapy**
505-A Tustin Avenue, suite 282
Santa Ana, CA 92705
phone: (714) 972-1725

**International Association of
Laryngectomees**
1599 Clifton Road, N.E.
Atlanta, GA 30329
phone: (404) 329-7650

International Myeloma Foundation
2120 Stanley Hills Drive
Los Angeles, CA 90046
phone: (800) 452-CURE or
(213) 654-3023 (in Los Angeles)

Leukemia Society of America
600 Third Avenue
New York, NY 10016
phone: (800) 955-4LSA (educational
materials) or (212) 573-8484 (general
information); fax: (212) 856-9686
website address: http://
www.leukemia.org

**Lymphoma Research Foundation of
America, Inc.**
8800 Venice Blvd., #207
Los Angeles, CA 90034
phone: (310) 204-7040;
fax: (310) 204-7043
e-mail address: LRFA@aol.com
website address: http://
www.lymphoma.org

Make Today Count
c/o Mid-America Cancer Center
1235 East Cherokee
Springfield, MO 65804-2263
phone: (800) 432-2273;
fax: (417) 888-7426

Make-A-Wish Foundation of America
100 W. Clarendon, suite 2200
Phoenix, AZ 85013-3518
phone: (800) 722-9474;
fax: 602-279-0855

Melanoma Foundation
c/o Richard Sagebiel, M.D.
UCSF/Mt. Zion Medical Center
2356 Sutter Street, 5th floor
San Francisco, CA 94120
phone: (415) 885-7546

**Mathews Foundation for Prostate
Cancer Research**
817 Commons Drive
Sacramento, CA 95825
phone: (800) 234-6284;
fax: (916) 927-5218
e-mail address: mathews@sna.com

**Mautner Project for Lesbians with
Cancer**
1707 L Street NW, suite 1060
Washington, D.C. 20036
phone: (202) 332-5536;
fax: (202) 265-6854
e-mail address: mautner@aol.com
website address: http://www.sirius.com/
~edisol/mautner/index.html

National Brain Tumor Foundation
785 Market Street, suite 1600
San Francisco, CA 94103
phone: (800) 934-CURE or (415) 284-
0208 (in San Francisco);
fax: (415) 284-0209
e-mail address: SSTF39B@prodigy.com

National Breast Cancer Coalition
1707 L Street NW, suite 1060
Washington, D.C. 20036
phone: (202) 296-7477;
fax: (202) 265-6854
website address: http://www.natlbcc.org

National Cancer Institute (NCI)
Cancer Information Service
9000 Rockville Pike, Building 31, room
10A19
Bethesda, MD 20892
website address: http://
cancernet.nci.nih.gov

**National Coalition for Cancer
Research (NCCR)**
426C Sweet, N.E.
Washington, D.C. 20002
phone: (202) 544-1880;
fax: (202) 543-2565

**National Coalition for Cancer
Survivorship (NCCS)**
1010 Wayne Avenue, suite 505
Silver Spring, MD 20910

phone: (888) 650-9127 (toll-free call);
fax: (301) 565-9670
website address: http://
www.access.digex.net/~mkragen/
cansearch.html

National Hospice Organization
1901 N. Moore Street, suite 901
Arlington, VA 22209
phone: (800) 658-8898 or
(703) 243-5900 (in Arlington)

National Kidney Cancer Association
1234 Sherman Avenue, suite 203
Evanston, IL 60202-1375
phone: (847) 332-1051;
fax: (847) 332-2978
BBS: (847) 332-1052
e-mail address: nkca@net100.com

National Leukemia Association, Inc.
585 Stewart Avenue, suite 536
Garden City, NY 11530
phone: (516) 222-1944

National Marrow Donor Program
3433 Broadway Street, NE, suite 500
Minneapolis, MN 55413
phone: (800) MARROW-2;
fax: (612) 627-8125
website address: http://
www.marrow.org

**National Patient Air Transport
Hotline (NPATH)**
P.O. Box 1940
Manassas, VA 22110
phone: (800) 296-1217;
fax: (703) 361-1792
e-mail address: npathmsg@aol.com
website address: www.npath.org

**Patient Advocates for Advanced
Cancer Treatments (PAACT)**
1143 Parmelee N.W.

Grand Rapids, MI 49504
phone: (616) 453-1477;
fax: (616) 453-1846

Physician Data Query (PDQ)
phone: (800) 4-CANCER
website address: http://
www.mcphu.edu/libraries/guides/
d15pdq.html

Planetree Health Resource Center
2040 Webster Street
San Francisco, CA 94115
phone: (415) 923-3680

R. A. Bloch Cancer Foundation, Inc.
The Cancer Hotline
4410 Main Street
Kansas City, MO 64111
phone: (816) 932-8453;
fax: (816) 931-7486

Share
817 Broadway, 6th floor
New York, NY 10016
phone: (212) 260-0580

The Life Extension Foundation
P.O. Box 229120
Hollywood, FL 33022-9120
phone: (800) 544-4440
website address: http://www.lifeorg/lef/
index.html

The Skin Cancer Foundation
245 Fifth Avenue, suite 2402
New York, NY 10016
phone: (212) 725-5176

The Skin Cancer Fund
P.O. Box 561
New York, NY 10156
phone: (800) SKIN-490;
fax: (212) 725-5751

Sunshine Foundation
4010 Levick Street
Philadelphia, PA 19135
phone: (800) 767-1976 or
(215) 335-2622 (in Philadelphia)

Sunshine Kids
2902 Ferndale Place
Houston, TX 77098
phone: (713) 524-1264

Support for People with Oral and Head and Neck Cancer, Inc.
P.O. Box 53
Locust Valley, NY 11560-0053
phone: (516) 759-5333;
fax: (516) 671-7637
e-mail address: spohnc@ix.netcom.com

Susan G. Komen Breast Cancer Foundation
5005 LBJ Freeway, suite 370
Dallas, TX 75244
phone: (800) I'M AWARE

United Ostomy Association
36 Executive Park, suite 120

Irvine, CA 92714
phone: (800) 826-0826 or (714) 660-8624 (in Irvine); fax: (714) 660-9262

Us-Too (for prostate cancer survivors)
930 North York Road, suite 50
Hinsdale, IL 60521-2993
phone: (800) 808-7866 or (630) 323-1002 (in Hinsdale); fax: (630) 323-1003

Wellness Community National Headquarters
2200 Colorado Avenue
Santa Monica, CA 90404-3506
phone: (800) PRO-HOPE or
(310) 453-2300 (in Santa Monica)

Y-Me
National Organization for Breast Cancer Information and Support, Inc.
18220 Harwood Avenue
Homewood, IL 60430-2104
phone: (800) 221-2141 or
(708) 799-8338 (in Homewood)
website address: http://www.y-me.org

APPENDIX III

State-by-State Guide to Cancer Research and Treatment Centers

ALABAMA

University of Alabama at Birmingham
Comprehensive Cancer Center
Basic Health Sciences Building, room
 108
1918 University Boulevard
Birmingham, AL 35294
phone: (205) 934-6612

University of South Alabama
USA Cancer Center, room 414
307 University Boulevard
Mobile, AL 36688
phone: (205) 460-7194

ALASKA

Virginia Mason Medical Center, RC-R1
1000 Seneca Street
Seattle, WA 98101
phone: (206) 223-6945

ARIZONA

The Arizona Cancer Center
University Medical Center at the
University of Arizona
1501 North Campbell Avenue
Tucson, AZ 85724
phone: (602) 626-6372

ARKANSAS

University Hospital of Arkansas
4301 West Markham Street
Little Rock, AR 72205
phone: (501) 686-7000

CALIFORNIA

The Kenneth Norris Jr. Comprehensive
Cancer Center
University of Southern California
1441 Eastlake Avenue
Los Angeles, CA 90033-0804
phone: (213) 226-2370

Jonsson Comprehensive Cancer Center
UCLA Breast Center
University of California Los Angeles
200 Medical Plaza
Los Angeles, CA 90027
phone: (213) 206-0278

City of Hope National Medical Center
Beckman Research Institute
1500 East Duarte Road
Duarte, CA 91010
phone: (818) 359-8111, ext. 2292

University of California San Diego
Cancer Center
225 Dickinson Street
San Diego, CA 92103
phone: (619) 543-6178

Stanford University Medical Center
Oncology Day Care Center
300 Pasteur Drive, room H0274
Stanford, CA 94305
phone: (415) 723-7621

COLORADO

University of Colorado Cancer Center
4200 East 9th Avenue, Box B190
Denver, CO 80262
phone: (303) 270-7235

CONNECTICUT

Yale University Comprehensive Cancer
Center
333 Cedar Street
P.O. Box 3333
New Haven, CT 06510
phone: (203) 785-6338

DISTRICT OF COLUMBIA

Lombardi Cancer Research Center
Georgetown University Medical Center
3800 Reservoir Road, N.W.
Washington, D.C. 20007
phone: (202) 687-2192

George Washington University Hospital
George Washington University
901 23rd Street, N.W.
Washington, D.C. 20037
phone: (202) 994-1000

Howard University Hospital
2041 Georgia Avenue, N.W.
Washington, D.C. 20060
phone (202) 865-6100

FLORIDA

Sylvester Comprehensive Cancer Center
University of Miami Medical School
1475 Northwest 12th Avenue
Miami, FL 33136
phone: (305) 548-4800

H. Lee Moffitt Cancer Center
University of South Florida
12902 Magnolia Drive
Tampa, FL 33682
phone: (813) 972-4673

Shands Hospital of the University of
Florida
1600 S.W. Archer Road
Gainesville, FL 32610
phone: (904) 395-0111

GEORGIA

Emory University Hospital
1364 Clifton Road, N.E.
Atlanta, GA 30322
phone: (404) 727-3456

St. Joseph's Hospital
5665 Peachtree Dunwoodie Road, N.E.
Atlanta, GA 30342
phone: (404) 252-9639

Medical College of Georgia Hospital
and Clinics
Georgia Radiation Therapy Center
1120 15th Street
Augusta, GA 30912
phone: (404) 721-2971

Grady Memorial Hospital
80 Butler Street, S.E.
Atlanta, GA 30335
phone: (404) 616-4885

HAWAII

Kaiser-Permanente Medical Center
32888 Moanaloa Road
Honolulu, HI
phone: (808) 834-5333

ILLINOIS

University of Chicago Cancer Research
Center
5841 South Maryland Avenue

Chicago, IL 60637
phone: (773) 702-9200
(800) 824-0200

Rush–Presbyterian–St. Luke's Medical
Center
1752 West Congress Parkway
Chicago, IL 60612
phone: (312) 942-5488

University of Illinois
840 South Wood Street, room 720 N
CSB
Chicago, IL 60612
phone: (312) 996-5985

Northwestern Memorial Hospital and
Prentice Women's Hospital
Superior Street and Fairbanks Court
Chicago, IL 60611
phone: (312) 908-5950

INDIANA

Indiana University Medical Center
1100 West Michigan Street
Indianapolis, IN 46223
phone: (317) 274-5000

Methodist Hospital of Indiana
Methodist Hospital Cancer Center
1701 North Senate Boulevard
Indianapolis, IN 46206
phone: (317) 927-5770

IOWA

University of Iowa Hospitals and Clinics
650 Newton Road
Iowa City, IA 52242
phone: (319) 356-1616

KANSAS

University of Kansas Hospital
39th and Rainbow Boulevard
Kansas City, KS 66103
phone: (913) 588-5000

KENTUCKY

University of Kentucky Hospital
Albert B. Chandler Medical Center
800 Rose Street
Lexington, KY 40526
phone: (606) 233-5000

LOUISIANA

Louisiana State University Hospital
P.O. Box 33932
1541 Kings Highway
Shreveport, LA 71361
phone: (318) 674-5000

Medical Center of Louisiana at New
Orleans
1532 Tulane Avenue
New Orleans, LA 70140
phone: (504) 568-2311

Tulane University
1430 Tulane Avenue
New Orleans, LA 70112
phone: (504) 588-5482

MARYLAND

Johns Hopkins Oncology Center
600 North Wolfe Street
Baltimore, MD 21205
phone: (301) 955-8638

Warren Grant Magnuson Clinical
Center
The National Institutes of Health
9000 Rockville Pike, Building 10
Bethesda, MD 20205
phone: (301) 496-4891

MASSACHUSETTS

Dana–Farber Cancer Institute
44 Binney Street
Boston, MA 02115
phone: (617) 732-3214

Massachusetts General Hospital
32 Fruit Street
Boston, MA 02114
phone: (617) 726-2000

The Breast Health Center
New England Medical Center
750 Washington Street
Boston, MA 02111
phone: (617) 956-5000

MICHIGAN

Meyer L. Prentis Comprehensive
Cancer Center of Metropolitan Detroit
110 East Warren Avenue
Detroit, MI 48201
phone: (313) 745-4329

Harper Hospital
3990 John R. Street
Detroit, MI 48201
phone: (313) 745-8040

Minority-Based Community Clinical
Oncology Program of Detroit
27211 Lahser Road, suite 2000
Southfield, MI 48034
phone: (313) 356-2828

University of Michigan Cancer Center
101 Simpson Drive
Ann Arbor, MI 48109-0752
phone: (313) 936-9583

Butterworth Hospital
Grand Rapids Clinical Oncology
Program
100 Michigan Street, N.E.
Grand Rapids, MI 49503
phone: (616) 774-1230

MINNESOTA

Mayo Comprehensive Cancer Center
200 First Street, S.W.
Rochester, MN 55905
phone: (507) 284-3413

MISSISSIPPI

University of Mississippi Medical
Center
University Hospitals and Clinics
2500 North State Street
Jackson, MS 39216
phone: (601) 984-4100

MISSOURI

Baptist Medical Center
Kansas City Clinical Oncology Program
6601 Rockhill Road
Kansas City, MO 64131
phone: (816) 276-7834

Barnes Hospital
Barnes Hospital Plaza
St. Louis, MO 63111
phone: (314) 362-5000

NEBRASKA

University of Nebraska Medical Center
Clinical Cancer Center
600 South 42nd Street
Omaha, NE 68198-1210
phone: (402) 559-5600

NEVADA

Southern Nevada Cancer Research
Foundation
501 South Rancho Drive, suite C-14
Las Vegas, NE 89106
phone: (702) 384-0013

NEW HAMPSHIRE

Norris Cotton Cancer Center
Dartmouth–Hitchcock Medical Center
1 Medical Center Drive
Lebanon, NH 03756
phone: (603) 650-5000

NEW JERSEY

Robert Wood Johnson University
Hospital

One Robert Wood Johnson Place
New Brunswick, NJ 08901
phone: (201) 828-3000

Newark Inner City Center for Medicine
and Immunology
1 Bruce Street
Newark, NJ 07103
phone: (201) 456-4600

University Hospital
University of Medicine and Dentistry of
New Jersey
150 Bergen Street
Newark, NJ 07103
phone: (201) 456-4300

NEW MEXICO

University Hospital
2211 Lomas Boulevard, N.E.
Albuquerque, NM 87106
phone: (505) 843-2111

NEW YORK

Memorial Sloan–Kettering Cancer
Center
1275 York Avenue
New York, NY 10021
phone: (800) 525-2225

Kaplan Comprehensive Cancer Center
New York University Medical Center
462 First Avenue
New York, NY 10016-9103
phone: (212) 263-6485

Columbia University Comprehensive
Cancer Center
Columbia University College of
Physicians and Surgeons
622 West 168th Street
New York, NY 10032
phone: (212) 305-2500

The Mount Sinai Medical Center
One Gustave Levy Place

New York, NY 10029
phone: (212) 650-6500

Albert Einstein College of Medicine
1300 Morris Park Avenue
Bronx, NY 10461
phone: (212) 920-4826

Kings County
State University of New York Health
Science Center
450 Clarkson Avenue
Brooklyn, NY 11203
phone: (718) 270-1552

Roswell Park Cancer Institute
Elm and Carlton Streets
Buffalo, NY 14263
phone: (716) 845-4400

University of Rochester Cancer Center
Strong Memorial Hospital
601 Elmwood Avenue
P.O. Box 704
Rochester, NY 14642
phone: (716) 275-4911

NORTH CAROLINA

Duke Comprehensive Cancer Center
(NCI)
P.O. Box 3814
Durham, NC 27710
phone: (919) 286-5515

Lineberger Comprehensive Cancer
Center
University of North Carolina
Department of Medicine
Chapel Hill, NC 27599
phone: (919) 966-4431

Cancer Center of Wake Forest
University at the Bowman Gray School
of Medicine
Medical Center Boulevard
Winston-Salem, NC 27157
phone: (919) 748-4464

OHIO

Ohio State University Comprehensive
Cancer Center
410 West 10th Avenue
Columbus, OH 43210
phone: (614) 293-8619

Case Western Reserve University
University Hospitals of Cleveland/
Ireland Cancer Center
2074 Abington Road
Cleveland, OH 44106
phone: (216) 844-5432

OKLAHOMA

Oklahoma Medical Center
800 N.E. 13th Street
Oklahoma City, OK 73104
phone: (405) 271-3700

St. Francis Hospital
Natalie Warren Bryant Cancer Center
6161 South Yale Avenue
Tulsa, OK 74136
phone: (918) 494-1234

OREGON

Oregon Health Sciences University
University Hospital
3181 S.W. Sam Jackson Park Road
Portland, OR 97201
phone: (503) 494-8311

PENNSYLVANIA

Fox Chase Cancer Center
7701 Burholme Avenue
Philadelphia, PA 19111
phone: (215) 728-2570

University of Pennsylvania Cancer
Center
Penn Tower Hotel
3400 Spruce Street, 6th floor
Philadelphia, PA 19104
phone: (215) 662-6364

Pittsburgh Cancer Institute
200 Meyran Avenue
Pittsburgh, PA 15213-2592
phone: (800) 537-4063

Presbyterian University Hospital
DeSoto at O'Hara Streets
Pittsburgh, PA 15213
phone: (412) 647-3325

Montefiore University Hospital
3459 5th Avenue
Pittsburgh, PA 15213
phone: (412) 648-6000

Milton S. Hershey Medical Center
Pennsylvania State University
P.O. Box 850
Hershey, PA 17033
phone: (717) 531-8521

RHODE ISLAND

Roger Williams Cancer Center
825 Chalkstone Avenue
Providence, RI 02908
phone: (410) 456-2071

SOUTH DAKOTA

Sioux Community Cancer Consortium
Central Plains Clinic, Ltd.
1000 East 21st Street, suite 2000
Sioux Falls, SD 57105
phone: (605) 331-3160

Rapid City Medical Center
P.O. Box 4097
Rapid City, SD 57709
phone: (803) 560-6812

TENNESSEE

Drew-Meharry-Morehouse Consortium
Cancer Center
1005 D. B. Todd Boulevard
Nashville, TN 37208
phone: (615) 327-6927

SOUTH CAROLINA

Medical Center of the Medical
University of South Carolina
171 Ashley Avenue
Charleston, SC 29425
phone: (803) 792-7616

Spartanburg Regional Medical Center
101 East Wood Street
Spartanburg, SC 29303
phone: (803) 560-6812

TEXAS

The University of Texas
M. D. Anderson Cancer Center
1515 Holcombe Boulevard
Houston, TX 77030
phone: (713) 792-3245

Institute for Cancer Research and Care
4450 Medical Drive
San Antonio, TX 78229
phone: (512) 616-5580

Sammons Cancer Center
Baylor University Medical Center
3500 Gaston Avenue
Dallas, TX 75246
phone: (214) 820-0111

Santa Rosa Hospital
519 West Houston Street
San Antonio, TX 78207
phone: (512) 224-6531

UTAH

Utah Regional Cancer Center
University of Utah Medical Center
50 North Medical Drive, room 2C10
Salt Lake City, UT 84132
phone: (801) 581-5052

VERMONT

Vermont Cancer Center
University of Vermont

1 South Prospect Street
Burlington, VT 05401
phone: (802) 656-4580

VIRGINIA

University of Virginia Medical Center
Cancer Center (BSC)
Jefferson Park Avenue
Box 334
Charlottesville, VA 22908
phone: (804) 924-0211

Massey Cancer Center
Virginia Commonwealth University
Medical College of Virginia
1200 East Broad Street
Richmond, VA 23298
phone: (804) 786-9641

Virginia Commonwealth University
Medical College of Virginia
P.O. Box 230, MCV Station
Richmond, VA 23298
phone: (804) 786-0450

WASHINGTON

Fred Hutchinson Cancer Research
Center
1124 Columbia Street
Seattle, WA 98104
phone: (206) 467-4675

The Cancer Center
University Hospital, University of
Washington
1959 Northeast Pacific Street
Seattle, WA 98195
phone: (206) 543-3300

WISCONSIN

Wisconsin Clinical Cancer Center
University of Wisconsin
600 Highland Avenue
Madison, WI 53792
phone: (608) 263-8090

Marshfield Medical Research
Foundation
Marshfield Clinic
1000 North Oak Avenue
Marshfield, WI 54449
phone: (715) 387-5134

APPENDIX IV

Brand-Name Food Products: Manufacturers' Addresses and Phone Numbers

Alpine Lace (Skim Milk Cheddar Cheese)
Alpine Lace Brands, Inc.
111 Dunnell Road
Maplewood, NJ 07040
phone: (201) 378-8600

Argo (Corn Starch)
phone: (800) 344-2746

Arrowhead Mills (Organic Whole Grain Soy Flour, Oat Flour, and Vital Wheat Gluten)
Arrowhead Mills
P.O. Box 2059
Hereford, TX 79045
phone: (806) 364-0730

Bertolli (Extra Light Olive Oil)
phone: (800) 908-9789

Bob's Red Mill (Stone Ground Golden Corn Masa Flour)
Bob's Red Mill Natural Foods, Inc.
5209 SE International Way
Milwaukee, OR 97222
phone: (503) 654-3215

Breakstone's (Fat Free Sour Cream)
phone: (800) 538-1998

Bush's (Chili Magic)
Bush Bros.
P.O. Box 52330, Department C
Knoxville, TN 37950-2330
phone: (423) 588-7685

Campbell's Soup Company (V-8 Picante Mild Flavor)
phone: (800) 257-8443

Classico (Tomato and Basil Pasta Sauce, Four Cheese Pasta Sauce)
phone: (800) 426-7336

Contadina (Protein Enriched Pasta, Tomato Sauce, and Tomato Paste)
Nestlé Consumer Services–BPP
P.O. Box 29055
Glendale, CA 91209-9055
phone: (818) 549-6000

Del Monte (Fresh Cut Peeled Diced Tomatoes)
phone: (800) 543-3090

ecoNugenics
65 Koch Road
Corte Madera, CA 94925
phone: (415) 454-6935

Edensoy (Original Organic Soy
Beverage)
Eden Foods, Inc.
701 Tecumseh Road
Clinton, MI 49236
phone: (517) 456-7424

Green Giant (Harvest Burgers For
Recipes, Harvest Burgers Original, and
Extra Sweet Niblets Corn)
phone: (800) 998-9996

Haelin Products Inc.
P.O. Box 7802
Metairie, LA 70010

Hain (Expeller Pressed Organic Canola
Oil)
Hain Consumer Affairs
50 Charles Lindbergh Boulevard
Uniondale, NY 11553
phone: (516) 237-6200

Healthy Choice (Fat Free Grated
Cheddar Cheese and Mozzarella
Cheese)
phone: (800) 323-9980

Heinz (Tomato Ketchup)
HJ Heinz General Office
1062 Progress Street
Pittsburgh, PA 15212
phone: (412) 456-5700

Hellman's (Low Fat Mayonnaise and
Dijonnaise)
phone: (800) 338-8831

Hershey's (Reduced Fat Chocolate
Chips)
phone: (800) 468-1714

Hunt's (Choice Cut Diced Tomatoes
With Roasted Garlic)
Hunt–Wesson, Inc.
P.O. Box 4800
Fullerton, CA 92834
phone: (714) 680-1000

Ivy Foods (Wheat Meat, Chicken Style)
7613 South Prospector Drive
Salt Lake City, UT 84121
phone: (801) 943-7664

Jell-O (Flan [Spanish-style custard])
phone: (800) 431-1001

Kame (Dark Sesame Oil, Oyster Sauce,
and Light Soy Sauce)
Kame
Liberty Richter, Inc.
400 Lyster Avenue
Saddle Brook, NJ 07663
phone: (201) 843-8900

Karo (Light Corn Syrup)
phone: (800) 338-8831

Kraft (Fat Free Singles, 2% Milk
Singles, and Whipped Cream Cheese
With Chives)
phone: (800) 634-1984

Land O'Lakes (Light Butter)
phone: (800) 328-4155

Lightlife (Meatless Smart Deli Country
Ham)
phone: (800) 274-6001

Manischewitz (Split Pea Soup Mix
With Barley)
The B. Manischewitz Company
Distributors
1 Manischewitz Plaza
Jersey City, NJ 07302
phone: (201) 333-3700

Morga (Vegetable Bouillon with Sea Salt)
Liberty-Richter, Inc.
400 Lyster Avenue
Saddle Brook, NJ 07663
phone: (201) 843-8900

Morningstar Farms (Breakfast Links, Breakfast Patties, Breakfast Strips, Chik Nuggets, and Deli Franks)
Worthington Foods
Worthington, OH 43085
phone: (614) 885-9511

Nasoya (Tofu, Egg Roll Wrappers, Won Ton Wrappers, and Nayonaisse)
phone: (800) 229-8638

Ocean Spray (Cranberry Juice Drink, and Ruby Red & Tangerine Juice Cocktail)
phone: (800) 662-3263

Old El Paso (Taco Sauce, Chopped Green Chilies, and Reduced Sodium Taco Seasoning Mix)
phone: (800) 300-8664

Pepperidge Farm (Light Style Wheat Bread and Very Thin Whole Wheat Bread)
Pepperidge Farm
595 Westport Avenue
Norwalk, CT 06856
phone: (203) 846-7000

Polly-O (Non Fat Ricotta Cheese)
Pollio Dairy Products
120 Mineola Boulevard
Mineola, NY 11501
phone: (516) 741-8000

Progresso (Black Beans, Garbanzo Beans, Pinto Beans, and Crushed Tomatoes with Added Puree)

Progresso
P.O. Box 555
Vineland, NJ 08360
phone: (609) 691-1565

Quaker (Old Fashioned Oats, Quick Grits, and Cornmeal)
The Quaker Oats Co.
P.O. Box 049003
Chicago, IL 60604-9003
phone: (312) 222-7111

Ralston Purina
Protein Technologies
Checkerboard Square
St. Louis, MO 63164
(314) 982-1000
(800) 325-1700

Rice Select (Teximati Brown Rice, Kasmati Rice, and Basmati Rice)
phone: (800) 229-RICE

Ronzoni (Curly Lasagne Noodles and Oven Ready Lasagna Noodles)
phone: (800) 468-1714

Soya Kaas (Monterey Jack Style Cheese Substitute)
American Natural Snacks
P.O. Box 1067
St. Augustine, FL 32085
phone: (904) 825-2039

Soyco (Lite & Less Grated Parmesan Cheese Alternative)
Soyco Foods
2441 Viscount Row
Orlando, FL 32809
phone: (407) 855-6600

Sunsweet (Lighter Bake Butter And Oil Replacement)
phone: (800) 417-2253

Thai Kitchen (Green Curry Paste, and Lite Coconut Milk)
Epicurean International, Inc.
155 Filbert Street, suite 252
Oakland, CA 94607
phone: (510) 268-0209

Tropicana (Pure Premium Orange Juice and Ruby Red Grapefruit Juice)
phone: (800) 237-7799

Twin Laboratories (Soy Cocktail, Phytonutrient Cocktail, Choline Cocktail II)

2120 Smithtown Avenue
Ronkonkoma, NY 11779
phone: (800) 645-5626

Westbrae (Westbrae Café Coffee Beverage, Westsoy Non-Fat Soy Beverage)
phone: (800) 769-6455

White Wave (Meatless Chicken Style Sandwich Slices and Silk)
White Wave, Inc.
1990 N. 57th Court
Boulder, CO 80301
phone: (303) 443-3470

SELECTED REFERENCES

Adams LL et al. "The Association of Lipoprotein Cholesterol with Vitamin A." *Cancer* 56 (1985): 2593–2597.

Adams LL et al. "Blood Pressure Determinants in a Middle-Class Black Population: the University of Pittsburgh Experience." *Preventive Medicine* 15 (1986): 232–243.

Aderounmu AF. "The Relative Importance of Genetic and Environmental Factors in Hypertension in Black Subjects." *Clinical and Experimental Hypertension* 3 (1981): 597–621.

Adler AI et al. "Is Diabetes Mellitus a Risk Factor for Ovarian Cancer? A Case-Control." *Cancer Causes and Control* 1996; 7:475–8.

Adlercreutz H, Markkanen H, Watanabe S. "Plasma Concentrations of Phyto-oestrogens in Japanese Men." *Lancet* 342 (1993): 1209–1210.

Alarcon et al. "Clinical Trial of Locally Available Mixed Diet or Lactose-Free Soy Formula for the Nutritional Therapy of Acute Diarrhea in Peruvian Children." In: *Proceedings of the XIVth International Congress on Nutrition* (Seoul, Korea, 1990), 87–88.

Albanes D et al. "Effects of Alpha-Tocopherol and Beta-Carotene Supplements on Cancer Incidence in the Alpha-Tocopherol Beta-Carotene Cancer Prevention Study." *American Journal of Clinical Nutrition* 62 (1995): 1427S–1430S.

Albini A et al. "Inhibition of Invasion, Gelatinase Activity, Tumor Take and Metastasis of Malignant Cells by *N*-Acetylcysteine." *International Journal of Cancer* 61 (1995): 121–129.

Amonette RA, Kaplan RJ. "Squamous-Cell and Basal-Cell Carcinomas in Black Patients." *Journal of Dermatol Surg* 2 (1976): 158–161.

Anderson JD. "Breast Feeding and Breast Cancer." *South African Medical Journal* 49 (1975): 479–482.

Anderson NB et al. "Type A Behavior, Family History of Hypertension, and Cardiovascular Responsivity among Black Women." *Health Psychology* 5 (1986): 393–406.

Anderson JJ, Rondano P, Holmes A. "Roles of Diet and Physical Activity in the Prevention of Osteoporosis." *Scandinavian Journal of Rheumatology Supplement* 103 (1996): 65–74.

Andersson SO et al. "Energy, Nutrient Intake and Prostate Cancer Risk: A Population-Based Case-Control Study in Sweden." *International Journal of Cancer* 68 (1996): 716–722.

Anthony MS et al. "Soybean Isoflavones Improve Cardiovascular Risk Factors without Affecting the Reproductive System of Peripubertal Rhesus Monkeys." *Journal of Nutrition* 126 (1996): 43–50.

Appel L et al. "A Clinical Trial of the Effects of Dietary Patterns on Blood Pressure. *New England Journal of Medicine* 336 (1997): 1117–1124.

Axtell LM, Myers MH. "Contrasts in Survival of Black and White Cancer Patients, 1960–73." *Journal of the National Cancer Institute* 60 (1978): 1209–1215.

Azuma J. "Therapeutic Effect of Taurine in Congestive Heart Failure: A Double-Blind Crossover Trial." *Clinical Cardiology* 8 (1985): 276–282.

Babain RJ et al. "Familial Patterns of Prostate Cancer: A Case-Control Analysis." *Journal of Urology* 145 (1991): 145–213.

Baekey PA et al. "Grapefruit Pectin Inhibits Hypercholesterolemia and Atherosclerosis in Miniature Swine." *Clinical Cardiology* 11 (1988): 597–600.

Bailey DG et al. "Interaction of Citrus Juices with Felodipine and Nifedipine." *Lancet* 337 (1991): 268–269.

Bailey DG et al. "Effect of Grapefruit Juice and Naringin on Nisoldipine Pharmacokinetics." *Clinical Pharmacology and Therapeutics* 54 (1993): 589–594.

Bailey DG et al. "Grapefruit juice–Felodipine Interaction: Reproductivity and Characterization with the Extended Release Drug Formulation." *British Journal of Clinical Pharmacology* 40 (1995): 135–140.

Bain RP, Greenberg RS, Whitaker JP. "Racial Differences in Survival of Women with Breast Cancer." *Journal of Chronic Diseases* 39 (1986): 631–642.

Bakth S et al. "Arrhythmia Susceptibility and Myocardial Composition in Diabetes." *Journal of Clinical Investigation* 1986; 77:382–395.

Balansky R et al. "Induction by Carcinogens and Chemoprevention by *N*-Acetylcysteine of Adducts to Mitochondrial DNA in Rat Organs." *Cancer Research* 56 (1996): 1642–1647.

Barker JE et al. "Glutathione Protects Astrocytes from Peroxynitrite-Mediated Mitochondrial Damage: Implications for Neuronal/Astrocytic Trafficking and Neurodegeneration." *Developmental Neuroscience* 18 (1996): 391–396.

Barnes, S et al. "Potential Role of Dietary Isoflavones in the Prevention of Cancer. *Advances in Experimental Medicine and Biology* 135 (1994): 135–147.

Barnes S, Peterson TG, Coward L. "Rationale for the Use of Genistein-Containing Soy Matrices in Chemoprevention Trials for Breast and Prostate Cancer." *Journal of Cellular Biochemistry* 22 (1995): 181–187.

Barrett-Connor E, Friedlander NJ. "Dietary Fat, Calories, and the Risk of Breast Cancer in Postmenopausal Women: A Prospective Population-Based Study." *Journal of the American College of Nutrition* 12 (1993): 390–399.

Bassett MT, Krieger N. "Social Class and Black–White Differences in Breast Cancer Survival." *American Journal of Public Health* 76 (1986): 1400–1403.

Beck SA, Smith KL, Tisdale MJ. "Anticachetic and Antitumor Effect of Eicosapentaenoic Acid and Its Effect on Protein Turnover." *Cancer Research* 51 (1991): 6089–6093.

Becker FF. "Inhibition of Spontaneous Hepatocarcinogenesis in C3H/HeN Mice by Edi Pro A, an Isolated Soy Protein." *Carcinogenesis* 2 (1981): 1213–1214.

Beier RC. "Natural Pesticides and Bioactive Components in Foods. *Reviews of Environmental Contamination and Toxicology* 113 (1990): 47–137.

Bellentani S et al. "Taurine Increases Bile Pool Size and Reduces Bile Saturation Index in the Hamster." *Journal of Lipid Research* 28 (1987): 1021–1027.

Belli DC et al. "The Influence of Taurine on the Bile Acid Maximum Secretory Rate in the Guinea Pig." *Pediatric Research* 24 (1988): 34–37.

Belli DC et al. "The Effect of Taurine on the Cholestatic Potential of Sulfated Lithocholate and Its Conjugates." *Liver* 11 162–169.

Benton RE et al. "Grapefruit Juice Alters Terfenadine Pharmacokinetics, Resulting in Prolongation of Repolarization on the Electrocardiogram." *Clinical Pharmacology and Therapeutics* 383–388.

Berlie J et al. ["Cancer of the Prostate: Epidemiologic Evaluation, Incidence, and Trends, Especially in France"] *Bulletin du Cancer* 72 (1985): 391–404.

Bertrand E et al. "Uric Acid: A Risk Factor for Coronary Heart Disease?" *Circulation* 59 (1979): 969–977.

Bhuvarahamurthy V, Balasubramanian N, Govindasamy S. "Effect of Radiotherapy and Chemoradiotherapy on Circulating Antioxidant System of Human Uterine Cervical Carcinoma." *Molecular and Cell Biochemistry* 158 (1996): 17–23.

Bird AP. "The Relationship of DNA Methylation to Cancer." *Cancer Surveys* 28 (1996): 87–101.

Birt DF, Pelling JC, Nair S, Lepley D. "Diet Intervention for Modifying Cancer Risk." *Progress in Clinical and Biological Research* 395 (1996): 223–234.

Bitonti AJ et al. "Depletion of Estrogen Receptor in Human Breast Tumor Cells by a Novel Substituted Indole That Does Not Bind to the Hormone Binding Domain." *Journal of Steroid Biochemistry and Molecular Biology* 58 (1996): 21–30.

Bloem LJ, Manatunga AK, Pratt JH. "Racial Difference in the Relationship of an Angiotensin I–Converting Enzyme Gene Polymorphism to Serum Angiotensin I–Converting Enzyme Activity." *Hypertension* 27 (1996): 62–66.

Bonham GS, Brock DB. "The Relationship of Diabetes with Race, Sex, and Obesity." *American Journal of Clinical Nutrition* 41 (1985): 776–783.

Bostick RM et al. "Relation of Calcium, Vitamin D, and Dairy Food Intake to Incidence of Colon Cancer Among Older Women: The Iowa Women's Health Study." *American Journal of Epidemiology* 137 (1993): 1302–1317.

Bougnoux P et al. "Alpha-Linolenic Acid Content of Adipose Breast Tissue: A Host Determinant of the Risk of Early Metastasis in Breast Cancer." *British Journal of Cancer* 70 (1994): 330–334.

Boutron MC et al. "Calcium, Phosphorus, Vitamin D, Dairy Products and Colorectal Carcinogenesis: A French Case Control Study." *British Journal of Cancer* 74 (1996): 145–151.

Bradlow HL et al. "Long-Term Responses of Women to Indole-3-Carbinol or a High Fiber Diet." *Cancer Epidemiology, Biomarkers and Prevention* 3 (1994): 591–595.

Bradlow HL et al. "Indole-3-Carbinol: A Novel Approach to Breast Cancer Prevention." *Annals of the New York Academy of Sciences* 768 (1995): 180–200.

Bradlow HL et al. "2-Hydroxyestrone: The 'Good' Estrogen." *Journal of Endocrinology* 150 (1996): S259–S265.

Brancati FL et al. "The Excess Incidence of Diabetic End-Stage Renal Disease among Blacks." *Journal of the American Medical Association* 268 (1992): 3079–3084.

Braun MM et al. "Prostate Cancer and Prediagnostic Levels of Serum Vitamin D Metabolites." *Cancer Causes and Control* 6 (1995): 235–239.

Brawley OW. "5-a-Reductase Inhibition and Prostate Cancer Prevention." *Cancer Epidemiology Biomarkers and Prevention* 3 (1994): 177–182.

Brenner RV et al. "The Antiproliferative Effect of Vitamin D Analogs on MCF-7 Human Breast Cancer Cells." *Cancer Letters* 92 (1995): 77–82.

Brickman AS et al. "Racial Differences in Platelet Cytosolic Calcium and Calcitropic Hormones in Normotensive Subjects." *Clinical Pharmacology and Therapeutics* 51 (1993): 495–500.

Brown LM et al. "Testicular Cancer in the United States: Trends in Incidence and Mortality." *International Journal of Epidemiology* 15 (1986): 164–170.

Bullock A et al. "Racial Differences in Prostate Cancer Detection and Staging." *Journal of Urology* 151 (1994): 292.

Buras RR et al. "Vitamin D Receptors in Breast Cancer Cells." *Breast Cancer Research and Treatment* 31 (1994): 191–202.

Burchfiel CM et al. "Cardiovascular Risk Factors and Impaired Glucose Tolerance: The San Luis Valley Diabetes Study." *American Journal of Epidemiology* 131 (1990): 57–70.

Cai Q, Wei H. "Effect of Dietary Genistein on Antioxidant Enzyme Activities in SENCAR Mice." *Nutrition and Cancer* 25 (1996): 1–7.

Canada et al. "Glutathione Depletion Increases the Cytotoxicity of Melphalan to PC-3, an Androgen-Insensitive Prostate Cancer Cell Line." *Cancer Chemotherapy and Pharmacology* 32 (1993): 73–77.

Cantafora A et al. "Effect of Taurine Administration on Liver Lipids in Guinea Pig." *Experientia* 42 (1986): 407–408.

Cantafora A et al. "Dietary Taurine Content Changes Liver Lipids in Cats." *Journal of Nutrition* 121 (1991): 1522–1528.

Cantrill R et al. "Concentration-Dependent Effect of Iron on Gamma-Linolenic Acid Toxicity in ZR-75-1 Human Breast Tumor Cells in Culture." *Cancer Letters* 72 (1993): 99–102.

Carroll KK et al. "Calcium and Carcinogenesis of the Mammary Gland." *American Journal of Clinical Nutrition* 54 (1991): 206S–208S.

Catalona WJ et al. "Measurement of Prostate-Specific Antigen in Serum as a Screening Test for Prostate Cancer." *New England Journal of Medicine* 324 (1991): 1156–1161.

Cerda JJ et al. "The Effects of Grapefruit Pectin on Patients at Risk for Coronary Heart Disease without Altering Diet or Lifestyle." *Clinical Cardiology* 589–594.

Chajès V et al. "Influence of n-3 Fatty Acids on the Growth of Human Breast Cancer Cells *in Vitro*: Relationship to Peroxides and Vitamin E." *Breast Cancer Research and Treatment* 34 (1995): 199–212.

Chaudry A. "Essential Fatty Acid Distribution in the Plasma and Tissue Phospholipids of Patients with Benign and Malignant Prostatic Disease." *British Journal of Cancer* 64 (1991): 1157–1160.

Chaudry AA et al. "Arachidonic Acid Metabolism in Benign and Malignant Prostatic Tissue *in Vitro*: Effects of Fatty Acids and Cyclooxygenase Inhibitors. *International Journal Cancer* 57 (1994): 176–180.

Chensney RW "Taurine: Its Biological Role and Clinical Implications." *Advances in Pediatrics* 32 (1985): 1–42.

Cho JH et al. "Increased Calcium Stories in Platelets from African Americans." *Hypertension* 25 (1995): 377–383.

Christakos S. "Vitamin D and Breast Cancer." *Advances in Experimental Medicine and Biology* 364:115–8.

Christensen JG, LeBlanc GA. "Reversal of Multidrug Resistance *in Vivo* by Dietary Administration of the Phytochemical Indole-3-Carbinol." *Cancer Research* 56 (1996): 574–581.

Christensen B. "Folate Deficiency, Cancer and Congenital Abnormalities. Is There a Connection?" *Tidsskrift for den Norske Laegeforening* 116 (1996): 250–254.

Chung FL et al. "New Potential Chemopreventive Agents for Lung Carcinogenesis of Tobacco-Specific Nitrosamine." *Cancer Research* 57 (1992): 2719S–2722S.

Clinton SK et al. "Cis-trans Lycopene Isomers, Carotenoids, and Retinol in the Human Prostate." *Cancer Epidemiology, Biomarkers and Prevention* 823–833.

Coalson DW et al. "Reduced Availability of Endogenously Synthesized Methionine for S-Adenosylmethionine Formation in Methionine-Dependent Cancer Cells." *Proceedings of the National Academy of Sciences of the United States of America* 79 (1982): 4248–5142.

Colette C et al. "Platelet Function in Type I diabetes: Effects of Supplementation with Large Doses of Vitamin E." *American Journal of Clinical Nutrition* 47 (1988): 256–261.

Colston KW et al. "Effects of Synthetic Vitamin D Analogues on Breast Cancer Cell Proliferation *in Vivo* and *in Vitro*." *Biochemical Pharmacology* 44 (1992): 693–702.

Comer PF et al. "Effect of Dietary Vitamin D3 (Cholecalciferol) on Colon Carcinogenesis Induced by 1,2-Dimethylhydrazine in Male Fischer 344 Rats." *Nutrition and Cancer* 19 (1993): 113–124.

Cooper R et al. "High-Density Lipoprotein Cholesterol and Angiographic Coronary Artery Disease in Black Patients." *American Heart Journal* 110 (1985): 1006–1011.

Cooper RS et al. "Survival Rates and Prehospital Delay during Myocardial Infarction among Black Persons." *American Journal of Cardiology* 57 (1986): 208–211.

Cooper RS et al. "Cell Cations and Blood Pressure in US Whites, US Blacks, and West African Blacks." *Journal of Human Hypertension* 4 (1990): 477–484.

Coovadia YM. "Primary Testicular Tumours among White, Black and Indian Patients." *South African Medical Journal* 54 (1978): 351–352.

Corder EH et al. "Vitamin D and Prostate Cancer: A Prediagnostic Study with Stored Sera." *Cancer Epidemiology, Biomarkers and Prevention* 2 (1993): 467–472.

Corder EH et al. "Seasonal Variation in Vitamin D, Vitamin D–Binding Protein, and Dehydroepiandrosterone: Risk of Prostate Cancer in Black and White Men." *Cancer Epidemiology, Biomarkers and Prevention* 4 (1995): 655–659.

Costa A et al. "Prostpects of Chemoprevention of Human Cancers with the Synthetic Retinoid Fenretinide." *Cancer Research* 54 (1994): 2032S–2037S.

Criqui MH et al. "Selenium, Retinol, Retinol-Binding Protein, and Uric Acid. Associations with Cancer Mortality in a Population-Based Prospective Case-Control Study." *Annals of Epidemiology* 1 (1991): 385–393.

Crowe JP Jr. et al. "The Interaction of Estrogen Receptor Status and Race in Predicting Prognosis for Stage I Breast Cancer Patients." *Surgery* 100 (1986): 599–605.

Crowell PL "Chemoprevention of Mammary Carcinogenesis by Hydroxylated Derivatives of D-Limonene." *Carcinogenesis* 13 (1992): 1261–1264.

Dabek J. "An Emerging View of Vitamin D." *Scandinavian Journal of Clinical and Laboratory Investigation Supplement* 201 (1990): 127–133.

Das UN. "Gamma-Linolenic Acid, Arachidonic Acid, and Eicosapentaenoic Acid as Potential Anticancer Drugs." *Nutrition* 6 (1990): 429–434.

Das UN. "Free Radicals: Biology and Relevance to Disease." *Journal of the Association of Physicians of India* 38 (1990): 495–498.

Das UN. "Tumoricidal Action of *cis*-Unsaturated Fatty Acids and Their Relationship to Free Radicals and Lipid Peroxidation." *Cancer Letters* 56 (1991): 235–243.

Das UN, Prasad VV, Reddy DR. "Local Application of Gamma-Linolenic Acid in the Treatment of Human Gliomas." *Cancer Letters* 94 (1995): 147–155.

Dashwood RH et al. "Anticarcinogenic Activity of Indole-3-Carbinol Acid Products: Ultrasensitive Bioassay by Trout Embryo Microinjection." *Cancer Research* 54 (1994): 3617–3619.

Daviglus ML et al. "Dietary Beta-Carotene, Vitamin C, and Risk of Prostate Cancer: Results from the Western Electric Study." *Epidemiology* 7 (1996) 472–477.

De Flora S et al. "Chemopreventive Properties and Mechanisms of N-Acetylcysteine. The Experimental Background." *Journal of Cell Biochemistry Supplement* 22 (1995): 33–41.

De Flora S et al. "Synergism between N-Acetylcysteine and Doxorubicin in the Prevention of Tumorigenicity and Metastatis in Murine Models." *International Journal of Cancer* 67 (1996): 842–848.

Decker EA. "The Role of Phenolics, Conjugated Linoleic Acid, Carnosine, and Pyrroloquinoline Quinone as Nonessential Dietary Antioxidants." *Nutrition Reviews* 53 (1995): 49–58.

DeLuca HF, Krisinger J, Darwish H. "The Vitamin D System: 1990." *Kidney International Supplement* 29 (1990): S2–S8.

Devesa SS. "Cancer Mortality, Incidence, and Patient Survival among American Women." *Women and Health* 11 (1986): 7–22.

Dimitriadis E et al. "Lipoprotein Composition in NIDDM: Effects of Dietary Oleic Acid on the Composition, Oxidisability and Function of Low and High Density Lipoproteins." *Diabetologia* 39 (1996): 667–676.

Donn AS, Muir CS. "Prostatic Cancer: Some Epidemiological Features." *Bulletin du Cancer* 72 (1985): 381–390.

Dorr RT. "Chemoprotectants for Cancer Chemotherapy." *Seminars in Oncology* 18 (1991): 48–58.

Dorvil NP et al. "Taurine Prevents Cholestasis Induced by Lithocholic Sulfate in Guinea Pigs." *American Journal of Clinical Nutrition* 37 (1983): 221–232.

du Toit PJ, van Aswegen CH, du Plessis DJ. "The Effect of Gamma-Linolenic Acid and Eicosapentaenoic Acid on Urokinase Activity." *Prostaglandins Leukotrienes and Essential Fatty Acids* 51 (1994): 121–124.

Durlach J et al. "Magnesium and Ageing. II. Clinical Data: Aetiological Mechanisms and Pathophysiological Consequences of Magnesium Deficit in the Elderly." *Magnesium Research* 6 (1993): 379–394.

Dwivedi C, Abu-Ghazaleh A, Guenther J. "Effects of Diallyl Sulfide and Diallyl Disulfide on Cisplatin-Induced Changes in Glutathione and Glutathione-S-Transferase Activity." *Anticancer Drugs* 7 (1996): 792–794

Dwyer JT et al. "Tofu and Soy Drinks Contain Phytoestrogens." *Journal of the American Dietetic Association* 94 (1994): 739–743.

Edgar B et al. "Acute Effects of Drinking Grapefruit Juice on the Pharmacokinetics and Dynamics of Felodipine—and Its Potential Clinical Relevance." *European Journal of Clinical Pharmacology* 42 (1992): 313–317.

Eichholzer M et al. "Prediction of Male Cancer Mortality by Plasma Levels of Interacting Vitamins: 17-Year Follow-Up of the Prospective Basel Study." *International Journal of Cancer* 66 (1996): 145–150.

Eisner GM. "Hypertension: Racial Differences." *American Journal of Kidney Diseases* 16 (1990): 35–40.

Ells GW et al. "Vitamin E Blocks the Cytotoxic Effect of Gamma-Linolenic Acid When Administered as Late as the Time of Onset of Cell Death—Insight to the Mechanism of Fatty Acid Induced Cytotoxicity." *Cancer Letters* 98 (1996): 207–211.

Emerson JC, Weiss NS. "Colorectal Cancer and Solar Radiation." *Cancer Causes and Control* 3 (1992): 95–99.

Erdman JW. "Control of Serum Lipids with Soy Protein." *New England Journal of Medicine* 333 (1995): 313–314.

Erickson JD. "Mortality in Selected Cities with Fluoridated and Nonfluoridated Water. *New England Journal of Medicine* 298 (1978): 1112–1116.

Ernster VL et al. "Race, Socioeconomic Status, and Prostatic Cancer." *Cancer Treat Reviews* 61 (1977): 187–191.

Ernster VL, Selvin S, Winkelstein W Jr. "Cohort Mortality for Prostatic Cancer among United States Nonwhites." *Science* 200 (1978): 1165–1166.

Ernster VL et al. "Prostatic Cancer: Mortality and Incidence Rates by Race and Social Class." *American Journal of Epidemiology* 107 (1978): 311–320.

Falconer JS et al. "Effect of Eicosapentaenoic Acid and Other Fatty Acids on the Growth *in Vitro* of Human Pancreatic Cancer Cell Lines." *British Journal of Cancer* 69 (1994): 826–832.

Feldman D, Skowronski RJ, Peehl DM. "Vitamin D and Prostate Cancer." *Advances in Experimental Medicine and Biology* 375 (1995): 53–63.

Fielding R. "The Role of Progressive Resistance Training and Nutrition in the Preservation of Lean Body Mass in the Elderly." *Journal of the American College of Nutrition* 14 (1995): 587–594.

Fisher WE, Boros LG, Schirmer WJ. "Reversal of Enhanced Pancreatic Cancer Growth in Diabetes by Insulin." *Surgery* 118 (1995): 453–457.

Flack JM et al. "Racial and Ethnic Modifiers of the Salt–Blood Pressure Response." *Hypertension* 27 (1991): 62–66.

Flagg EW, Coates RJ, Greenberg, RS. "Epidemiologic Studies of Antioxidants and Cancer in Humans." *Journal of the American College of Nutrition* 14 (1995): 419–427.

Fleming ID et al. "Skin Cancer in Black Patients." *Cancer* 35 (1975): 600–605.

Forman MR et al. "Overweight Adults in the United States: The Behavioral Risk Factor Surveys." *American Journal of Clinical Nutrition* 44 (1986): 410–416.

Franceschi S et al. "Tomatoes and Risk of Digestive Tract Cancers." *International Journal of Cancer* 59 (1994): 181–184.

Franconi F. "Plasma and Platelet Taurine Are Reduced in Subjects with Insulin-Dependent Diabetes Mellitus: Effects of Taurine Supplementation." *American Journal of Clinical Nutrition* 61 (1995): 1115–1119.

Franke AA, Custer LJ. "Daidzein and Genistein Concentrations in Human Milk and Soy Consumption." *Clinical Chemistry* 42 (1996): 955–964.

Friedewald WT, Thom TJ. "Decline of Coronary Heart Disease Mortality in the United States." *Israel Journal of Medical Sciences* 22 (1986): 307–312.

Fuhr U, Klittich K, Staib AH. "Inhibitory Effect of Grapefruit Juice and Its Bitter Principal, Naringenin, on CYP1A2 Dependent Metabolism of Caffeine in Man." *British Journal of Clinical Pharmacology* 35 (1993): 431–436.

Fuhr U, Kummert AL. "The Fate of Naringin in Humans: A Key to Grapefruit Juice–Drug Interactions." *Clinical Pharmacology and Therapeutics* 58 (1995): 365–373.

Fujimori A et al. "Silencing and Selective Methylation of the Normal Topoisomerase I Gene in Camptothecin-Resistant CEM/C2 Human Leukemia Cells." *Oncology Research* 8 (1996): 295–301.

Fushimi H et al. "Zinc Deficiency Exaggerates Diabetic Osteoporosis." *Diabetes Research and Clinical Practice* 20 (1993): 191–196.

Gann PH et al. "Circulating Vitamin D Metabolites in Relation to Subsequent Development of Prostate Cancer." *Cancer Epidemiology, Biomarkers and Prevention* 5 (1996): 121–126.

Garland C et al. "Dietary Vitamin D and Calcium and Risk of Colorectal Cancer: A 19-Year Prospective Study in Men." *Lancet* 1 (1985): 307–309.

Gerber M et al. "Oxidant-Antioxidant Status Alternations in Cancer Patients." *Journal of Nutrition* 126 (1996): 1201S–1207S.

Ghoshal AK, Farber E. "The Induction of Liver Cancer by Dietary Deficiency of Choline and Methionine without Added Carcinogens." *Carcinogenesis* 5 (1984): 1367–1370.

Giovannucci E et al. "Folate, Methionine, and Alcohol Intake and Risk of Colorectal Adenoma." *Journal of the National Cancer Institute* 85 (1993): 875–884.

Giovannuci E et al. "Alcohol, Low-Methionine–Low-Folate diets, and Risk of Colon Cancer in Men." *Journal of the National Cancer Institute* 87 (1995): 265–273.

Giovannuci E et al. "Intake of Carotenoids and Retinol in Relation to Risk of Prostate Cancer." *Journal of the National Cancer Institute* 87 (1995): 1767–1776.

Giovannuci E. "How Is Individual Risk for Prostate Cancer Assessed?" *Hematology/Oncology Clinics of North America* 10 (1996): 537–548.

González CA et al. "Borage Consumption as a Possible Gastric Cancer Protective Factor." *Cancer Epidemiology, Biomarkers and Prevention* 2 (1993): 157–158.

Gorham ED, Garland FC, Garland CF. "Sunlight and Breast Cancer Incidence in the USSR." *International Journal of Epidemiology* 19 (1990): 820–824.

Gorwitz K, Dennis R. "On the Decrease in the Life Expentancy of Black Males in Michigan." *Public Health Reports* 91 (1976): 141–145.

Goseki N et al. "Synergistic Effect of Methionine-Depleting Total Parenteral Nutrition with 5-Fluorouracil on Human Gastric Cancer: A Randomized, Prospective Clinical Trial." *Japanese Journal of Cancer Research* 86 (1995): 484–89.

Gould MN. "Prevention and Therapy of Mammary Cancer by Monoterpenes." *Journal of Cellular Biochemistry Supplement* 22 (1995): 139–144.

Gould MN, Wacker WD, Maltzman TH. "Chemoprevention and Chemotherapy of Mammary Tumors by Monoterpenoids." *Progress in Clinical and Biological Research* 347 (1990): 255–268.

Gould MN et al. "Limonene Chemoprevention of Mammary Carcinoma Induction Following Direct *in Situ* Transfer of v-Ha-ras." *Cancer Research* 54 (1994): 3540–3543.

Grammatikos SI et al. "n-3 and n-6 Fatty Acid Processing and Growth Effects in Neoplastic and Non-cancerous Human Mammary Epithelial Cell Lines." *British Journal of Cancer* 70 (1994): 219–227.

Grubbs CJ et al. "Chemoprevention of Chemically-Induced Mammary Carcinogenesis by Indole-3-Carbinol." *Anticancer Research* 15 (1995): 709–716.

Guertin F et al. "Liver Membrane Composition after Short-Term Parenteral Nutrition with and without Taurine in Guinea Pigs: The Effect of Taurine." *Proceedings of the Society for Experimental Biology and Medicine* 203 (1993): 418–423.

Guo HY, Hoffman RM, Herrera H. "Unchecked DNA Synthesis and Blocked Cell Division Induced by Methionine Deprivation in a Human Prostate Cancer Cell Line" [letter]. *In Vitro Cellular and Developmental Biology Animal* 29A (1993): 359–361.

Haag JD, Lindstrom MJ, Gould MN. "Limonene-Induced Regression of Mammary Carcinomas." *Cancer Research* 52 (1992): 4021–4026.

Haag JD, Gould MN. "Mammary Carcinoma Regression Induced by Perillyl Alcohol, a Hydroxylated Analog of Limonene." *Cancer Chemotherapy and Pharmacology* 34 (1994): 477–483.

Haffner SM et al. "Cardiovascular Risk Factors in Confirmed Prediabetic Individuals: Does the Clock for Coronary Heart Disease Start Ticking before the Onset of Clinical Diabetes?" *Journal of the American Medical Association* 263 (1990): 2893–2898.

Hagenfeldt Y et al. "Effects of Orchidectomy and Different Modes of High Dose

Estrogen Treatment on Circulating 'Free' and Total 1,25-Dihydroxyvitamin D in Patients with Prostatic Cancer." *Journal of Steroid Biochemistry and Molecular Biology* 39 (1991): 155–159.

Hammarqvist F et al. "Skeletal Muscle Glutathione Is Depleted in Critically Ill Patients." *Critical Care Medicine* 25 (1997): 78–84.

Hanai T et al. "Comparison of Prostanoids and Their Precursor Fatty Acids in Human Hepatocellular Carcinoma and Noncancerous Reference Tissues." *Journal of Surgical Research* 54 (1993): 57–60.

Hanchette CL, Schwartz GG. "Geographic Patterns of Prostate Cancer Mortality. Evidence for a Protective Effect of Ultraviolet Radiation." *Cancer* 70 (1992): 2861–2869.

Hanigan MH, Gallagher BC, Taylor PT Jr. "Cisplatin Nephrotoxicity: Inhibition of Gamma-Glutamyl Transpeptidase Blocks the Nephrotoxicity of Cisplatin without Reducing Platinum Concentrations in the Kidney." *American Journal of Obstetrics and Gynecology* 175 (1996): 270–273.

Harding JJ, Blakytny R, Ganea E. "Glutathione in Disease." *Biochemical Society Transactions* 24 (1996): 881–884.

Hawrylewicz EJ, Zapata JJ, Blair WH. "Soy and Experimental Cancer: Animal Studies." *Journal of Nutrition* 125 (1995): 698S–708S.

Hayashi Y et al. "Anticancer Effects of Free Polyunsaturated Fatty Acids in an Oily Lymphographic Agent Following Intrahepatic Arterial Administration to a Rabbit Bearing VX-2 Tumor." *Cancer Research* 52 (1992): 400–405.

Hayes RB et al. "Serum Retinol and Prostate Cancer." *Cancer* 62 (1988): 2021–2026.

Hayes K. "Taurine Modulates Platelet Aggregation in Cats and Humans." *American Journal of Clinical Nutrition* 49 (1989): 1211–1216.

Heaney RP, Weaver CM, Fitzsimmons ML. "Soybean Phytate Content: Effect on Calcium Absorption." *American Journal of Clinical Nutrition* 53 (1991): 745–747.

Heby O. "DNA Methylation and Polyamines in Embryonic Development and Cancer." *International Journal of Developmental Biology* 39 (1995): 737–757.

Hecht SS. "Chemoprevention of Lung Cancer by Isothiocyanates." *Advances in Experimental Medicine and Biology* 401 (1996): 1–11.

Hedlund TE, Moffatt KA, Miller GJ. "Vitamin D Receptor Expression Is Required for Growth Modulation by 1 Alpha-25-Dihydroxyvitamin D3 in the Human Prostatic Carcinoma Cell Line." *Journal of Steroid Biochemistry and Molecular Biology* 58 (1996): 277–288.

Heilbrun LK, Nomura A, Stemmermann GN. "Black Tea Consumption and Cancer Risk: A Prospective Study." *British Journal of Cancer* 54 (1986): 677–683.

Hendrich S et al. "Defining Food Components as New Nutrients." *Journal of Nutrition* 124 (1994): 1789S–1792S.

Herlitz H et al. "Grapefruit Juice: A Possible Source of Variability in Blood Concentration of Cyclosporin A." *Nephrology, Dialysis, Transplantation* 8 (1993): 375.

Herring BD. "Cancer of the Prostate in Blacks." *Journal of the National Medical Association* 69 (1977): 165–167.

Hertog M et al. "Antioxidant Flavonols and Ischemic Heart Disease in a Welsh Population of Men: The Caerphilly Study." *American Journal of Clinical Nutrition* 65 (1995): 1489–1494.

Hietanen E et al. "Diet and Oxidative Stress in Breast, Colon and Prostate Cancer Patients: A Case-Control Study." *European Journal of Clinical Nutrition* 48 (1994): 575–586.

Hoffman RM. "Altered Methionine Metabolism and Transmethylation in Cancer." *Anticancer Research* 5 (1985): 1–30.

Hollander AA et al. "The Effect of Grapefruit Juice on Cyclosporine and Prednisone Metabolism in Transplant Patients." *Clinical Pharmacology and Therapeutics* 57 (1995): 318–324.

Hollman P et al. "Absorption and Dietary Quercetin Glycosides and Quercetin in Healthy Ileostomy Volunteers." *American Journal of Clinical Nutrition* 62 (1995): 1276–1282.

Honig PK et al. "Grapefruit Juice Alters the Systemic Bioavailability and Cardiac Repolarization of Terfenadine in Poor Metabolizers of Terfenadine." *Journal of Clinical Pharmacology* 36 (1996): 345–351.

Honorle EK et al. "Soy Isoflavones Enhance Coronary Vascular Reactivity in Athero-sclerotic Female Macaques." *Fertility and Sterility* 67 (1997): 148–154.

Hopewell JW et al. "The Modulation of Radiation-Induced Damage to Pig Skin by Essential Fatty Acids." *British Journal of Cancer* 68 (1993): 1–7.

Hopewell JW et al. "Amelioration of Both Early and Late Radiation-Induced Damage to Pig Skin by Essential Fatty Acids." *International Journal of Radiation Oncology, Biology, Physics* 30 (1994): 1119–1125.

Horrobin DF. "Nutritional and Medical Importance of Gamma-Linolenic Acid." *Progress in Lipid Research* 31 (1992): 163–194.

Hoshiya Y et al. "Methionine Starvation Modulates the Efficacy of Cisplatin on Human Breast Cancer in Nude Mice." *Anticancer Research* 16 (1996): 3515–3517.

Hrelia S et al. "Gamma-Linolenic Acid Supplementation Can Affect Cancer Cell Proliferation via Modification of Fatty Acid Composition." *Biochemical and Biophysical Research Communications* 225 (1996): 441–447.

Hsieh TC, Wu JM. "Changes in Cell Growth, Cyclin/Kinase, Endogenous Phospho-proteins and nm23 Gene Expression in Human Prostatic JCA-1 Cells Treated with Modified Citrus." *Biochemistry and Molecular Biology International* 37 (1995): 833–841.

Hubbard NE, Erickson KL. "Role of Dietary Oleic Acid in Linoleic Acid–Enhanced Metastasis of a Mouse." 1991.

Huggins C, Hodges CV. "Studies on Prostate Cancer 1: The Effect of Castration, of Estrogen and of Androgen Injection on Serum Phosphatases in Metastatic Carcinoma of the Prostate." *Cancer Research* 1 (1941): 293–297.

Hutchins AM, Slavin JL, Lampe JW. "Urinary Isoflavonoid Phytoestrogen and Lignan Excretion after consumption of Fermented and Unfermented Soy Products." *Journal of the American Dietetic Association* 95 (1995): 545–551.

Ingram D. "Diet and Subsequent Survival in Women with Breast Cancer." *British Journal of Cancer* 69 (1995): 592–595.

Inohara H, Raz A. "Effects of Natural Complex Carbohydrate (Citrus Pectin) on Murine Melanoma Cell Properties Related to Galectin-3 Functions." *Glycoconjugate Journal* 11 (1994): 527–532.

Isaacs WB. "Molecular Genetics of Prostate Cancer." *Cancer Surveys* 25 (1995): 357–379.

Isaacs WB et al. "Genetic Alterations in Prostate Cancer." *Cold Spring Harbor Symposia on Quantitative Biology* 59 (1994): 653–659.

Isaacs WB et al. "Molecular Biology of Prostate Cancer." *Seminars in Oncology* 21 (1994): 514–521.

Isaacs WB et al. "Molecular Biology of Prostate Cancer Progression." *Cancer Surveys* 23 (1995): 19–32.

Isaacson C. "The Changing Pattern of Liver Disease in South African Blacks." *South African Medical Journal* 53 (1978): 365–368.

Isaacson C et al. "The Iron Status of Urban Black Subjects with Carcinoma of the Oesophagus." *South African Medical Journal* 67 (1985): 591–593.

Israel K, Sanders BG, Kline K. "RRR-Alpha-Tocopheryl Succinate Inhibits the Proliferation of Human Prostatic Tumor Cells with Defective Cell Cycle/Differentiation Pathways." *Nutrition and Cancer* 24 (1995): 161–169.

Issa JP, Baylin SB, Belinsky SA. "Methylation of the Estrogen Receptor CpG Island in Lung Tumors Is Related to the Specific Type of Carcinogen Exposure." *Cancer Research* 56 (1996): 3655–3658.

Izzotti A et al. "Chemoprevention of Carcinogen-DNA Adducts and Chronic Degenerative Diseases." *Cancer Research* 54 (1994): 1994S–1998S.

Jackson MA et al. "Characterization of Prostatic Carcinoma among Blacks: A Preliminary Report." *Cancer Chemotherapy Report* 59 (1975): 3–15.

Jackson MA et al. "Characterization of Prostatic Carcinoma among Blacks: A Continuation Report." *Cancer Treatment Report* 61 (1977): 167–172.

James SY, Mackay AG, Colston KW. "Vitamin D Derivatives in Combination with 9-*cis* Retinoic Acid Promote Active Cell Death in Breast Cancer Cells." *Journal of Molecular Endocrinology* 14 (1995): 391–394.

James SY, Mackay AG, Colston KW. "Effects of 1,25-Dihydroxyvitamin D_3 and Its Analogues on Induction of Apoptosis in Breast Cancer Cells." *Journal of Steroid Biochemistry and Molecular Biology* 58 (1996): 395–401.

Jarrard DF, Bova GS, Isaacs WB. "DNA Methylation, Molecular Genetic, and Linkage Studies in Prostate Cancer." *Prostate Supplement* 6 (1996): 36–44.

Jarrett R et al. "Glucose Tolerance and Blood Pressure in Two Population Samples: Their Relation to Diabetes Mellitus and Hypertension." *International Journal of Epidemiology* 7 (1978): 15–24.

Jarrett RJ. "Type 2 (Non–Insulin-Dependent) Diabetes Mellitus and Coronary Heart Disease: Chicken, Egg or Neither?" *Diabetologia* 26 (1984): 99–102.

Jenkins DJA, Jenkins AL. "The Glycemic Index, Fiber and the Dietary Treatment of Hypertriglyceridemia and Diabetes." *Journal of the American College of Nutrition* 6 (1987): 11–17.

Jennings E. "Folic Acid as a Cancer-Preventing Agent." *Medical Hypotheses* 45 (1995): 297–303.

Jenski LJ, Zerouga M, Stillwell W. "Omega-3 Fatty Acid-Containing Liposomes in Cancer Therapy." *Proceedings of the Society for Experimental Biology and Medicine* 210 (1995): 227–233.

Jiang WG et al. "Regulation of the Expression of E-Cadherin on Human Cancer Cells by Gamma-Linolenic Acid (GLA)." *Cancer Research* 55 (1995): 5043–5048.

Joannic J et al. "How the Degree of Unsaturation of Dietary Fatty Acids Influences the Glucose and Insulin Responses to Different Carbohydrates in Mixed Meals." *American Journal of Clinical Nutrition* 65 (1996): 1427–1433.

Johnson JL et al. "Cardiovascular Disease Risk Factors and Mortality among Black Women and White Women aged 40–64 Years in Evans County, Georgia." *American Journal of Epidemiology* 123 (1986): 209–220.

Jones PA. "DNA Methylation and Cancer." *Cancer Research* 46 (1986): 461–466.

Jones PA et al. "Methylation, Mutation and Cancer." *Bioessays* 14 (1992): 33–36.

Jones PA. "DNA Methylation Errors and Cancer." *Cancer Research* 56 (1996): 2463–2467.

Joossens JV, Geboers J. "Nutrition and Cancer." *Biomedicine and Pharmacotherapy* 40 (1986): 127–138.

Kaiser U et al. "Expression of Vitamin D Receptor in Lung Cancer." *Journal of Cancer Research and Clinical Oncology* 122 (1996): 356–359.

Kannel WB, McGee DL. "Diabetes and Cardiovascular Disease: The Framingham Study." *Journal of the American Medical Association* 241 (1979): 2035–2038.

Kapadia GJ et al. "Carcinogenicity of *Camellia Sinensis* (Tea) and Some Tannin-Containing Folk Medicinal Herbs Administered Subcutaneously in Rats." *Journal of the National Cancer Institute* 57 (1976): 207–209.

Kapadia GJ et al. "Carcinogenicity of Some Folk Medicinal Herbs in Rats." *Journal of the National Cancer Institute* 60 (1978): 683–686.

Karlson J et al. "Inhibition of Tumor Cell Growth by Monoterpenes *in Vitro:* Evidence of a *Ras*-Independent Mechanism of Action." *Anticancer Drugs* 7 (1996): 422–429.

Karmali RA, Adams L, Trout JR. "Plant and Marine n-3 Fatty Acids Inhibit Experimental Metastasis of Rat Mammary Adenocarcinoma Cells." *Prostaglandins Leukotrienes and Essential Fatty Acids* 48 (1993): 309–314.

Kass DH et al. "Examination of DNA Methylation of Chromosomal Hot Spots Associated with Breast Cancer." *Anticancer Research* 13 (1993): 1245–1251.

Katdare M et al. "Prevention of Mammary Preneoplastic Transformation by Naturally-Occurring Tumor Inhibitors." *Cancer Letters* 111 (1997): 141–147.

Kaul L et al. "The Role of Diet in Prostate Cancer." *Nutrition and Cancer* 9 (1987): 123–128.

Kearney J et al. "Calcium, Vitamin D, and Dairy Foods and the Occurrence of Colon Cancer in Men." *American Journal of Epidemiology* 143: (1996): 907–917.

Keler T, Barker CS, Sorof S. "Specific Growth Stimulation by Linoleic Acid in Hepatoma Cell Lines Transfected with the Target Protein of a Liver Carcinogen." *Proceedings of the National Academy of Sciences of the United States of America* 89 (1992): 4830–4834.

Kelloff GJ et al. "Chemoprevention Clinical Trials." *Mutation Research* 267 (1992): 291–295.

Kennedy AR. "The Evidence for Soybean Products as Cancer Preventive Agents." *Journal of Nutrition* 125 (1995): 733S–743S.

Kew MC, Dibisceglie AM, Paterson AC. "Smoking as a Risk Factor in Hepatocellular Carcinoma. A Case-Control Study in Southern African Blacks." *Cancer* 56 (1985): 2315–2317.

Kim YI et al. "Global DNA Hypomethylation Increases Progressively in Cervical Dysplasia." *Cancer* 74 (1994): 893–899.

Kim JD et al. "Exercise and Diet Modulate Cardiac Lipid Peroxidation and Antioxidant Defenses." *Free Radical Biology and Medicine* 20 (1996): 83–88.

Kim YI, Mason JB. "Nutrition Chemoprevention of Gastrointestinal Cancers: A Critical Review." *Nutrition Reviews* 54 (1996): 259–279.

Kim YI et al. "Folate Deficiency in Rats Induces DNA Strand Breaks and Hypomethylation within the p53 Tumor Suppressor Gene." *American Journal of Clinical Nutrition* 65 (1997): 46–52.

King RA, Broadbent JL, Head RJ. "Absorption and Excretion of the Soy Isoflavone Genistein in Rats." *Journal of Nutrition* 126 (1996): 176–182.

Klatsky AL, Armstrong MA, Friedman GD. "Racial Differences in Cerebrovascular Disease Hospitalizations." *Stroke* 22 (1991): 229–304.

Kobrinsky NL et al. "Treatment of Advanced Malignancies with High-Dose Acetaminophen and *N*-Acetylcysteine Rescue." *Cancer Investigation* 14 (1996): 202–210.

Kojima T, Tanaka T, Mori H. "Chemoprevention of Spontaneous Endometrial Cancer in Female Donryu Rats by Dietary Indole-3-Carbinol." *Cancer Research* 54 (1994): 1446–1449.

Kolonel LN et al. "Relationship of Dietary Vitamin A and Ascorbic Acid Intake to the Risk for Cancers of the Lung, Bladder, and Prostate in Hawaii." *National Cancer Institute Monographs* 69 (1985): 137–142.

Kolonel LN, Hankin JH, Nomura AM. "Multiethnic Studies of Diet, Nutrition, and Cancer in Hawaii." *Princess Takamatsu Symposia* 16 (1985): 29–40.

Kolonel LN, Hankin JH, Yoshizawa CN. "Vitamin A and Prostate Cancer in Elderly Men: Enhancement of Risk." *Cancer Research* 47 (1987): 2982–2985.

Kolonel LN. "Nutrition and Prostate Cancer." *Cancer Causes and Control* 7 (1996): 78–44.

Konety BR et al. "The Role of Vitamin D in Normal Prostate Growth and Differentiation." *Cell Growth and Differentiation* 7 (1996): 1563–1570.

Laird PW, Janenisch R. "DNA Methylation and Cancer." *Human Molecular Genetics* (1994): 3 Spec 1487–1495.

Laird PW, Jaenisch R. "The Role of DNA Methylation in Cancer Genetics and Epigenetics." *Annual Review of Genetics* 30 (1996): 441–464.

Lamartiniere CA et al. "Genistein Suppresses Mammary Cancer in Rats." *Carcinogenesis* 16 (1995): 2833–2840.

Larson DL, Bennett JE. "Chimney Sweeper's Disease Revisited: First Case Reported in a Black. Case Report." *Plast and Reconstructive Surgery* 61 (1978): 281–283.

Lee YS et al. "Grapefruit Juice and Its Flavonoids Inhibit 11 Beta-Hydroxysteroid Dehydrogenase." *Clinical Pharmacology and Therapeutics* 59 (1996): 62–71.

Lertratanangkoon K, Orkiszewski RS, Scimeca JM. "Methyl-Donor Deficiency Due to Chemically Induced Glutathione Depletion." *Cancer Research* 56 (1996): 995–1005.

Leskinen-Kallio S et al. "Uptake of 11C-Methionine in Breast Cancer Studied by PET. An Association with the Size of S-Phase Fraction." *British Journal of Cancer* 64 (1991): 1121–1124.

Liao S. "Androgen Action: Molecular Mechanism and Medical Application." *Journal of the Formosan Medical Association* 93 (1994): 741–751.

Lipkin M, Newmark H. "Calcium and the Prevention of Colon Cancer." *Journal of Cellular Biochemistry Supplement* 22 (1995): 65–73.

Lips P. "Vitamin D Deficiency and Osteoporosis: The Role of Vitamin D Deficiency and Treatment with Vitamin D and Analogues in the Prevention of Osteoporosis-Related Fractures." *European Journal of Clinical Investigation* 26 (1996): 436–442.

Lockwood K et al. "Apparent Partial Remission of Breast Cancer in 'High Risk' Patients Supplemented with Nutritional Antioxidants, Essential Fatty Acids and Coenzyme Q_{10}." *Molecular Aspects of Medicine* 15 (1994): 231S–2340S.

Lockwood K, Moesgaard S, Folkers K. "Partial and Complete Regression of Breast Cancer in Patients in Relation to Dosage of Coenzyme Q_{10}." *Biochemical and Biophysical Research Communications* 199 (1994): 1504–1508.

Lu-Yao GL, Greenberg ER. "Changes in Prostate Cancer Incidence and Treatment in USA." *Lancet* 343 (1994): 251–254.

Lundahl J et al. "Relationship between Time and Intake of Grapefruit Juice and Its Effect on Pharmacokinetics and Pharmacodynamics of Felodipine in Healthy Subjects." *European Journal of Clinical Pharmacology* 49 (1995): 61–67.

Maasilta P et al. N-Acetylcysteine in Combination with Radiotherapy in the Treatment of Non–Small Cell Lung Cancer: A Feasibility Study." *Radiotherapy and Oncology* 25 (1992): 192–195.

Madhavi N, Das UN. "Effect on n-6 and n-3 Fatty Acids on the Survival of Vincristine Sensitive and Resistant Human Cervical Carcinoma Cells *in Vitro*." *Cancer Letters* 84 (1994): 31–41.

Maish WA et al. "Influence of Grapefruit Juice on Caffeine Pharmacokinetics and Pharmacodynamics." *Pharmacotherapy* 16 (1996): 1046–1052.

Malvy D, Amédée-Manesme O. ["Vitamin A: An Indirect Factor in the Prevention of Cancer"]. *Presse Medicale* 16 (1987): 1087–1089.

Manson JE et al. "A Prospective Study of Maturity-Onset Diabetes Mellitus and Risk of Coronary Heart Disease and Stroke in Women." *Archives of Internal Medicine* 151 (1991): 1141–1147.

McCarty M. "Anabolic Effects of Insulin on Bone Suggest a Role for Chromium Picolinate in Preservation of Bone Density." *Medical Hypotheses* 45 (1995): 241–246.

McCarty MF. "Fish Oil May Impede Tumour Angiogenesis and Invasiveness by

Down-Regulating Protein Kinase C and Modulating Eicosanoid Production." *Medical Hypotheses* 46 (1996): 107–115.

McPhillips JB, Barrett-Connor E, Wingard DL. "Cardiovascular Disease Risk Factors Prior to the Diagnosis of Impaired Glucose Tolerance and Non–insulin-Dependent Diabetes Mellitus in a Community of Older Adults." *American Journal of Epidemiology* 131 (1990): 443–453.

Mehlman MA. "Dangerous and Cancer-Causing Properties of Products and Chemicals in the Oil-Refining and Petrochemical Industry—Part XXII: Health Hazards from Exposure to Gasoline Containing Methyl Tertiary Butyl Ether: Study of New Jersey Residents." *Toxicology and Industrial Health* 12 (1996): 613–627.

Mehta RG et al. "Cancer Chemopreventive Activity of Brassinin, a Phytoalexin from Cabbage." *Carcinogenesis* 16 (1995): 399–404.

Mengeaud V et al. "Effects of Eicosapentaenoic Acid, Gamma-Linolenic Acid and Prostaglandin E1 on Three Human Colon Carcinoma Cell Lines." *Prostaglandins Leukotrienes Essential Fatty Acids* 47 (1992): 313–319.

Merkel U, Sigusch H, Hoffmann A. "Grapefruit Juice Inhibits 7-Hydroxylation on Coumarin in Healthy Volunteers." *European Journal of Clinical Pharmacology* 46 (1994): 175–177.

Messina MJ et al. "Soy Intake and Cancer Risk: A Review of the *in Vitro* and *in Vivo* Data." *Nutrition and Cancer* 21 (1994): 113–131.

Meydani S et al. "Vitamin E Supplementation and *in Vivo* Immune Response in Healthy Elderly Subjects." *Journal of the American Medical Association* 227 (1997): 1380–1386.

Michnovicz JJ, Bradlow HL. "Induction of Estradiol Metabolism by Dietary Indole-3-Carbinol in Humans" [see comments]. *Journal of the National Cancer Institute* 82 (1990): 947–949.

Michnovicz JJ, Bradlow HL. "Dietary and Pharmacological Control of Estradiol Metabolism in Humans." *Annals of the New York Academy of Sciences* 595 (1990): 291–299.

Min DI et al. "Effect on Grapefruit Juice on Cyclosporine Pharmacokinetics in Renal Transplant Patients." *Transplantation* 62 (1996): 123–125.

Morse MA et al. "Effects of Indole-3-Carbinol on Lung Tumorigenesis and DNA Methylation Induced by 4-(Methylnitrosamino)-1-(3-Pyridyl)-1-Butanone (NNK) and on the Metabolism and Disposition of NNK in A/J Mice." *Cancer Research* 50 (1990): 2613–2617.

Morton RA Jr. "Racial Differences in Adenocarcinoma of the Prostate in North American Men." *Urology* 44 (1994): 637–645.

Morton RA Jr. et al. "Hypermethylation of Chromosome 17P Locus D17S5 in Human Prostate Tissue." *Journal of Urology* 156 (1996): 512–516.

Nakashima T, Taniko T, Kuriyama K. "Therapeutic Effect of Taurine Administration on Carbon Tetrachloride-Induced Hepatic Injury." *Japanese Journal of Pharmacology* 32 (1982): 583–589.

Narisawa T et al. "Inhibitory Effect of Dietary Perilla Oil Rich in the n-3 Polyunsaturated Fatty Acid Alpha-Linolenic Acid on Colon Carcinogenesis in Rats." *Japanese Journal of Cancer Research* 82 (1991): 1089–1096.

Narisawa T et al. "Colon Cancer Prevention with a Small Amount of Dietary Perilla Oil High in Alpha-Linolenic Acid in an Animal Model." *Cancer* 73 (1994): 2069–2075.

Natarajan N et al. "Race-Related Differences in Breast Cancer Patients. Results of the 1982 National Survey of Breast Cancer by the American College of Surgeons." *Cancer* 56 (1985): 1704–1709.

Nayeri S et al. "The Anti-proliferative Effect of Vitamin D_3 Analogues Is Not Mediated by Inhibition of the AP-1 Pathway, but May Be Related to Promoter." *Oncogene* 11 (1953): 1853–1858.

Nelson RG et al. "Low Incidence of Fatal Coronary Heart Disease in Pima Indians Despite High Prevalence of Non–insulin-Dependent Diabetes." *Circulation* 81 (1990): 987–995.

Nelson JB et al. "Methylation of the 5'CpG Island of the Endothelin B Receptor Gene Is Common in Human Prostate Cancer." *Cancer Research* 57 (1997): 35–37.

Neoptolemos JP et al. "Arachidonic Acid and Docosahexaenoic Acid Are Increased in Human Colorectal Cancer." *Gut* 32 (1991): 278–281.

Newberne PM, Rogers AE. "The Role of Nutrients in Cancer Causation." *Princess Takamatsu Symposia* 16 (1985): 205–222.

Newell GR, Lynch HK, Carr DT. "Decreasing Lung Cancer Deaths among Young Men in Texas." *Texas Medicine* 81 (1985): 29–31.

Newmark HL, Lipkin M. "Calcium, Vitamin D, and Colon Cancer." *Cancer Research* 52 (1992): 2067S–2070S.

Ng PC et al. "Mixed Estrogenic and Anti-estrogenic Activities of Yuehchukene—a bis-Indole Alkaloid." *European Journal of Pharmacology* 264 (1994): 1–12.

Ni A. "Obesity and Cardiovascular Disease Risk Factors in Black and White Girls: The NHLBI Growth and Health Study." *American Journal of Public Health* 82 (1992): 1613–1620.

Niwa T, Swaneck G, Bradlow HL. "Alterations in Estradiol Metabolism in MCF-7 Cells Induced by Treatment with Indole-3-Carbinol and Related Compounds." *Steroids* 59 (1994): 523–527.

Nomura A, Kolonel LN. "Shedding New Light on the Etiology of Prostate Cancer?" [editorial; comment]. *Cancer Epidemiology, Biomarkers Prevention* 2 (1993): 409–410.

Norman AW. "The Vitamin D Endocrine System: Manipulation of Structure–Function Relationships to Provide Opportunities for Development of New Cancer." *Journal of Cellular Biochemistry Supplement* 22 (1995): 218–225.

Ocké MC et al. "Average Intake of Anti-oxidant (Pro)vitamins and Subsequent Cancer Mortality in the 16 Cohorts of the Seven Countries Study." *International Journal of Cancer* 61 (1995): 480–484.

Ohta H et al. "Mechanism of the Protective Action of Taurine against Isoprenaline Induced Myocardial Damage." *Cardiovascular Research* 22 (1988): 407–413.

Omenn GS. "Micronutrients (Vitamins and Minerals) as Cancer-Preventive Agents." *IARC Scientific Publications: Micronutrients* 139 (1996): 33–45.

Ownby HE et al. "Racial Differences in Breast Cancer Patients." *Journal of the National Cancer Institute* 75 (1985): 55–60.

Pagliacci MC et al. "Growth-Inhibitory Effects of the Natural Phyto-oestrogen Genistein in MCF-7 Human Breast Cancer Cells." *European Journal of Cancer* 30A (1994): 1675–1682.

Palli D et al. "Plasma Pepsinogens, Nutrients, and Diet in Areas of Italy at Varying Gastric Cancer Risk." *Cancer Epidemiology, Biomarkers and Prevention* 1 (1991): 45–50.

Pan WH et al. "Relationship of Clinical Diabetes and Asymptomatic Hyperglycemia to Risk of Coronary Heart Disease Mortality in Men and Women." *American Journal of Epidemiology* 123 (1986): 504–516.

Pandalai PK et al. "The Effects of Omega-3 and Omega-6 Fatty Acids on *in Vitro* Prostate Cancer Growth." *Anticancer Research* 16 (1996): 815–820.

Pasquali D, Thaller C, Eichele G. "Abnormal Level of Retinoic Acid in Prostate Cancer Tissues." *Journal of Clinical Endocrinology Metabolism* 81 (1996): 2186–2191.

Peehl DM. "Cellular Biology of Prostatic Growth Factors." *Prostate Supplement* 6 (1996): 74–78.

Pegoraro RJ et al. "Clinical Patterns of Presentation of Breast Cancer in Women of Different Racial Groups in South Africa." *South African Medical Journal* 68 (1985): 808–810.

Pegoraro RJ et al. "Estrogen and Progesterone Receptors in Breast Cancer among Women of Different Racial Groups." *Cancer Research* 46 (1986): 2117–2120.

Pegoraro RJ et al. "Breast Cancer Prognosis in Three Different Racial Groups in Relation to Steroid Hormone Receptor Status." *Breast Cancer Research and Treatment* 7 (1986): 111–118.

Peterson G, Barnes S. "Genistein Inhibits Both Estrogen and Growth Factor–Stimulated Proliferation of Human Breast Cancer Cells." *Cell Growth and Differentiation* 7 (1996): 1345–13451.

Petrakis NL et al. "Stimulatory Influence of Soy Protein Isolate on Breast Secretion in Pre- and Postmenopausal Women." *Cancer Epidemiology, Biomarkers and Prevention* 5 (1996): 785–794.

Pienta KJ et al. "Inhibition of Spontaneous Metastasis in a Rat Prostate Cancer Model by Oral Administration of Modified Citrus Pectin" [see comments]. *Journal of the National Cancer Institute* 87 (1995): 348–353.

Pierson HF, Fisher JM, Rabinovitz M. "Modulation by Taurine of the Toxicity of Taumustine, a Compound with Antitumor Activity." *Journal of the National Cancer Institute* 75 (1985): 905–909.

Pillay SP, Angorn IB, Baker LW. "Colorectal Carcinoma in Young Black Patients: A Report of Eight Cases." *Journal of Surgical Oncology* 10 (1978): 125–132.

Pinard MF et al. "Functional Aspects of Membrane Folate Receptors in Human Breast Cancer Cells with Transport-Related Resistance to Methotrexate." *Cancer Chemotherapy and Pharmacology* 38 (1996): 281–288.

Piva R et al. "Different Methylation of Oestrogen Receptor DNA in Human Breast

Carcinomas with and without Oestrogen Receptor." *British Journal of Cancer* 61 (1990): 270–275.

Platt D, Raz A. "Modulation of the Lung Colonization of B16-F1 Melanoma Cells by Citrus Pectin." *Journal of the National Cancer Institute* 84 (1992): 438–442.

Polednak AP. "Breast Cancer in Black and White Women in New York State." *Cancer* 58 (1986): 807–815.

Potter SM. "Soy Protein and Serum Lipids." *Current Opinion in Lipidology* 7 (1996): 260–264.

Pratt JH et al. "Racial Differences in Aldosterone Excretion: A Longitudinal Study in." 1993.

Prieto JG. "Eye Color in Skin Cancer." *International Journal of Dermatology* 16 (1977): 406–407.

Pritchard RS, Baron JA, Gerhardsson de Verdier M. "Dietary Calcium, Vitamin D, and the Risk of Colorectal Cancer in Stockholm, Sweden." *Cancer Epidemiology, Biomarkers and Prevention* 5 (1996): 897–900.

Purasiri P et al. "Modulation of Cytokine Production *in Vivo* by Dietary Essential Fatty Acids in Patients with Colorectal Cancer." *Clinical Science* 87 (1994): 711–717.

Qu YH, et al. "Genotoxicity of Heated Cooking Oil Vapors." *Mutatation Research* 298 (1992): 105–111.

Raines EW, Ross R. "Biology of Atherosclerotic Plaque Formation: Possible Role of Growth Factors in Lesion Development and the Potential Impact of Soy." *Journal of Nutrition* 125 (1995): 624S–630S.

Ramón JM et al. "Nutrient Intake and Gastric Cancer Risk: A Case-Control Study in Spain." *International Journal of Epidemiology* 22 (1993): 983–988.

Rao GN. "Influence of Diet on Tumors of Hormonal Tissues." *Progress in Clinical and Biological Research* 394 (1996): 41–56.

Reaven PD, Barrett-Connor EL, Browner DK. "Abnormal Glucose Tolerance and Hypertension." *Diabetes Care* 13 (1990): 119–124.

Reddy BS et al. "Chemoprevention of Colon Carcinogenesis by Organosulfur Compounds." *Cancer Research* 53 (1993): 3493–3498.

Reichman ME et al. "Serum Vitamin A and Subsequent Development of Prostate Cancer in the First National Health and Nutrition Examination Survey Epidemiologic Follow-Up." *Cancer Research* 50 (1990): 2311–2315.

Reinli K, Block G. "Phytoestrogen Content of Foods—a Compendium of Literature Values." *Nutr and Cancer* 26 (1996): 123–148.

Ren Z, Gould MN. "Inhibition of Ubiquinone and Cholesterol Synthesis by the Monoterpene Perillyl Alcohol." *Cancer Letters* 76 (1994): 185–190.

Richter F et al. "Inhibition of Western–Diet Induced Hyperproliferation and Hyperplasia in Mouse Colon by Two Sources of Calcium." *Carcinogenesis* 16 (1995): 2685–2689.

Robbins RC, Martin FG, Roe JM. "Ingestion of Grapefruit Lowers Elevated Hematocrits in Human Subjects." *International Journal for Vitamin and Nutrition Research* 58 (1988): 414–417.

Rohan TE et al. "Dietary Factors and Risk of Prostate Cancer: A Case-Control Study in Ontario, Canada." *Cancer Causes and Control* 6 (1995): 145–154.

Rojas C et al. "Increase in Heart Glutathione Redox Ratio and Total Antioxidant." *Free Radical Biology and Medicine* 21 (1996): 907–915.

Rose DP, Cohen LA. "Effects of Dietary Menhaden Oil and Retinyl Acetate on the Growth of DU 145 Human Prostatic Adenocarcinoma Cells Transplanted into Athymic Nude Mice." *Carcinogenesis* 9 (1988): 603–605.

Rose DP, Connolly JM, Liu XH. "Effects of Linoleic Acid and Gamma-Linolenic Acid on the Growth and Metastasis of a Human Breast Cancer Cell Line in Nude Mice and on Its Growth." *Nutrition and Cancer* 24 (1995): 33–45.

Ross R et al. "Serum Testosterone Levels in Healthy Young Black and White Men." *Journal of the National Cancer Institute* 76 (1986): 45–48.

Ross RK et al. "Case-Control Studies of Prostate Cancer in Blacks and Whites in Southern California." *Journal of the National Cancer Institute* 78 (1987): 869–874.

Rouleau T et al. "Dietary Supplementation with Taurine Increases Bile Acid Synthesis in Guinea Pigs." *Pediatric Research* 31 (1992): 116A.

Runkel M, Tegtmeier M, Legrum W. "Metabolic and Analytical Interactions of Grapefruit Juice and 1,2-Benzopyrone (Coumarin) in Man." *European Journal of Clinical Pharmacology* 50 (1996): 225–230.

Saad MF et al. "Insulin and Hypertension: Relationship to Obesity and Glucose Tolerance in Pima Indians." (Diabetes 39 (1990): 1430–1435.

Saad MF et al. "Racial Differences in the relation between Blood Pressure and Insulin Resistance." *New England Journal of Medicine* 324 (1991): 733–739.

Saintot M, Astre C, Pujol H, Gerber M. "Tumor Progression and Oxidant-Antioxidant Status." *Carcinogenesis* 17 (1996): 1267–1271.

Salyers AA et al. "Neutral Steroid Concentrations in the Faeces of North American White and South African Black Populations at Different Risks for Cancer of the Colon. SB:M." *South African Medical Journal* 51 (1977): 823–827.

Sasaki H, Fukushima M. "Prostaglandins in the Treatment of Cancer." *Anticancer Drugs* 5 (1994): 131–138.

Satariano WA, Belle SH, Swanson GM. "The Severity of Breast Cancer at Diagnosis: A Comparison of Age and Extent of Disease in Black and White Women." *American Journal of Public Health* 76 (1986): 779–782.

Sauer LA, Dauchy RT. "The Effect of Omega-6 and Omega-3 Fatty Acids on 3H-Thymidine Incorporation in Hepatoma 7288CTC Perfused *in Situ*." *British Journal of Cancer* 66 (1992): 297–303.

Schreurs WH et al. "The Influence of Radiotherapy and Chemotherapy on the Vitamin Status of Cancer Patients." *International Journal for Vitamin and Nutrition Research* 55 (1985): 425–432.

Schubert W et al. "Inhibition of 17 Beta-Estradiol Metabolism by Grapefruit Juice in Ovariectomized Women." *Maturitas* 20 (1994): 155–163.

Schulz S, F Bü, Ansorge S. "Prenylated Proteins and Lymphocyte Proliferation: Inhibition by D-Limonene Related Monoterpenes." *European Journal of Immunology* 24 (1994): 301–307.

Schwartz GG, Hulka BS. "Is Vitamin D Deficiency a Risk Factor for Prostate Cancer? (Hypothesis)." *Anticancer Research* 10 (1990): 1307–1311.

Schwartz GG. "Multiple Sclerosis and Prostate Cancer: What Do Their Similar Geographies Suggest?" *Neuroepidemiology* 11 (1992): 244–254.

Schwartz GG et al. "Human Prostate Cancer Cells: Inhibition of Proliferation by Vitamin D Analogs." *Anticancer Research* 14 (1994): 1077–1081.

Schwartz GG et al. "1,25-Dihydroxy-16-ene-23-yne-Vitamin D_3 and Prostate Cancer Cell Proliferation *in Vivo.*" *Urology* 46 (1995): 365–269.

Sengelov H et al. "Inter-relationships between Single Carbon Units' Metabolism and Resting Energy Expenditure in Weight-Losing Patients with Small Cell Lung Cancer." *European Journal of Cancer* 30A (1994): 1616–1620.

Shabahang M et al. "The Effect of 1,25-Dihydroxyvitamin D_3 on the Growth of Soft-Tissue Sarcoma Cells as Mediated by the Vitamin D Receptor." *Annals of Surgical Oncology* 3 (1996): 144–149.

Sharif SI, Ali BH. "Effect of Grapefruit Juice on Drug Metabolism in Rats." *Food and Chemical Toxicology* 32 (1994): 1169–1171.

Shields PG et al. "Mutagens from Heated Chinese and U.S. Cooking Oils." *Journal of the National Cancer Institute* 87 (1995): 836–841.

Simard A, Vobecky J, Vobecky JS. "Vitamin D Deficiency and Cancer of the Breast: An Unprovocative Ecological Hypothesis." *Canadian Journal of Public Health* 82 (1991): 300–303.

Simboli-Campbell M et al. "1,25-Dihydroxyvitamin D_3 Induces Morphological and Biochemical Markers of Apoptosis in MCF-7 Breast Cancer Cells." *J Steroid Biochemistry and Molecular Biology* 58 (1996): 367–376.

Sitrin MD et al. "Dietary Calcium and Vitamin D Modulate 1,2-Dimethylhydrazine-Induced Colonic Carcinogenesis in the Rat." *Cancer Research* 51 (1991): 5608–5613.

Skowronski RJ, Peehl Dm, Feldman D. "Vitamin D and Prostate Cancer: 1,25-Dihydroxyvitamin D_3 Receptors and Actions in Human Prostate Cancer Cell Lines." *Endocrinology* 132 (1993): 1952–1960.

Skowronski RJ, Peehl DM, Feldman D. "Actions of Vitamin D_3, Analogs on Human Prostate Cancer Cell Lines: Comparison with 1,25-Dihydroxyvitamin D_3." *Endocrinology* 136 (1995): 20–26.

Slonim AE et al. "Modification of Chemically Induced Diabetes in Rats by Vitamin E: Supplementation Minimizes and Depletion Enhances Development of Diabetes." *Journal of Clinical Investigation* 71 (1983): 1282–1288.

Sminia P et al. "Hyperthermia, Radiation Carcinogenesis and the Protective Potential of Vitamin A and *N*-Acetylcysteine." *Journal of Cancer Research and Clinical Oncology* 1996; 122:343–350.

Snowdon DA. "Animal Product Consumption and Mortality Because of All Causes Combined, Coronary Heart Disease, Stroke, Diabetes, and Cancer in Seventh-Day Adventists." *American Journal of Clinical Nutrition* 48 (1988): 739–748.

So FV et al. "Inhibition of Human Breast Cancer Cell Proliferation and Delay of Mammary Tumorigenesis by Flavonoids and Citrus Juices." *Nutrition and Cancer* 26 (1996): 167–181.

Southgate J, Pitt E, Trejdosiewicz LK. "The Effects of Dietary Fatty Acids on the Proliferation of Normal Human Urothelial Cells *in Vitro.*" *British Journal of Cancer* 74 (1996): 728–734.

Spitz; MR et al. "Incidence and Descriptive Features of Testicular Cancer among United States Whites, Blacks, and Hispanics, 1973–1982." *Cancer* 58 (1986): 1785–1790.

Sridevi K, Rao KP. "Modification of Genetic Damage by Dihomo-Gamma-Linolenic Acid." *Bulletin of Environmental Contamination of Toxicology* 52 (1994): 457–464.

Stamler J. "The Marked Decline in Coronary Heart Disease Mortality Rates in the United States, 1968–1981; Summary of findings and Possible Explanations." *Cardiology* 72 (1985): 11–22.

Stern MP, Haffner SM. "Body Fat Distribution and Hyperinsulinemia as Risk Factors for Diabetes and Cardiovascular Disease." *Arteriosclerosis* 6 (1986): 123–130.

Stevens J et al. "Cancer of the Pancreas in Blacks: A Ten-Year Experience." *Journal of the National Medical Association* 69 (1977): 249–251.

Stoewsand GS. "Bioactive Organosulfur Phytochemicals in *Brassica oleracea* Vegetables—a Review." *Food and Chemical Toxicology* 33 (1995): 537–543.

Strange C et al. "Platelets Attenuate Oxidant-Induced Permeability in Endothelial." *Journal of Applied Physiology* 81 (1996): 1701–1706.

Struewig J et al. "The Risk of Cancer Associated with Specific Mutations of BRAC1 and BRAC2 among Ashkenazi Jews." *New England Journal of Medicine* 336 (1997): 1401–1408.

Suchocka Z, Kobylílnska K, Pachecka J. "Activity of Glutathione-Dependent Enzymes in Long Term Diabetes." *Acta Poloniae Pharmaceutica* 52 (1995): 213–217.

Summerson JH, Konen JC, Dignan MB. "Racial Differences in Lipid and Lipoprotein Levels in Diabetes." *Metabolism* 41 (1992): 851–855.

Swain R, Kaplan B. "Vitamins as Therapy in the 1990s." *Journal of the American Board of Family Practice* 8 (1995): 206–216.

Swanson GM, Belle SH, Satariano WA. "Marital Status and Cancer Incidence: Differences in the Black and White Populations." *Cancer Research* 45 (1985): 5883–5889.

Synderwine EG. "The Food-Derived Heterocyclic Amines and Breast Cancer: A 1995 Perspective." *Recent Results in Cancer Research* 140 (1996): 17–25.

Szarka CE, Grana G, Engstrom PF. "Chemoprevention of Cancer." *Current Problems in Cancer* 18 (1994): 6–79.

Szyf M. "The DNA Methylation Machinery as a Target for Anticancer Therapy." *Pharmacology and Therapeutics* 70 (1996): 1–37.

Takeda S et al. "Lipid Peroxidation in Human Breast Cancer Cells in Response to Gamma-Linolenic Acid and Iron." *Anticancer Research* 12 (1992): 329–333.

Takeda, Horrobin SD, Manku M. "The Effect of Gamma-Linolenic Acid on Human Breast Cancer Cell Killing, Lipid Peroxidation and the Production of Schiff-Reactive Materials." *Medical Science Research* 20 (1992): 203–205.

Takeda S et al. "Mechanism of Lipid Peroxidation in Cancer Cells in Response to Gamma-Linolenic Acid (GLA) Analyzed by GC-MS(I): Conjugated Dienes with Peroxyl (or Hydroperoxyl) Groups and Cell-Killing Effects." *Anticancer Research* 13 (1993): 193–199.

Tang W et al. "Racial Differences in Coronary Calcium Prevalence among High-Risk Adults." (1995).

Tew BY et al. "A Diet High in Wheat Fiber Decreases the Bioavailability of Soybean Isoflavones in a Single Meal Fed to Women." *Journal of Nutrition* 126 (1996): 871–877.

Thomas MG, Tebbutt S, Williamson RC. "Vitamin D and Its Metabolites Inhibit Cell Proliferation in Human Rectal Mucosa and a Colon Cancer Cell Line." *Gut* 33 (1992): 1660–1663.

Thompson IM et al. "Chemoprevention of Prostate Cancer." *Seminars in Urology* 13 (1995): 122–129.

Tisdale MJ. "Inhibition of Lipolysis and Muscle Protein Degradation by EPA in Cancer Cachexia." *Nutrition* 12 (1996): S31–S33.

Tiwari RK et al. "Selective Responsiveness of Human Breast Cancer Cells to Indole-3-Carbinol, a Chemopreventive Agent." *Journal of the National Cancer Institute* 86 (1994): 126–131.

Tolosa de Talamoni N et al. "Glutathione Plays a Role in the Chick Intestinal Calcium." *Comparative Biochemistry and Physiology* 115 (1996): 127–132.

Trizna Z, Hsu TC, Schantz SP. "Protective Effects of Vitamin E Against Bleomycin-Induced Genotoxicity in Head and Neck Cancer Patients *in Vitro*." *Anticancer Research* 12 (1992): 325–327.

Trowell H. "Hypertension, Obesity, Diabetes Mellitus, and Coronary Heart Disease." In *Western Diseases: Their Emergence and Prevention* (1981), 24. Harvard University Press, Cambridge, MA.

Tzonou A et al. "Diet and Ovarian Cancer: A Case-Control Study in Greece." *International Journal of Cancer* 55 (1993): 411–414.

Van Aswegen CH, Du Plessis DJ. "Can Linoleic Acid and Gamma-Linolenic Acid Be Important in Cancer Treatment?" *Medical Hypotheses* 43 (1994): 415–417.

van der Merwe CF et al. "The Effect of Gamma-Linolenic Acid, an *in Vitro* Cytostatic Substance Contained in Evening Primrose Oil, on Primary Liver Cancer. A Double-Blind Placebo Controlled Trial." *Prostaglandins Leukotrienes and Essential Fatty Acids* 40 (1990): 199–202.

van der Westhuyzen J. "Methionine Metabolism and Cancer." *Nutrition and Cancer* 7 (1985): 179–183.

van Zandwijk N. "N-Acetylcysteine for Lung Cancer Prevention." *Chest* 107 (1995): 1437–1441.

Vernon SW et al. "Ethnicity, Survival, and Delay in Seeking Treatment for Symptoms of Breast Cancer." *Cancer* 55 (1985): 1563–1571.

Voors AW, Webber LS, Berenson GS. "Racial Contrasts in Cardiovascular Response Tests for Children from a Total Community." *Hypertension* 2 (1980): 686–694.

Wagenknecht LE et al. "Racial Differences in Serum Cotinine Levels among Smokers in the Coronary Artery Risk Development in (Young) Adults Study" [see comments]. *Hypertension* 15 (1990): 188–192.

Wainfan E, Poirier LA. "Methyl Groups in Carcinogenesis: Effects on DNA Methylation and Gene Expression." *Cancer Research* 52 (1992): 2071S–2077S.

Walker AR et al. "Low Survival of South African Urban Black Women with Cervical Cancer." *British Journal of Obstetrics and Gynaecology* 92 (1985): 1272–1278.

Walker AR. "Prostate Cancer—Some Aspects of Epidemiology, Risk Factors, Treatment and Survival." *South African Medical Journal* 69 (1986): 44–47.

Walker, AR et al. "Survival of Black Men with Prostatic Cancer in Soweto, Johannesburg, South Africa." *Journal of Urology* 135 (1986): 58–59.

Wang TT, Sathyamoorthy N. Phang JM. "Molecular Effects of Genistein on Estrogen Receptor Mediated Pathways." *Carcinogenesis* 17 (1995): 271–275.

Waterfield CJ et al. "Taurine: A Possible Urinary Marker of Liver Damage. A Study of Taurine Excretion in Carbon Tetrachloride Treated Rats." *Archives of Toxicology* 65 (1991): 548–555.

Weber A et al. "Can Grapefruit Juice Influence Ethinylestradiol Bioavailability?" *Contraception* 53 (1996): 41–47.

Weinberger MH. "Racial Differences in Renal Sodium Excretion: Relationship to Hypertension." *American Journal of Kidney Diseases* 21 (1993): 41–45.

Weiss NS, Peterson AS. "Racial Variation in the Incidence of Ovarian Cancer in the United States." *American Journal of Epidemiology* 107 (1978): 91–95.

Welsh J. "Induction of Apoptosis in Breast Cancer Cells in Response to Vitamin D and Antiestrogens." *Biochemistry and Cell Biology* 72 (1994): 537–545.

West DW et al. "Adult Dietary Intake and Prostate Cancer Risk in Utah: A Case-Control Study with Special Emphasis on Aggressive Tumors." *Cancer Causes and Control* 2 (1991): 85–94.

Wigmore SJ et al. "The Effect of Polyunsaturated Fatty Acids on the Progress of Cachexia in Patients with Pancreatic Cancer." *Nutrition* 12 (1996): S27–S30.

Wilczek H, Vachalovsky. "Importance of Vitamin D in Prostatic Carcinoma." *Casopis Lekaru Ceskych* 135 (1996): 716–718.

Willett WC, Hunter DJ. "Vitamin A and Cancers of the Breast, Large Bowel, and Prostate: Epidemiologic Evidence." *Nutrition Reviews* 52 (1994): S53–S59.

Wingard DL, Barrett-Connor E. "Family History of Diabetes and Cardiovascular Disease Risk Factors and Mortality among Euglycemic, Borderline Hyperglycemic, and Diabetic Adults." *American Journal of Epidemiology* 125 (1987): 948–958.

Wyndham CH. "A Comparison of Mortality Rates from Cancer in White, Indian and Coloured Adults in 1970 and 1980." *South African Medical Journal* 67 (1985): 709–711.

Xu X et al. "Bioavailability of Soybean Isoflavones Depends upon Gut Microflora in Women." *Journal of Nutrition* 125 (1995) 2307–2315.

Yam D, Eliraz A, Berry EM. "Diet and Disease—the Israeli Paradox: Possible Dangers of a High Omega-6 Polyunsaturated Fatty Acid Diet." *Israel Journal of Medical Sciences* 32 (1996): 1134–1143.

Yamamoto J, Horie T, Awazu S. "Amelioration of Methotrexate-Induced Malabsorption by Vitamin A." *Cancer Chemotherapy and Pharmacology* 39 (1997): 239–244.

Yamanaka Y et al. "Effect of Dietary Taurine on Cholesterol Gallstone Formation and Tissue Cholesterol Contents in Mice." *Journal of Nutrition Science and Vitaminology* 31 (1985): 225–232.

Yan C et al. "Transport and Function of Taurine in Mammalian Cells and Tissues." *Acta Toxicology and Therapeutics* 12 (1991): 277–298.

Yan C, Bravo CE, Cantafora A. "Effect of Taurine Levels on Liver Lipid Metabolism: An *in Vivo* Study in the Rat." *Proceedings of the Society of Experimental Biology and Medicine* 202 (1993): 88–96.

Yao K, Latta M, Bird RP. "Modulation of Colonic Aberrant Crypt Foci and Proliferative Indexes in Colon and Prostate Glands of Rats by Vitamin E." *Nutrition and Cancer* 26 (1996): 99–109.

Yavelow J et al. "Bowman-Birk Soybean Protease Inhibitor as an Anticarcinogen." *Cancer Research* 43 (1983): 2454S–2459S.

Yee GC et al. "Effect of Grapefruit Juice on Blood Cyclosporin Concentration." *Lancet* 345 (1995): 955–956.

Yip I, Aronson W, Heber D. "Nutritional Approaches to the Prevention of Prostate Cancer Progression." *Advances in Experimental Medicine and Biology* 399 (1996): 173–181.

Young, MR. "Eicosanoids and the Immunology of Cancer." 1994.

Zaidan E, Sims NR. "Alterations in the Glutathione Content of Mitochondria Following Short-Term Forebrain Ischemia in Rats." *Neurosciences Letters* 218 (1996): 75–78.

Zaidi NH et al. "Tissue and Cell Specific Methylation, Repair and Synthesis of DNA in the Upper Gastrointestinal Tract of Wistar Rats Treated with *N*-Methyl-*N'*-Nitro-*N*-Nitrosoguanidine via the Drinking Water." *Carcinogenesis* 14 (1991): 1991–2001.

Zeller K et al. "Effect of Restricting Dietary Protein in Patients with Insulin-Dependent Diabetes Mellitus." *New England Journal of Medicine* 324 (1991): 78–84.

Ziegler RG. "Epidemiologic Studies of Vitamins and Cancer of the Lung, Esophagus, and Cervix." *Advances in Experimental Medicine and Biology* 206 (1986): 11–26.

Ziegler RG. "Alcohol-Nutrient Interactions in Cancer Etiology." *Cancer* 58 (1986): 1942–1948.

Zugmaier G et al. "Growth-Inhibitory Effects of Vitamin D Analogues and Retinoids on Human Pancreatic Cancer Cells." *British Journal of Cancer* 73 (1996): 1341–1346.

Zureik M et al. "Fatty Acid Proportions in Cholesterol Esters and Risk of Premature Death from Cancer in Middle Aged French Men" [see comments]. *British Medical Journal* 311 (1995): 1251–1254.

INDEX

Acetyl-L-carnitine (ALC), 150
Adult-onset (type 2) diabetes, 14, 21, 49, 100, 149, 150, 155, 167, 212
    incidence of, 146–47
    insulin insensitivity, 146
    insulin-resistant, 152
    racial/ethnic differences, 145
    risk factors for, 148
Aflatoxin, 67
African men, prostate cancer, 138
Africans
    and heart disease, 161–62
ALA (alpha-linolenic acid), 70
Alcohol, 76–77
    and breast cancer, 121
    and heart disease, 189–92
    and osteoporosis, 220
    and prostate cancer, 142–43
Alcohol dehydrogenase, 189
Allicin, 185
Alliin, 185
Allylic sulfides, 49
Alpha-carotene, 55, 180
Alpha-lipoic acid (ALA), 149–50, 188
American black men
    prostate cancer, 5, 28, 126, 137–38
American black women
    breast cancer, 97, 108–10
    smoking, 197–98
    testosterone levels, 138
American blacks, 4–5, 28–29
    diabetes, 145, 156–57
    hypertension, 193–94
    retinopathy, 156–57
American Cancer Society (ACS), 46, 97, 124
American diet, 50, 105, 204
    exercise and, 196–97
    and temporary diabetics, 145
American Heart Association (AHA), 48, 167
American Hispanics, 145, 156–57
American Indians, 145
Amino-acid profiles, 93, 126, 171
    comparison of soybeans and beef, 171–72, 172f

Amino acids, 90, 93, 151
    sulfur-containing, 171, 208, 216
Amputations, 144, 146, 149
Angina pectoris, 77, 177, 183–84, 186, 195
    experimental formula for, 199t
    experimental protocol for, 198
Angiogenesis, 15, 16, 214
    soy foods/beverages and, 81–83
Angiogenesis research, 83–84
Angioplasty, 20, 21
Angiostatin, 83
Animal foods, 105, 116, 126, 205, 216
    fats in, 125, 167
Animal protein, 50, 93, 162, 171, 205, 209–10
Antiadhesives, 18
Antioxidants, 17, 22, 68, 73, 150, 151, 153, 174, 188, 196
    "packaging," 166
Apoptosis, 40, 43, 107
Appetizers (recipes), 239–47
Apple-shaped obesity pattern, 99, 102, 156
Arachidonic acid, 121, 142, 143
Artery damage/blockage, 20–21
    homocysteine and, 172–74
Ascorbic acid, 55
Ashkenazi Jewish women, 28, 43
Atherosclerosis, 17, 92, 172, 180, 181, 183, 187
    experimental diet and protocol, 198–202, 200–01t, 202t, 216
    monoclonal origin of, 174–75

B-complex vitamin supplement, 152, 173
B vitamins, 173
Bailar, John, 19
BCG (bacille Calmette-Guérin), 47, 114
Bellantoni, Michele, 203
Benign prostatic hyperplasia (BPH), 126, 128, 130–31, 191
Berger, Peter, 174
Beta-carotene, 55, 56, 180, 183
Beta-HCH (beta-hexachlorocyclohexane), 106, 107
Bifidobacteria, 87
Bile acids, 87, 90–91

Biochemotherapy, 24–25
Bioflavonoids, 65
Biological differences
    breast cancer, 108–10, 108*t*
    prostate cancer, 138
Bis (maltolato) oxovanadium (BMOV), 132
Bisphenol-A, 106
Bladder cancer, 46–47
Blender Drinks (recipes), 331–38
Bleomycin, 22
Blindness, 144, 146, 156
Blood cholesterol level, 175, 187
    soy in lowering, 90–92, 93–94, 126
Blood clots/clotting, 18, 68, 73, 169, 179, 190
Blood insulin levels
    and breast cancer, 99, 100–01, 105
Blood sugar levels, 18, 60, 144, 145, 147–48,
        149, 151, 152, 153, 154, 157
    lowering, 188–89
Blood vessel growth blockers, 15–16
Bone health, 205, 212
Bone loss, 203, 206, 209, 212
    calcium supplements and, 210
    stopping, 204–05
Bones
    foods and nutrients for, 213–14
Boron, 212
Bowman-Birk inhibitor (BBI), 89
BRAC1/2 genes, 43, 105
Brachytherapy, 135–36
Brain, 151
Breads (recipes), 259–70
Breakfasts (recipes), 231–38
Breast cancer, 34, 43, 57, 58, 59, 62, 69,
        96–122, 214
    alcohol consumption and, 143, 189–90
    American black women, 5, 28
    assessing risk of, 98*t*
    biological differences in blacks and whites,
        108–10, 108*t*
    experimental diet and protocol, 116–22,
        118–20*t*
    fats and, 71
    foods fighting, 110–12
    hormone replacement therapy and, 215
    phyto-foods fighting, 103*f*
    phytonutrients and estrogens and, 101–02,
        106–07
    risk factors for, 98, 99
    risk of, 97–110
    soy and, 78, 81, 87
    vitamin D and, 107–08, 131
Butyrate, 63
Bypass surgery, 5, 20–21, 73

Cachexia, 53, 72
Calcipotriol, 214
Calcium, 22, 153, 180, 204, 205, 212, 213
    food sources, 207–08
Calcium absorption, 210–11

Calcium content (selected foods), 209*t*
Calcium intake, 208
Calcium loss, 75–76, 93, 190, 209–10, 216
    alcohol and, 220
    through diet, 205–06
Calcium-magnesium supplement, 211
Calcium sources, 211
Calcium supplements, 204, 207, 210–11
Calories, 69, 100
    burned through exercise, 122, 143, 195*t*
Cancer(s), 3–4, 5, 10, 11, 12–14, 29, 30,
        49, 169
    alcohol and, 190
    American blacks, 28, 29
    carotenoids and, 56–58
    categories of, 37, 38*t*
    connection with heart disease, 174–75
    fats and, 69
    genistein fighting, 89*t*
    how it arises, 38–39
    how it spreads, 39–40
    incidence of, 19
    insulin overproduction in, 146, 147
    milk products and, 208
    new remission therapies for, 24–25
    new standard for a cure, 31–45
    nutrients and, 22
    permanent remissions, 11–12
    phytonutrients and, 15–18, 48–49, 58–60,
        62–77
    reversing, 6–7
    role of genetics in, 40–43
    soy and, 78, 80–89, 94–95
    survival rates, 44*t*
    vitamin D and, 214
    what it is, 37–38
    see also Conventional cancer treatment
Cancer associations and support groups (list),
        351–56
Cancer cells, 15–16, 17, 18, 25–26, 32–33, 37,
        48, 49
    immortality of, 43–44
    in metastasis, 40
Cancer death rate, 29
Cancer research and treatment centers (list),
        357–64
Cancer treatment outcomes
    suggested classification of, 33*t*
Cancer treatments, 4, 12
    failure of, 5
    phytonutrients with, 13–14
    vitamins and minerals and, 22, 23*t*
    see also Conventional cancer treatments
Canola oil, 70, 94, 121, 142
Carbohydrate science, 18
Carbohydrates, 153
Carcinogen detoxifiers, 17
Carcinogens, 10, 38, 67
Cardiovascular disease, 73, 161–202
Carnosine, 150, 180–81

Carotenoid-rich foods, 55–56
Carotenoids, 22, 48, 53, 56–57, 129, 166
  with heart disease, 180
  research on, 57–58
Case histories, 10
  cancer, 34–37, 113–16, 133–37
  heart disease, 162–64, 157–77, 192–93
Cellular suicide, 43
Centers for Disease Control and Prevention
    (CDC), 46, 198
Chemotherapeutic drugs, 58, 60, 84, 112
Chemotherapy, 4, 10, 13, 17, 20, 32–33,
    49, 58
  antioxidant defenses against, 121
  nutrients and phytonutrients for use with,
    23t
  omega-3 fatty acids and, 72–73
  and soy foods, 84
Cheresh, David A., 84
China/Chinese, 99, 161
Chinese men, 126, 138
Chlorogenic acid, 55
Cholesterol, 72, 125, 166
  converted to oxysterols, 169–70
  in selected foods, 168t
  soy and, 90–92
  why it matters, 164–67
Cholesterol intake, 167
Cholesterol level, 176, 177, 207
  reduced by soy protein, 179
Choline, 185
Choline-rich foods, 186t
Chromium, 212
Chromium picolinate, 150–51
Cisplatin, 22, 121
Citric acid, 64, 130
Citrus fruits, 64–66, 111
CLA (conjugated linoleic acid), 71–72
Coenzyme Q$_{10}$, 183–84
Colon cancer, 5, 57, 60, 63, 75, 107, 208
  insulin in, 101
  soy and, 87, 94
  vitamin D and, 131
Computer software, 29–30, 349
Conventional cancer treatments, 16, 31, 49
  and nutrition, 115
  phytonutrients and, 19–20, 49
  shortcomings, of, 44–45
  ways to boost, 25–26
Conventional medical treatments, 6, 10, 12
  dietary strategies and, 13
  heart disease, 20
  prostate cancer, 137
Corn oil, 39, 74
Coronary Artery Surgery Study, 20
Creatine kinase, 196
Cure
  for cancer, 31–45
  new definition of, 32–34
Cysteine, 98, 171

Dairy products, 50, 205, 206–07
  and breast cancer, 121
  low-fat, 94, 207, 208
  and prostate cancer, 143
Davis, Devra Lee, 106–07
Degenerative diseases, 5, 11, 29
Desserts (recipes), 323–30
DHA (docosahexanoic acid), 70, 72, 73
DHEA-S (dehydroepiandrosterone-sulfate),
    212
Diabetes, 3, 4, 5, 11, 29, 30, 49, 73, 77, 101
  American black women, 28
  chromium and, 212
  experimental diet and protocol, 157, 159t,
    160t
  fats and, 69
  homocysteine and, 173
  nutrients that fight, 22, 149–53
  permanent remissions, 12
  preventing/reversing, 13
  phytonutrients and, 18
  soy and, 78, 94
  testing for, 147–49
  see also Adult onset (type 2), diabetes;
    Juvenile (type 1) diabetes
Diabetes insipidus, 144
Diabetes mellitus, 4, 144–60
  reversing, 6–7
Diabetes risk
  minority groups and, 147, 156–57
Diabetics, temporary, 145
Diabetics' food exchange guide, 157–58
Diet
  atherosclerosis, 178t, 198–99, 202t
  breast (and ovarian) cancer, 99–100, 105,
    116–22, 120t
  in/and cancer, 34
  in cancer treatment, 25–26, 114, 116
  and degenerative disease, 5, 12
  and diabetes, 145, 146, 147, 155, 157
  guidelines, 164t
  and heart disease, 161–62, 163–64
  high-fat, 87
  high-protein, 170–71, 172, 173, 174, 205
  and hypertension, 193
  Masai, 161–62
  osteoporosis, 216, 219t
  in permanent remissions, 14
  and prostate cancer, 125–29, 134–35, 141t
  samples, 135t, 178t
Dietary cholesterol levels, 175
Dietary fat(s), 25–26, 98
  American blacks, 138
  and prostate cancer, 127
Dietary strategies, 13
  to prevent breast cancer, 99–101
Dietary supplements, 47, 56, 71
  with diabetes, 145, 146, 147, 149, 150, 153
  and disease, 3–4
  doctor's permission/supervision needed, 72,

116, 133, 149, 152, 153, 181, 182, 186, 187, 188, 199
garlic, 185
omega-3 fat, 70
omega-3 fatty acids, 73
Dietary treatment strategies, 6, 10, 12
for cancer, 44–45
Dihydroepiandrosterone (DHEA), 153, 215
Dihydrotestosterone (DHT), 126, 130, 131
Disease prevention/reversal, 5–7
diet in, 14, 27
food and dietary supplements in, 3–4
phytonutrients in, 11, 17
DNA (deoxyribonucleic acid), 17, 39, 67, 196
Dormancy, 83, 84
Doxorubicin, 26, 58
Dressings/Sauces/Dips (recipes), 287–94
Drugs, 10, 17, 20, 58

Eat to Succeed (Haas), 93
Eat to Win (Haas), 4, 164–65
Eating, new way of, 10, 22–24
Edema, 75, 77
Egg yolks, 121, 143
Endometrial cancer, 87, 101
Environmental carcinogens, 39, 43, 102–07, 175
Environmental toxins, 102, 121, 130
Entrées (recipes), 295–311
EPA (eicosapentanoic acid), 70, 72, 73–74
Estradiol, 17, 58, 59, 88, 102, 111, 121, 189
Estradiol metabolism, 104*f*
Estrogen(s), 16, 96, 98–99, 101, 210
and breast cancer, 101–02, 106–07
circulating level of, 122
and osteoporosis, 215
protecting from heart attack, 174
soy mimics, 87–88
Exercise, 105, 107, 109
with atherosclerosis, 199
and bone loss, 204
and cancer, 121–22, 143
dangers in, 195, 196–97
with diabetes, 145, 146, 147, 148, 155, 157
doctor's permission needed, 155, 157, 195, 220
and heart disease/stroke, 194–96
and hypertension, 193–94
and osteoporosis, 220
Experimental Atherosclerosis Reversal Protocol, 163, 200*t*
Extending dormancy, 16
External-beam radiation, 135–36
Eye damage (diabetes), 147, 149
Eyre, Haron, 13

Fat, why it matters, 167–70
Fat intake, 155–56
Fats, 100
effect on lipoprotein cholesterol levels, 170*t*

friendly, 68–74, 181
friendly/unfriendly ratio, 99, 101, 105
limiting intake of, 73–74
Fatty acids, 39, 138, 167–69
Fiber, 62–63, 75, 90, 188–89
5-alpha-reductase, 126, 130
5-year survival rates, 31, 44, 97, 110
Fixx, Jim, 197
Flavonoids, 53, 111
Flaxseed, 70, 130, 169
Folic acid, 64–65, 174
Folkman, Judah, 16, 83, 84
Food exchange guide
diabetics, 157–58
Food guide pyramid (USDA), 45, 49–50
Food products
biodesigned, 49
brand-name, 365–68
new, 5–6
Foods, 3–4
calcium content, 209*t*
calcium-rich, 205, 207–08, 211
cholesterol content of, 168*t*
containing carotenoids, 180
containing choline, 185, 186*t*
containing coenzyme Q$_{10}$, 184
containing L-Taurine, 184
containing proanthocyanidins, 186–87
containing selenium, 183
derived from soybean, 85*t*
high in zinc, 132
magnesium-rich, 213
phytonutrient-rich, 48, 49
with protease inhibitors, 89
for strong bones, 213–14
sugar in, 155
that fight breast cancer, 110–12
vitamin C–rich, 214
vitamin D–rich, 107, 132, 214
Foods to avoid
with breast cancer, 116–21
with osteoporosis, 216
with prostate cancer, 142–43
Framingham Heart Study, 176
Free-radical blockers, 17
Free radicals, 39, 48, 55, 65, 68, 73, 149, 151, 165, 174, 175, 196
vitamin C and, 181, 183
"French paradox," 76, 142–43
Fruits, 53, 64–66, 75
Functional foods, 49, 57

Garlic, 66–68, 184–85
Genetic predisposition
to diabetes, 147, 156
to obesity, 156
Genetics
in racial differences in disease rates, 28–29
role of, in cancer, 40–43, 98

Genistein, 59, 72, 81, 83, 85, 86, 87, 111, 137, 179
  fighting cancer, 89f
Gestational diabetes, 147
Giovannucci, Edward, 129
GLA (gamma linolenic acid), 71, 73–74
Glucose, 147, 149, 150, 152, 153, 212
Glucose tolerance, impaired, 212
Glucose tolerance test, 148
Glycemic index, 154, 155
Glycemic index values, 154t
Gonzales, Nicholas, 34–35, 36, 116
Gonzales regimen, 117t
Greece, 57, 70
Green tea, 188

Health Professionals Follow-Up Study, 127, 129
Heart attack, 4, 14, 20, 48, 73, 175
  estrogen protection from, 174
  exercise and, 195–96, 197
  plaque and, 166
  risk factors for, 166t
  soy preventing, 92
Heart disease, 3, 5, 11, 20–21, 29, 30, 49, 64, 77
  alcohol and, 143, 189–92
  connection with cancer, 174, 175
  diabetes and, 144, 146, 147, 156
  diet and, 161–62, 163–64
  exercise and, 194–96
  fats and, 69
  garlic protects against, 68
  homocysteines in, 173
  milk and, 208
  nutrients that fight, 22, 179–89
  permanent remissions, 12
  phytonutrients and, 18
  preventing/reversing, 6–7, 13, 175–77
  soy and, 78, 80, 90–92, 94
High blood pressure, 4, 147, 192–93
  see also Hypertension
High-density lipoprotein (HDL) cholesterol, 90, 181, 187, 190, 191
High-density lipoproteins (HDL), 165
Homocysteine, 171, 172–74, 185
Hormone blockers, 16
Hormone replacement therapy, 98, 102, 215–16
Hyperinsulinemia, 99, 100–01
Hypertension, 3, 75, 190
  American blacks, 4–5, 28, 193–94
Hyperthermia, 26

Immune boosters, 17
Indole-3-carbinol, 58, 112
Indoles, 48
Insulin, 98, 145, 151, 152, 153, 190, 212, 215
Insulin injections, 145, 147
Insulin insensitivity, 21, 146

Insulin-like growth factors (IGF–I, –II), 100, 101
Insulin resistance, 4, 99, 100–01, 148, 156, 167
Insulin sensitivity, 149, 152, 153, 157
Interferons, 24, 34
Interleukins, 24, 25
Ishii, Douglas, 148–49
Isoflavones, 59, 79, 80t, 81t, 84, 88, 90, 91, 111, 128, 136
  dietary intake, 86–87
Isoflavonoids, 49, 179
Isothiocyanates, 48, 49

Japan, 57, 87, 161
Japanese diet, 59–60, 78, 94–95, 100, 127, 181, 188
Japanese men
  prostate cancer, 33–34, 59–60, 126–27, 136, 138
Japanese women
  breast cancer rate, 99–100
Juvenile (type 1) diabetes, 144–45, 149

Kidney function/disease, 93, 144, 146
Klatsky, Arthur, 191
Koop, Everett C., 27–28
Korda, Michael, 137

L-Carnitine, 185–86
Lectins, 18
Legumes, 60, 128, 207, 208
L-Glutamine, 151
L-Glutathione, 151
Limonene, 65
Lin, Robert, 68
Lindane, 106
Linoleic acid, 121, 170
Lipoprotein cholesterol levels
  effects of fats and oils on, 170t
Lipoproteins, 165
Liver cancer, 5, 94, 143
Low-density lipoprotein (LDL) cholesterol, 39, 68, 165, 170, 179, 180, 182–83, 185, 189
  soy and, 90, 92–93
Low-density lipoproteins (LDL), 165, 166, 188
L-Taurine, cardiovascular effects of, 184, 184t
Lung cancer, 5, 20, 34, 55, 56, 57, 60, 94, 97, 208
Lycopene, 11, 55, 56, 57–58, 112, 129, 166, 180, 183

Magnesium, 39, 212, 213
Man to Man (Korda), 137
Marine oils, 169–70
Masai, 161–62
Medical therapies, experimental, 24–25
Mediterranean diet, 55, 57, 169, 181
  alcohol in, 191, 192
  olive oil in, 69

Men, and alcohol, 190–91
Menarche, age of, 96, 98
Menopause, 96, 174
Metastasis, 39–40, 49, 121
   modified citrus pectin interfering with,
      132–33
   patterns of, 42*f*
Metastasis sites
   tumor type and, 41*t*
Methionine, 93, 171, 172–73
Methionine-rich foods, 116–21, 216
Milk, 93–94, 131, 208, 211
   health risks of, 206–07
Mills, James, 174
Minerals, 22, 39, 148
Minority groups
   and diabetes risk, 147, 156–57
Modified citrus pectin (MCP), 18, 66, 132–33
Monoclonal origin of atherosclerosis, 174–75
Monounsaturated fatty acids, 101
Monounsaturated oils, 169
MRFIT (Multiple Risk Factor Intervention
   Trial), 3
Multivitamins, 22, 46–48, 182
Mussalo-Rauihamaa, Helena, 107

N-acetyl-cysteine (NAC), 151
Naringenin, 65, 111
National Academy of Sciences
   Institute of Medicine, 208
National Cancer Institute (NCI), 19, 47
   Black/White Cancer Survival Study, 108,
      109
   Diet and Cancer Branch, 6, 9, 24, 48, 49,
      57
National Research Council (NRC)
   Food and Nutrition Board, 46
Nerve damage, 146, 149, 152
Nerve disorders, 148–49
Neural-tube defects, 174
Neuropathies, 148–49, 150
Niacin, 187
Nonylphenol, 106
Nurses' Health Study, 148
Nutrient formulas, new, 5–6
Nutrients
   protecting from homocysteine damage, 171
   for strong bones, 213–14
   that fight diabetes, 149–53
   that fight heart disease, 179–89
   that fight osteoporosis, 211–13
   that fight prostate cancer, 130–33, 138
   for use with chemotherapy and radiotherapy,
      23*t*
   see also Phytonutrients; Supplementary
      nutrients
Nutrition
   and cancer, 114–15
   in cancer treatment, 25–26

doctors' lack of training in, 3, 26–28, 124,
   146
and medicine, 6
Nutritional strategies, 5

Obesity, 69, 98, 169
   American blacks, 28, 156
   and breast cancer, 98–99, 102
   diabetes and, 146, 147, 148
Oils
   effect on lipoprotein cholesterol levels, 170*t*
Olive oil, 69–70, 74, 101, 121, 142, 169, 170
   and breast cancer, 112
   and heart disease, 181
Omega-3 fatty acids, 25–26, 50, 70, 72–73,
   101, 169, 184
   and cancer, 112, 130
   and heart disease, 181
Omega-3 marine oils
   and cancer, 121, 142
Omega-6 fatty acids, 101
Oncogenes, 40
Onions, 66–68
O'Reilly, Michael S., 83
Osborne, Michael, 107
Osteoclasts, 204–05
Osteoporosis, 3, 4, 5, 11, 14, 29, 49, 77,
   203–20
   experimental diet and protocol, 216–20,
      217*t*, 218*t*, 219*t*
   milk products and, 207
   nutrients that fight, 22, 211–13
   permanent remissions, 12
   phytonutrients and, 19
   preventing/reversing, 6–7, 13
   risk for developing, 208–10
   soy and, 78, 93
Ovarian cancer, 5, 43, 57, 58, 78, 87, 101
   experimental diet and protocol, 116–22,
      118–20*t*
   nutritional principles, 96*n*
Oxysterols, 170

p53 gene, 43, 175
P-coumaric acid, 55
Pancreas, 145, 146, 149, 153
Pancreatic cancer, 5, 100, 143
Parathyroid hormone, 210
Pasteur, Louis, 184–85
Pear-shaped women, 99
Pecta-Sol, 133
Pectin, 66, 132, 189
Percent body fat, 98
Permanent remissions, 11–12, 14, 24, 35, 77
   angiogenesis research in, 83–84
   theory of, 15–18
   vitamins and minerals in, 22
Permanent Remissions diet, 29
Permanent Remissions Registry, 7
Pesticides, 98, 105

Phytic acid, 63, 81*t*, 87
Phytochemicals, 44–45, 47
Phytoestrogen-rich foods, 128
Phytoestrogens, 88
Phytofood group
  for prostate health, 127–29
Phytofood products
  that fight breast/ovarian cancer, 110*t*
  that fight prostate cancer, 128*t*
Phytofood Pyramid Guide, 45, 49–77, 51*f*
  how to use, 50–54
  level one, 55–58
  level two, 59–60
  level three, 62–63
  level four, 64–66
  level five, 66–68
  level six, 68–74
Phytofood Servings Guide, 53*t*
Phytofoods
  with diabetes, 148
  and heart disease, 173, 177, 180, 188–89
  that fight breast cancer, 103*f*
  that fight prostate cancer, 140*f*
Phytonutrient Activity Chart, 54*t*
Phytonutrient Food Guide Pyramid, 77, 100
Phytonutrient-rich foods
  and heart disease, 161, 166, 175, 192–93,
    199
  for osteoporosis, 216, 217*t*
Phytonutrients, 3, 9, 10–11, 174
  and breast cancer, 99–100, 101–02, 106–07
  and cancer, 174, 175
  in cancer remissions, 48–49
  in conjunction with conventional
    treatments, 13–14, 19–20
  in cure for cancer, 32–37, 39, 40, 43
  fighting disease, 18–19
  and heart disease, 174–75, 179, 189, 191
  in permanent remissions, 14, 15–18
  in plant foods, 48, 49
  in preventing/reversing prostate cancer, 124,
    125–29, 133–37, 138
  in prevention, 77
  and smoking, 198
  in soy foods/beverages, 81*t*, 87, 208
  twenty-first-century vitamins, 46–77
  for use with chemotherapy and radiotherapy,
    23*t*
Phytosterols, 81*t*
Pineal gland, 151
Plant foods, 196
  phytonutrients in, 48, 49
Plaque, 4, 14, 48, 60, 90, 91, 165, 166, 170,
    174, 175, 179
  exercise and, 196, 197
Plastic containers, 105–06
Polycarbonate, 105–06
Polyphenols, 48, 76
Polyunsaturated fat, 142
Polyunsaturated vegetable oils, 167–69

Pregnancy, 98, 147, 173, 204
Prevention, 5–6, 27
  phytonutrients in, 77
  prostate cancer, 124–25
Proanthocyanidins, 186–87
Progesterone, 215–16
Prostaglandins, 67, 71
Prostate cancer, 19, 33–34, 57, 66, 78, 123–43
  American black men, 5, 28, 126, 137–38
  experimental diet and protocol, 138–43,
    139*t*, 141*t*
  Japanese men, 33–34, 59–60, 126–27, 136,
    138
  lycopene and, 57–58
  soy and, 87
Protease inhibitors, 81*t*, 87, 88–89, 136
Protein
  in calcium loss, 205–06
  why it matters, 170–72

Quercetin, 65, 111

Racial differences
  in disease rates, 28–29
  in hypertension, 193
Radiotherapy, 4, 10, 13, 17, 20, 33, 49, 112
  antioxidant defenses against, 121
  damage from, 150, 180
  nutrients and phytonutrients for use with,
    23*t*
  and soy foods, 84
Recipe hints, 223–26
Recipes, 227–338
  Ambrosia, 323
  Annato Vinaigrette, 287
  Apple Cinnamon Oatmeal, 231
  Avocado Dressing Dip, 288
  "Bacon" Cheese "Burger," 249–50
  Aunt Jean's Zucchini Bread, 259–60
  "Beefy" Bacon Burrito, 251
  Berry Tofu Smoothie, 331
  Biscuits 'n' "Sausage," 232–33
  Black-Eyed Salsa, 279
  Broccoli and Tofu Lo Mein with "Chicken,"
    295–96
  Buttermilk Biscuits, 261
  Buttermilk Pancakes with Banana, 234
  Café Espressoy Shake, 332
  Cajun Coleslaw (and Dressing), 280–81
  Cheddar Jalapeño Corn Muffins, 262
  Cheese Grits, 235
  Chewy Oatmeal Chocolate Chip Cookies,
    324
  "Chicken" Nuggets, 239
  Chili Con "Carne," 297
  Chocolate Bundt Cake with Fruit Ribbon
    and Mocha Frosting, 325–26
  Creamy Garlic Dip, 289
  "Creamy" Pink Tomato Sauce, 290
  Deluxe Refried Beans, 313

Double Chocolate Malt, 333
Dreemsicle Shake, 334
Egg "Fu" Salad Sandwiches, 252
Festive Kasmati Rice, 314
Fruit Yogurt Crunch, 236
Hearty Lasagne, 298–99
Honey Mustard Dip, 291
Horseradish-Encrusted Salmon, 300–01
Hummus, 240
list of, 227–30
Lobster Malabar, 302
Mandarin Orange Muffins, 263
Marzipan Cheese Tart, 327–28
"Meatball" Oven Grinder Subs, 253–54
Menopause Muffins, 264–65
Mexican "Beef," 315
Mrs. B's Chilies Rellenos, 303
Nothing Lost Tartar Sauce, 292
Oat Bread (Baguettes and Rolls), 266–68
Pasta e Fagiole, 271–72
Pigs in the Blanket, 237
Pink Citrus Ice, 329
Pita Salad Sandwich, 282
Po' Boy Sandwich ("Chicken" Style), 255
Potstickers ("Pork" Dumplings), 241–42
Pure Fruit Smoothie, 335
Ravioli di Liguria, 304–05
Red Beans and Rice, 316–17
Red Lentil Soup (Right Away), 273
Rigatoni with Garlic, Tomatoes and Basil, 306
Rio Grande Pinto Bean Soup, 274–75
Robert's Favorite Omelet, 238
"Sausage" Ratatouille à la Ann, 307–08
Scalloped Potatoes, 318
Shrimp and "Scallops" Creole, 309–10
Shrimp Wrapped in "Bacon," 243
Snappy Cocktail Sauce, 293
Southwestern Corn Chowder, 276
Soy Milk Blend, 294
Special Restaurant Salsa, 244
Spicy Couscous with Tomatoes, 319
Spinach Pita Puffs, 245
Spinach Salad with Warm "Bacon" Dressing, 283
Strawberries and "Cream," 330
Strawberry Banana Shake, 336
Super Soy Power Shake, 82t, 337
Sweet Carrot Side, 320
Sweet-and-Sour Cabbage Soup with "Beef," 277
Taco Salad, 284–85
Thai Noodles, 246–47
Tangy Collard Greens, 321
Tex-Mex Brown Rice, 322
Tomato Rice Soup, 278
Tricolor Pasta with Salmon (Skillet Dinner), 311
Tropical Fruit Shake, 338
Tuna Dijon Salad, 286

Triple-Decker Club, 256–57
Tuscan Garlic Bread, 269
Whole-Wheat Croutons, 270
Recommended daily allowance (RDA), 131
Recommended dietary allowances (RDAs), 46, 47
Red meat, 127, 142, 205–06
Remission therapies for cancer, 24–25
Remissions, 10, 14
see also Permanent remissions
Report on Nutrition and Health (Koop), 27–28
Reproductive hormones, 97, 98 101–02
Retinoids, 22, 48
Retinopathy, 146, 151–52, 156–57
Robinson, Killian, 173
Rosenberg, Steven A., 13

Safflower oil, 39, 74
Salads (recipes), 279–86
Salt, 50, 75–76, 192, 193
Sanders, Charles L., 26–27
Saponins, 81t, 87, 161, 179
Saturated fats, 72, 101, 167
Saw palmetto, 130–31
Seafood, 70, 73, 130, 169
Selenium, 22, 39, 47, 66, 183
Sex hormones, 125, 213
Shalala, Donna, 31
Side dishes (recipes), 313–22
Sirtori, Cesare, 91
16-alpha-hydroxyestrone, 102
Skim milk, 60, 94, 121, 143, 207, 208
Smoking, 183, 197–98
Snacks and sandwiches (recipes), 249–57
Sodium, 193, 206, 220
Soups (recipes), 271–78
Soy, 78–95
    amino-acid profile, 171, 172f
    amount needed, 84–87
    and heart diseases, 90–92
    mimics estrogen, 87–88
    and osteoporosis, 93
Soy-based meat replacers, 53, 60, 61t, 78, 79
Soy foods/beverages, 29, 53, 59–60, 72, 82t
    and angiogenesis, 81–83, 84
    and breast cancer, 111
    calcium from, 207–08
    cocktail, 72, 135–37
    drinks/drink mixes, 79–81, 81t
    phytonutrients in, 81t, 87
    and prostate cancer, 127, 128
    types of, 90
Soy milk, 60, 90, 93–94
Soy phytonutrients, 179
Soy products, 16
    brand-name, 86t
    and breast cancer, 99, 100
    choosing, 79
Soy protein, 126, 210, 213
Soy protein sources, 111t, 180t

Soybeans, 16
    foods derived from, 85t
Spontaneous remissions, 14
Sphingolipids, 208
Steinmetz, Rosemary, 106
Stomach cancer, 19, 60, 94
Strength training, 204, 220
Stroke, 4, 20, 14, 49, 73, 166, 175
    alcohol and, 190
    diabetes and, 144, 146
    exercise and, 194–96, 196, 197
    homocysteine and, 173
    risk factors for, 166t
    soy preventing, 92
Sugar, 50, 74–75, 100, 144, 153–55
    in soy foods, 87
Sulfonylurea, 147
Supplementary nutrients
    angina pectoris, 199t
    doctor's supervision required, 138, 157, 216
    see also Dietary supplements
Surgery, 10, 13, 17, 20, 32, 49
Sweet and Dangerous (Yudkin), 74

Tamoxifen, 59, 88, 100–01, 115
Teicher, Beverly A., 84
Telomerase (enzyme), 44
Telomere(s), 44
Testosterone, 16, 130, 138, 143, 216
Testosterone/DHEA ratio, 153
Testosterone-estrogen ratio, 125–26
Thymus, 151
Thyroxin, 91
Tobacco consumption, 197–98
Tofu, 60, 87, 90
Tomato-concentrate products, 129
Tomato sauces/tomatoes, 55, 57–58, 112
Toxicity
    niacin, 187
    vitamins, 131, 153, 214
Trichopoulos, Dimitrios, 70, 112
Triglycerides, 152, 153, 169, 181, 187
Tumor growth, 15–16, 33, 68, 83, 167
    homocysteine in, 173
    protease inhibitors and, 88–89
Tumor-suppressor genes, 43
Tumor types
    general classification of, 38t
    and metastasis sites, 41t
Tumors, 37–38
    cell types in, 84
2-hydroxyestrone, 102
Type 2 diabetes
    see Adult onset (type 2) diabetes

U.S. Department of Agriculture (USDA), 173
    Food Guide Pyramid, 49–50, 52f

U.S. Food and Drug Administration (FDA),
    18, 64, 94

Vanadyl sulfate, 152
Vegetable oils, 39, 105
    and cancer, 121, 142
    health risk in, 167
    oxidized, 170
    polyunsaturated, 167–69
Vegetable protein, 171
Vegetables, 53, 216
    calcium from, 207, 208
    carotenoid, 56–58
    cruciferous, 17, 58, 112
Vinblastine, 58
Vitamin B₆, 151–52
Vitamin C, 22, 47, 66, 73, 149, 166, 188
    with diabetes, 152
    and heart disease, 181–83
    and strong bones, 213–14
Vitamin D, 210
    and breast cancer, 107–08
    in milk, 211
    new forms of, 214
    and prostate cancer, 131–32
    and strong bones, 214
Vitamin D₃, 153, 212
Vitamin E, 22, 47, 56, 73, 166, 188
    natural form of, 153, 181, 182–83
    and heart disease, 181–83
    and prostate cancer, 132
Vitamin E Quinone, 182
Vitamin K, 22, 182
Vitamin supplements, 108, 132
Vitamins, 22
    and diabetes, 148
    industrial-strength, 10–11
    megadoses of, 47

Walking, 147, 155, 157, 220
War on cancer, 20, 31
Weight cycling, 106–07
Weight lifting, 204, 220
Weight loss, 148, 155
Weight-loss diets, 162
Whole grains and cereals, 53, 62–63
Wine, 76, 77, 142–43, 187, 191, 192
Women
    and alcohol, 189–90
    and smoking, 197–98
    see also American black women

Xenobiotics, 17, 58
Xenoestrogens, 97, 102–07

Yo-yo dieting, 98, 106–07
Yudkin, John, 74

Zinc, 39, 132